Dr Sarah Brewer gre graduated from Caml Scientist in 1980 and Cambridge Clinical Sc 1983.

Although her first love is medicine, her major passion is writing, for which she has won three awards. She is the author of two previous books and, as a freelance journalist, her work has appeared in several magazines and journals, including *Woman's Weekly*, *Woman's Realm*, *Slimmer* and *BBC Good Health*. She is now actively pursuing a career in medical journalism and is resident doctor to the *Daily Mirror*, the *Birmingham Evening Mail* and the *North West Evening Mail*.

Sarah Brewer lives in London and is currently working on several projects, including two medical thrillers.

THE BODY
AWARENESS
PROGRAMME

Dr Sarah Brewer

BANTAM BOOKS
LONDON · NEW YORK · TORONTO · SYDNEY · AUCKLAND

THE BODY AWARENESS PROGRAMME
A BANTAM BOOK : 0 553 40654 X

First publication in Great Britain

PRINTING HISTORY

Bantam edition published 1994

This book is not intended as a substitute for the medical advice of a
personal physician. The reader should regularly consult a physician in
matters relating to his or her health and particularly in respect of any
symptoms which may require diagnosis or medical attention.

Set in Bembo and Helvetica by
Phoenix Typesetting, Ilkley, West Yorkshire.

Bantam Books are published by Transworld Publishers Ltd,
61–63 Uxbridge Road, Ealing, London W5 5SA,
in Australia by Transworld Publishers (Australia) Pty Ltd,
15–25 Helles Avenue, Moorebank, NSW 2170,
and in New Zealand by Transworld Publishers (NZ) Ltd,
3 William Pickering Drive, Albany, Auckland.

Reproduced, printed and bound in Great Britain by
Cox & Wyman Ltd, Reading, Berks.

Dedication

This book is dedicated to everyone, everywhere, who cares about their h alth and what they eat.

With special thanks to: Keith Floyd who first got me hooked into fish; Steve Barrett of Plymouth for his culinary and artistic vision; Rick Stein for running the ultimate seafood restaurant in Padstow, Cornwall; *The Good Food Guide* for identifying the best fish restaurants in any locale; Robert Lenkiewicz for widening my horizons and immortalizing me in oils; Richard Marchant for cooking, testing, tasting and perfecting the many recipes in this book – and for uncorking all that wine; Holmes Place of London for running an excellent, professional gymnasium; for assessing my fitness level, prescribing a fitness regime and gently bullying me into keeping it; Britannia Healthcare for providing information on anti-oxidant vitamins; Serafina Clarke for surpassing her role as agent; Bantam Books for publishing the most up-to-date concepts on healthy eating and successful slimming; Australia for exporting such delicious, oaky wines.

Contents

Foreword

Experts in nutrition now recommend a Mediterranean-style diet: lots of garlic, olive oil, seafood, bread, pasta, fresh fruit and vegetables, herbs and red wine.

It sounds idyllic and much more attractive than the stodgy pastry and chip diet many Westerners follow.

If we take a tip from the Eskimos and reinforce the Mediterranean diet with increased amounts of fish, it's possible to improve our health almost miraculously – merely by cutting down on saturated fats and meat.

Recent research emphasizes the importance of certain dietary supplements – especially betacarotene, vitamins C and E, plus gammalinolenic acid found in evening primrose oil.

These super nutrients are especially important when our body-fat stores are raided whilst losing weight. The slimming process releases many harmful, partially hydrogenated, trans-fatty acids and free radicals.

These chemicals are associated with increased stickiness of the blood and increased oxidation of cholesterol. Both lead to furring up of the arteries in a process called atherosclerosis.

By combining modern, healthy-eating concepts with relaxation and regular exercise, it's possible to improve your

chances of a longer, healthier, more creative and rewarding life.

That's what the *Body Awareness Programme* is all about.

This book contains three healthy-eating packages which
are tailored to suit everyone from ages 11 to 99:

Body Awareness Food Exchange Diet

This allows anyone who is overweight to mix-and-match
their foods within predetermined portion levels. The
number of portions you can eat depend on:

- your age
- how overweight you are
- whether you are male or female
- how active you are

Body Awareness Mediterranean Slim Diet

This is a predetermined eating regime which provides an
average of 1,200 kcals per day. It incorporates all the latest
nutritional advice and is based around a Mediterranean-
style diet. It is low in fat – especially saturated fat – and
high in carbohydrate, fibre and antioxidants. This diet
provides:

- 20 per cent of energy as protein
- 20 per cent as fat
- 55 per cent as carbohydrate
- 5 per cent as red wine
- over 30g of fibre per day

If you drink red grape juice instead of red wine, your
carbohydrate intake will increase to 60 per cent.

Body Awareness Maintenance Plan

This diet is suitable for readers who:
- are at the right weight for their height but want to eat more healthily
- have recently lost weight on a calorie-restricted diet and want to keep if off

The maintenance plan advises on the number of calories or food exchange portions to eat every day in order to maintain your weight. It also includes a selection of over 160 delicious, Mediterranean-style recipes. Just work out how much you can eat within your calorie allowance and tuck in.

The Modern View of a Healthy Diet

Whole forests have been decimated to produce the reams of dietary advice issued over the last half century.

Much of this advice has been contradictory, ludicrous or downright dangerous. It's not so long ago that the idea of a healthy diet involved foods rich in saturated fat (e.g. eggs, butter, steak) and a lack of wholemeal bread, potatoes, pasta or rice.

Only fruit and vegetables (perhaps with the exception of the avocado and banana, banned in many slimming regimes) have gained recognition down the ages as healthy and good for us.

The cynical can be forgiven for sighing and thinking that any new dietary advice is likely to be as controversial or inaccurate as that given a decade ago.

We are, however, now much closer to understanding the complex workings of our body machinery. Hormones and tissue factors unheard of even a few years ago are now understood and have had their molecular structure unravelled.

In many cases, the geographical position of the genes' coding for these enzymes and proteins has been traced and artifical, 'recombinant' versions – often synthesized by genetically engineered microbes – are used to treat disease.

Modern science is at last qualified to pronounce on what is good and what is bad when it comes to diet.

The mathematical science of epidemiology is on our side too. By identifying which parts of the world have problems with particular diet-related conditions (e.g. coronary heart disease) we can analyse what is wrong with the local diet.

Conversely, by studying parts of the world where diet-related diseases are scarce, we can draw conclusions about what a healthy diet and lifestyle entail. There are four outstanding areas in the world where dietary links to health have excited epidemiologists. These are:
- the Mediterranean
- Toulouse and surrounding areas in France
- Greenland – in particular the diet of the Eskimos
- coastal regions of Japan inhabited by fisherfolk

By adopting the lessons learned in these regions and combining them with other scientific evidence, we have finally come up with a natural, healthy diet that will see us safely into the twenty-first century and beyond.

Changing the eating habits of a lifetime is not going to be easy. But I can promise you it will be interesting.

You will be exposed to exciting new taste experiences. You will lose your cravings for simple sugars and stodgy snacks high in saturated fat. You will lose any excess weight easily and painlessly and, most importantly, your risk of developing or dying from diseases that are the scourge of Western life today will be significantly lowered.

Aims of the Body Awareness Programme

The three Body Awareness diets all have similar aims:

1. To eliminate as much processed and pre-packed foods (jumping with additives) as possible. The diets are based on natural wholefoods filled with minerals, vitamins and fibre.

2. To increase your carbohydrate intake to 55–60 per cent. The World Health Organization recommends that unrefined carbohydrates supply 50–70 per cent of daily calories. Most of us obtain less than 40 per cent of our energy from this source.

3. To increase your intake of fresh fruit, salads and vegetables to 400–800g daily. For maximum health, we need to eat over 500g of fruit and vegetables per day. This may sound a lot, but it's surprisingly easy. Fruits and vegetables are high in antioxidants and help protect against coronary heart disease and cancer – especially tumours of the gut and bladder.

4. To decrease the amount of dietary fat, especially saturated fat that you eat. Fats should make up no more than 30 per cent of daily calories. That's around 75g for men and 53g for women. Most of us eat around 100g of fat per day which is far too high. The Mediterranean Slim Diet contains only 20 per cent fat for fast weight loss, of which the majority is derived from fish oils or olive oil for optimum health.

5. To decrease the amount of red meat and eggs in your diet. When following the Mediterranean Slim Diet, meat is only eaten once a week, with red and white meat alternating. On other days, you eat as a vegetarian or a fish-itarian. This automatically reduces the amount of saturated fat in your diet.

6. To increase the amount of fish you eat. Fish contains Omega-3 oils which are beneficial for your heart and

cholesterol balance. Fish is also an excellent source of protein.

7. To increase the amount of pulses, seeds and nuts in your diet. The World Health Organization recommends that we include 30g of nuts or seeds in our daily diet. This is especially important for those who don't eat meat. Nuts and seeds are high in essential fatty acids.

8. To reduce the amount of simple sugars and sweets you eat. These provide refined carbohydrates which are rapidly absorbed and cause detrimental sugar fluctuations in the blood.

9. To enable you to enjoy the beneficial effects of wine. Wine – especially red wine – is good for health in moderation. Many studies have shown that a moderate intake of wine can reduce the risk of death from coronary heart disease by a massive 40 per cent.

   Red grape juice is thought to be as beneficial as red wine itself. The Mediterranean Slim Diet allows you to choose between one glass of good red wine or red grape juice per day.

10 To include food supplements which are essential for maximum health, especially during weight loss:

- Gammalinolenic acid (oil of evening primrose; starflower oil) to provide essential fatty acids and maintain your skin quality and hormonal balance. This is especially important on a low-fat slimming diet.
- Vitamins C, E and betacarotene – powerful antioxidants that help prevent cell damage from free radical reactions. Free radicals are released in higher numbers as you raid your fat stores whilst losing weight. A supplement such as Vital 3 is recommended.

Readers suffering from fatigue, stress and tiredness – or with a tendency towards anaemia – may wish to take an iron supplement as well.

Exercise

Exercise is essential to improve your health and speed up weight loss. It:

- converts flabby tissues to muscle so you look toned and slim more quickly
- improves the stamina and efficiency of your heart
- increases the rate at which your body uses oxygen
- increases your basal metabolic rate so you burn fat more rapidly

Relaxation

Relaxation is essential to improve your self-esteem and decrease levels of stress hormones. Flotation therapy is especially beneficial to a weight-loss regime. By stimulating the creative side of your brain, flotation therapy expands your mental capacity and allows you to become more 'body aware'.

Introduction

A recent government report reached a rather frightening conclusion – almost half the adults in the United Kingdom have put their health at risk through being overweight.

The 1990 study into dietary and nutritional habits showed that in the last decade, although the average calorie intake was *below* the recommended level, the incidence of obesity has risen from 8 per cent to 12 per cent in women and from 6 per cent to 8 per cent in men.

In addition, 36 per cent of women and 35 per cent of men fall into the overweight category without yet being obese. Spot the significant word 'yet'. As a nation we are on an ever-increasing spiral of fat accumulation despite the plethora of dietary advice books and exercise programmes available.

Half the women in the UK claim to be 'on a diet' at any one time and the consumer, who is busy consuming in all senses of the word, spends around £6 million every week on diet foods alone – without counting what is spent on diet-related health books, slimming magazines and wonder treatments. If these are included, the figure reached is a staggering £1,000 million per year.

Why is none of it working? Increasing numbers of people are dying or becoming unwell from weight-related diseases.

Disorders Related to Overweight and Unhealthy Diet

Circulatory
- Angina
- Atherosclerosis (hardening of the arteries)
- Cerebro-vascular accidents (strokes)
- Hypertension (high blood pressure)
- Myocardial infarction (heart attack)
- Peripheral vascular disease (poor circulation)
- Varicose veins

Metabolic
- Diabetes
- Hyperlipidaemia (high blood cholesterol/fats)
- Gout

Gastro-intestinal
- Acid reflux (heartburn)
- Cholelithiasis (gall stones)
- Cirrhosis and other diseases of the liver
- Diverticular disease
- Inflammatory bowel disease
- Irritable bowel syndrome

Respiratory
- Breathlessness
- Hypoventilation (under-breathing)
- Sleep apnoea (snoring; lack of oxygen at night)

Musculo-skeletal
- Back pain
- Osteoarthritis
- Joint pains

Immunological
- Auto-immune disease
- Eczema
- Frequent infections

Malignancy
- Cancer of the bladder
- Cancer of the breast
- Cancer of the cervix
- Cancer of the endometrium (womb lining)
- Cancer of the gastro-intestinal tract
- Cancer of the ovary
- Cancer of the pancreas
- Cancer of the prostate
- Cancer of the rectum

Gynaecological
- Cyclical breast pain
- Dysmenorrhoea (painful periods)
- Menorrhagia (heavy periods)
- Premenstrual syndrome
- Thrush
- Urinary tract infection

Pregnancy
- Gestational diabetes
- High blood pressure in pregnancy
- Pre-eclampsia (and toxaemia)
- Sub-fertility

Psychological
- Alcohol abuse
- Anxiety and stress
- Depressive illness
- Lethargy
- Obsessive/compulsive eating disorders

If we include minor niggles like haemorrhoids and constipation, the drain on the NHS, and our health, is staggering.

Our Diet Is the Main Problem

Our Western diet is essentially unhealthy. Combined with a stressful and sedentary lifestyle, it contains all the ingredients needed for early death through coronary heart disease. Add in obesity and cigarette smoking and you might as well get your coffin measured now.

Coronary heart disease is one of the biggest killers in the Western world. In the USA, over 1.5 million people have heart attacks per year and another 80 million are investing in one through elevated cholesterol levels and deposits.

In the UK, 180,000 people die every year from coronary heart disease. Two-thirds of us have blood cholesterol levels above the recommended upper limit of 5.2 mmol/l.

We eat more convenience food than the rest of Europe and, on average, get over 40 per cent of our daily energy requirements from saturated fats. This figure is dangerously high.

Our government is sufficiently worried to suggest that we reduce our total fat intake to no more than 35 per cent of daily calories. American guidelines go even further, suggesting a healthier fat intake is 30 per cent of energy intake.

Unless you have consciously lowered the amount of fat in your diet – it's probably slowly killing you.

The Baddy

The most dangerous type of fat is saturated fat. This is readily converted by the liver into an undesirable form of cholesterol linked with hardening and furring up of the arteries (low density LDL-cholesterol).

British guidelines recommend we reduce our saturated fat intake to less than 11 per cent of total energy intake. For Americans, the corresponding figure is less than 10 per cent. Unfortunately, the British currently obtain as much as 15 per cent of energy from saturated fat.

Our eating and lifestyle habits need changing – and fast. Otherwise, doctors will soon be writing 'food' as a cause of death on most certificates.

Changing Our Habits

One problem with dieting is that changes made whilst attempting to lose weight are subconsciously labelled as 'temporary'.

As soon as weight is lost, and in most cases even before the goal is met, old eating habits creep back with a vengeance. In go the chocolates, cakes and biscuits and on go the yo-yoing pounds.

The dieting cycle *can* be broken; overweight *can* be conquered. Positive and realistic attitudes are needed – but most of all, you must be prepared for dietary changes to permeate your life. For ever.

Be aware of your diet and your body at all times. Nurture it, like a delicate flower – don't treat it harshly and leave it to struggle like a weed.

Body awareness means thinking slim, healthy, beautiful and self-confident for ever. It means being aware of how your body works and providing it with the nutrients and lifestyle it craves for optimum healthy functioning.

Healthy eating and exercise should be with you for the rest of your life; and you will live longer to enjoy it as a result.

Follow the Body Awareness Programme and improve

your total health – weight, looks, mind, creativity, fitness, sex-drive and self-esteem.

Learn to relax, diffuse away that stress, think positively and as a consequence you will improve two of the most important attributes you possess – your fitness and your health.

For Slimmers

If you need to lose weight, use the Body Awareness Food Exchange or Mediterranean Slim diets to shed those excess pounds – scientifically, healthily and safely.

Retain these principles with the Body Awareness Maintenance Plan and you need never fight your battle of the bulge again.

Weight Maintenance

If your weight is normal and you want to eat more healthily, or you have recently lost weight on a calorie-restricted diet and want to keep it off, the Body Awareness Maintenance Plan is the one for you.

A healthy diet plus exercise can significantly improve the physiological and biochemical processes occurring in your body right now. They have been proved to:
- lower the stickiness of blood
- reduce blood levels of harmful LDL-cholesterol
- reduce the secretion of stress hormones
- correct steroid hormone imbalances
- reduce blood pressure
- maintain normal blood glucose
- help to reverse atherosclerosis
- lower your risk of coronary artery disease
- lower your risk of certain cancers

- improve your fertility
- encourage positive thought
- improve your mental functions
- prevent recurrent depression
- improve the texture of skin
- increase the density of bone
- improve your overall fitness and well-being

The Body Awareness Programme will show you how.

CHAPTER 1

The Principles of Body Awareness

The Body Awareness Programme is based on scientific principles. It harnesses and combines natural, life-enhancing factors to improve your overall health. These involve:

- beneficial dietary changes
- healthy exercise
- relaxation techniques
- creative thought
- improved self-esteem

Beneficial Dietary Changes

The nutritional programme is based largely on the Mediterranean diet with a little Eskimo and Japanese thrown in. It also recommends dietary supplements of gammalinolenic acid (oil of evening primrose; starflower oil), betacarotene, and vitamins E and C. These have beneficial effects on the way our body metabolizes fats and feeds into certain biochemical pathways.

Enzyme blocks are overcome, damaging free radicals are mopped up and essential dietary oils are not excessively oxidized before their positive effects are enjoyed.

If you are not comfortable with increasing the amount of fish in your diet, don't despair. Fish oil supplements (1g Omega-3 fatty acids per day or 3g fish oil containing one-third fatty acids) will have the same beneficial effects.

Introducing the Mediterranean Diet

The biggest killer in both the UK and USA is coronary heart disease. In contrast, experiments have shown that people following a diet high in:
- olive oil
- garlic
- unrefined carbohydrates
- fish
- lean white meat
- red wine
- fresh fruit
- fresh vegetables
- fresh herbs and spices

have the lowest incidence of coronary heart disease in the Western world. This is particularly true of those living around the Mediterranean, despite the fact that their diet is high in saturated fats.

Saturated fats usually raise blood cholesterol levels and hasten hardening and furring up of the arteries. Yet something in the diet or lifestyle of Mediterranean people seems to protect them against the harmful effects of their fatty diet.

This protection does not stem from an inherited, genetic trait. If people native to the Mediterranean area move away and change their diet and lifestyle – for example to that of the Scots – their risk of developing coronary heart disease rapidly soars.

It's now thought that a combination of vitamin C, E and betacarotene, certain substances found in red wine and grapes, plus some aspects of the Mediterranean lifestyle play an important role in this protective effect.

Introducing the Eskimo Diet

The Japanese and the Eskimos also have a low incidence of coronary heart disease. They eat a diet high in fish oils and reap the benefits of a substance called eicosapentanoic acid (EPA). This is produced by plankton, eaten by fish and concentrated in marine body oils.

When incorporated into our diet, EPA from fish discourages clotting of blood and lowers our blood cholesterol levels. This dramatically reduces our risk of death from coronary heart disease.

The Body Awareness Diet

The Body Awareness Diet brings together all the scientifically proven benefits of both the Mediterranean diet and the Eskimo diet. It incorporates the cholesterol-lowering properties of garlic, olive oil, walnuts, fish oils, red wine, exercise and profound relaxation.

Oil of evening primrose (rich in gammalinolenic acid) and vitamin E are added to balance and protect our dietary fats. This offsets common, low-fat dieting problems such as dry skin, menstrual disturbances and cyclical breast pain. Exciting new research also suggests that both gammalinolenic acid and EPA (eicosapentanoic acid) can also protect against certain cancers (*see Chapter 8*).

Healthy Exercise

Exercise has a number of beneficial effects on the body,

one of the most important being its cholesterol-lowering effect. The Body Awareness Programme allows you to assess your current fitness level, which is likely to be lower than you expected.

A suggested fitness regime is included. This is not arduous, or boring, and will definitely improve your health. It will build up your strength, stamina and suppleness and, most importantly, improve the condition of your heart.

The exercise programme is scientifically based. It uses your pulse rate to fine-tune exercise levels and to achieve the maximum cardiovascular benefit.

If you are not keen on counting your pulse rate or doing sums, don't worry – these aren't essential. They merely provide a deeper element of body awareness if required.

Relaxation Techniques

Total health and fitness encompass mental balance too. Stress is a major killer and needs to be combated with effective relaxation techniques. These include aromatherapy, massage, meditation, flotation and REST (restricted environment stimulation therapy). Everyone should try at least one float in their lifetime. Don't be surprised if you get hooked.

Again, this isn't an essential component of body awareness, though it is a very desirable one. For those unwilling, or unable to undertake a flotation programme, alternative relaxation techniques are suggested.

Creative Thought

Combined with a balanced diet and improved fitness,

effective relaxation frees the creative and intellectual aspects of your brain. You will become:

- more empathic
- more responsive
- more creative
- more inquisitive
- more self-confident
- less stressed

As well as helping you to achieve a new silhouette, body awareness encourages you to find a new inner self. You will actively seek new goals, new ways to stretch your mind and accomplish new achievements. You will contribute more to life and, as a consequence, you will receive more back.

Improved Self-esteem

As you lose weight and become more body aware, your self-confidence, self-esteem and peak performance will soar. Your stress levels will plummet and your risk of coronary heart disease will significantly reduce.

Getting Started

We're going to tackle the Body Awareness Programme in the best traditions of an experienced trouble-shooter. First, you need to assess:

- where you are (body awareness assessment phase)
- where you want to be (target weight and fitness)
- how you're going to get there (your personal body awareness programme)

At the end of each week, whilst following the body awareness regime, regularly up-date your Body Awareness

Self-assessment Chart (*see Appendix 9*). This will provide a complete record of your achievements in:

- losing weight
- losing inches
- re-sculpting your shape
- improving your fitness index

CHAPTER 2

Where You Are Now

Body Awareness Assessment Phase

Work through the following chapter and fill out the self-assessment questionnaires.

An initial, accurate assessment of your overall fitness is important. This will help to indicate:

- how poor your health is now
- how overweight you are
- your risk of dying from a weight-related disease
- how much your heart is struggling
- how supple you are
- how quickly you can regain optimum fitness

Most importantly of all, an honest assessment of where you are now will raise your body awareness. It will focus your mind on the positive steps you can take to improve yourself and increase your enjoyment of life.

How Overweight Are You?

Everyone has at some time or another glanced at a height versus 'desirable' weight chart and wondered if they needed to diet. The tables were drawn up by insurance companies who loaded certain premiums against the risks of ill–health from obesity.

These charts were based on population norms but unfortunately, it's now almost normal to be overweight. Apart from anything else, these charts entailed assigning oneself arbitrarily to frame columns headed Large, Medium or Small – and allowed too much leeway for cheating. How easy to massage those figures and claim an enormous frame despite having sparrow–sized bones.

By far the best and most modern way of calculating excess body fat is Quetelet's Body Mass Index (BMI). Quetelet was a Belgian researcher who noted that, for normal weight people, there is a more or less constant relationship between weight and the square of a person's height.

$$\text{BMI} = \frac{\text{weight (kg)}}{\text{height (m)} \ \text{x} \ \text{height (m)}}$$

For example, if we take a mythical woman whose weight is 70kg (11 st) and height 1.7m (5ft 7ins) her BMI can be obtained by dividing 70 by 1.7 twice:

$$70 \div 1.7 \div 1.7 = 24.22.$$

BMI is useful as it can be used to grade obesity as follows:

Body Mass Index	Weight Band	Grade
<20	Underweight	–
20–24.9	Healthy	0
25–29.9	Overweight	I
30–39.9	Obese	II
>40	Morbidly obese	III

Write your initial BMI here ....
Write your initial weight band here...
Write your initial grade of obesity here ....

For men, a healthy BMI falls within the range of 20 to 24.9. A slightly lower BMI of 18.7 to 23.8 is better for women because our muscle:fat ratio is necessarily different to allow for feminine curves.

A few gremlins can affect results, e.g. if your muscle mass is significantly above normal (e.g. body builders/weight-lifters) or if your body has retained an excessive amount of fluid (e.g. serious heart failure or kidney disease).

BMI is unlikely to mislead the averagely unfit participant of the Body Awareness Programme.

If you think you are retaining water, try pressing your thumb into the flesh just above your ankle. Maintain a good pressure for at least 10 seconds. If a noticeable 'pit' in your flesh results, this can indicate oedema (excess fluid). Consult your doctor for a check-up.

Is Your Excess Weight Tempting Fate?

BMI calculation confirms that almost half the British population is overweight, with a BMI of greater than 25kg/m^2.

When you've worked out your BMI, plot it on the Risk of Death chart overleaf and work out the extent to which your excess fat is killing you.

Write the increased risk of death for your BMI here ......

The higher your BMI rises above 25, the higher your percentage of body fat – and the more your health is at risk.

At a BMI of 30, risk of death is 50 per cent above that expected for the non-overweight. At a BMI of 35, your risk of death is doubled, mostly due to diseases associated with excess fat.

TABLE 1: Mortality Index Chart

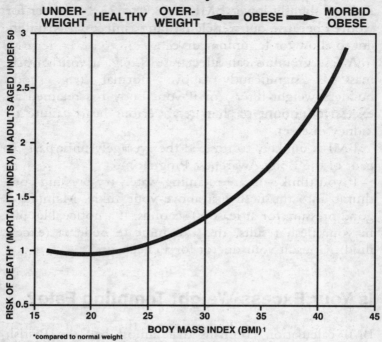

UNDER-WEIGHT   HEALTHY   OVER-WEIGHT   ◄ OBESE ►   MORBID OBESE

RISK OF DEATH* (MORTALITY INDEX) IN ADULTS AGED UNDER 50

BODY MASS INDEX (BMI)[1]

*compared to normal weight

CLASSIFICATION	ACCEPTABLE	OVER-WEIGHT	OBESE	MORBID OBESE
BODY MASS[1] **INDEX (BMI)** 1. Adapted from BRAY G.A. *Int. J. Obesity*, 1978; 2;99 –114	20 – 24.9	25 – 29.9	30 – 40	> 40
HEALTH RISK[2] **CLASSIFICATION** 2. Adapted from BRAY G.A. *In Human Obesity*, 1985; 222 –234	HEALTHY	LOW	MODERATE	HIGH
GARROW GRADE[3] **OF OBESITY** 3. Adapted from GARROW JS. *In Treat Obesity Seriously*, 1981; 1 –5	0	I	II	III

Used with the permission of Servier Laboratories (UK) Limited

The BMI of 24.22 we calculated earlier for our mythical woman is just about OK as far as health goes, though above the recommended 23.8 upper limit for women. She may want to lose a few more kilograms to lower her BMI to nearer 22. At this level, she will look and feel her best.

Skinfold Measurement

Whilst BMI is more accurate than old-fashioned weight for height charts, it does have limits. It is based on measuring the amount of fat in your body, but cannot differentiate between how much weight is fat or how much is muscle and bone.

A good way of assessing the percentage of fat in your body is to have skinfold thicknesses measured. Most high-tech health clubs and a few GP surgeries can do this for you.

Body fat is pinched between special callipers and fat thickness measured. This is done at the back of the arms, the top of the arms, above the hip, beneath the shoulder blade and at the front of the thighs. It is quick and relatively simple, but does nip a little.

The assessment relies heavily on the accuracy of the person taking the measurement, so to minimize discrepancies, three consecutive readings are taken and the average value used. The results are analysed by computer or assessed from charts.

Write your initial skin fold thicknesses here:
1. Back of the arms (triceps)   = ... mm
2. Above the hip (suprailiac)   = ... mm
3. Front of the thighs   = ... mm
Sum of skinfold thickness 1,2 & 3 = ... mm

How Much Spare Flesh to Lose?

It's an encouraging exercise to measure the amount of flesh you are losing. When dieting, the scales frequently measure no weekly loss at all. Despite sticking rigidly to your eating regime, and despite feeling fitter in yourself, the scales stubbornly refuse to budge. There are many reasons for this (*see Chapter 4*).

One is that muscle weighs more than adipose tissue (fat). You have converted flab to lean flesh and your percentage of body fat has fallen. Weight loss may not record this change, but contour measurement will. Your silhouette is trimmer. By measuring yourself, and recording flesh loss, you will maintain your positive attitude to dieting.

For accuracy, use a non–stretch, paper tape measure and get someone else to measure for you. If you can't face someone else knowing your innermost secrets, self–assessment is OK. You can improve accuracy by marking the position of the tape on your skin with an indelible ink pen. Then, each time you re-measure, ensure the tape is in the same place. It's best to use centimetres rather than inches – these will show a greater reduction over time.

Write your initial body dimensions here:

Bust .... cm

Chest (below bust) .... cm

Left upper arm .... cm

Right upper arm .... cm

Waist .... cm

Hips.. cm

Left thigh .... cm

Right thigh .... cm

Sum total of above = ... cm

Are You an Apple or a Pear?

Using a tape measure, work out both your waist and hip measurements. You can either use centimetres or inches as long as the same measurement is taken for both readings. Now divide your waist measurement by your hip measurement to get the ratio.

$$\frac{\textbf{waist}}{\textbf{hip}} = \textbf{ratio}$$

If the ratio is greater than 0.85 for women (0.95 for men), you are an apple or android shape. If your ratio is less, you are a pear, or gynoid shape.

Your waist/hip ratio is important. Those with a central (apple) deposition of adipose tissue are at a greater risk of coronary heart disease, stroke, high blood pressure, atherosclerosis, high blood cholesterol and diabetes than those with a more peripheral, pear-shaped distribution of fat. The reason for this is not fully understood, but may be related to altered metabolism of intra-abdominal adipose tissue (brown fat). See page 402.

If you have a BMI over 30 and are also apple-shaped, you are significantly at risk of coronary heart disease; even more so if it runs in your family.

Write your body shape here: Waist/hip ratio = ...
I am apple/pear-shaped.

Are You an Ectomorph, an Endomorph, or a Mesomorph?

Body shape can be loosely divided into three main types which will help to determine your metabolic rate:

Ectomorphs tend to be tall for their weight, with long,

thin limbs and muscles. Their skeletal frame is narrow and they have a naturally high metabolic rate. They have a high ratio of lean to fatty tissue and can cope with a large calorie intake without putting on weight.

Ectomorphs also have a relatively high amount of brown fat which can uncouple the metabolism of food from the production of energy-rich storage molecules. Excess energy is expended as heat and by constantly moving or fidgeting.

Endomorphs tend to be overweight, shorter than average and not at all athletic. They have a high ratio of fatty tissue to lean muscle and are often described as 'cuddly'. As fatty tissue burns calories more slowly than lean tissue, endomorphs have a lower metabolic rate than either ectomorphs or mesomorphs and have a constant problem battling against their tendency to put on weight.

Mesomorphs are of average build, with well-developed, plump muscles. They tend to be robust and athletic. Mesomorphs may weigh as much as, or more than, an endomorph of the same height but they look thinner because of the higher proportion of lean muscle to fat.

Their silhouettes are more attractive because they are well toned rather than flabby. As lean tissue burns calories faster than fatty tissue, mesomorphs have a relatively high basal metabolic rate.

Most people can recognize bits of each body type in themselves, but one type will tend to predominate.

Ectomorphs will naturally gravitate towards the lower end of the healthy BMI range for their height. Mesomorphs will tend towards the middle to upper ranges of the healthy BMI for their height. They have a greater amount of muscle mass which weighs more than fat. Endomorphs may have difficulty losing weight and in keeping it off once they've done so. They will naturally gravitate towards the upper limit of their BMI range and often exceed it.

It's most important for endomorphs to stick rigidly to the Body Awareness Maintenance Plan once they've reached a healthy weight.

If you are an endomorph, weigh yourself at least once a week. Take immediate remedial measures if you find you've gained even a few extra pounds. Otherwise, the excess weight will acquire an unpleasant tendency to multiply rapidly into an excess stone of flesh.

Write your predominant body type here ....

At this point you have a pretty good idea of where you are as regards body fat and body shape. Now let's start to formulate our body awareness goals.

CHAPTER 3

Where You Want To Be

When you take the plunge and start to slim, you need to know where you're going. It's tempting to set too strict a goal which turns out to be unrealistic or downright impossible.

Achieving your optimum body weight means losing some, but not necessarily all, of your excess fat. The Body Mass Index (BMI) range that you should initially aim at is one which is optimal for your health and your heart. This is called **coarse tuning**.

Once you are within your optimum BMI range, you can decide how much further you wish to go. This is called **fine tuning**. You may still have visible rolls of fat you wish to re-sculpt, especially if you haven't followed a regular and effective exercise regime.

For women, being fit and healthy doesn't mean having a beanpole model's shape. You can look and feel good while still being overtly feminine.

It is important to realize that at a BMI of less than 20 for men (18.7 for women), health is again at risk; this time through being underweight. That is the trap into which victims of anorexia nervosa fall. They have a higher risk of death from heart disease because their heart muscle is undernourished and easily tires.

How Much Should You Weigh?

There's no single ideal weight for each individual height. Using our knowledge of BMI, it's possible to work backwards and calculate a range of desirable, healthy weights to aim for. If your weight falls within the BMI range for your height, your risk of dying from a weight-related disease is at an optimal low.

TABLE 2: Optimum Body Weight For Males
Coarse Tuning Males – based on BMI of 20–25

HEIGHT		OPTIMUM BODY WEIGHT RANGE	
Metres	Feet/inches	Kilograms	Stones/pounds
1.47	4ft 10ins	43–53	6st 10lb–8st 6lb
1.50	4ft 11ins	45–56	7st 1lb–8st 11lb
1.52	5ft	46–58	7st 4lb–9st 1lb
1.55	5ft 1ins	48–60	7st 7lb–9st 5lb
1.57	5ft 2ins	49–61	7st 10lb–9st 8lb
1.60	5ft 3ins	51–64	8st 1lb–10st
1.63	5ft 4ins	53–66	8st 5lb–10st 5lb
1.65	5ft 5ins	55–68	8st 8lb–10st 9lb
1.68	5ft 6ins	56–70	8st 12lb–11st
1.70	5ft 7ins	58–72	9st 1lb–11st 4lb
1.73	5ft 8ins	60–75	9st 6lb–11st 10lb
1.75	5ft 9ins	61–76	9st 9lb–12st
1.78	5ft 10ins	63–79	9st 13lb–12st 6lb
1.80	5ft 11ins	65–81	10st 3lb–12st 9lb
1.83	6ft	67–83	10st 7lb–13st 1lb
1.85	6ft 1in	69–85	10st 11lb–13st 5lb
1.88	6ft 2ins	71–88	11st 2lb–13st 12lb
1.90	6ft 3ins	72–90	11st 5lb–14st 2lb
1.93	6ft 4ins	75–93	11st 10lb–14st 8lb

TABLE 3: Optimum Body Weight For Women
Coarse Tuning Females – based on BMI of 18.7–23.8

HEIGHT		OPTIMUM BODY WEIGHT RANGE	
Metres	Feet/inches	Kilograms	Stones/pounds
1.47	4ft 10ins	40–51	6st 4lb–8st
1.50	4ft 11ins	42–54	6st 8lb–8st 7lb
1.52	5ft	43–55	6st 11lb–8st 9lb
1.55	5ft 1in	45–57	7st 1lb–8st 13lb
1.57	5ft 2ins	46–59	7st 3lb–9st 4lb
1.60	5ft 3ins	48–61	7st 8lb–9st 8lb
1.63	5ft 4ins	50–63	7st 12lb–9st 13lb
1.65	5ft 5ins	51–65	8st–10st 3lb
1.68	5ft 6ins	53–67	8st 5lb–10st 7lb
1.70	5ft 7ins	54–69	8st 7lb–10st 12lb
1.73	5ft 8ins	56–71	8st 11lb–11st 2lb
1.75	5ft 9ins	57–73	8st 13lb–11st 7lb
1.78	5ft 10ins	59–75	9st 4lb–11st 11lb
1.80	5ft 11ins	61–77	9st 8lb–12st 1lb
1.83	6ft	63–80	9st 13lb–12st 8lb

You may be surprised at the weight range for each height, but remember:
- This BMI range gives you the optimum weight range for your health.
- At this level, your relative risk of dying from a weight-related disease is minimal.
- Once you are within this healthy BMI band, you can fine tune your weight depending on how you feel in yourself and on whether you are an ectomorph, mesomorph or endomorph.

Write your optimum weight range for health here ....

Most women feel at their best around a BMI of 21 to 22;

most men at a BMI of 22 to 23. Out of interest, let's see how much this narrows our BMI target range:

TABLE 4:
Fine Tuning Males – based on BMI of 22–23

HEIGHT		OPTIMUM BODY WEIGHT RANGE	
Metres	Feet/inches	Kilograms	Stones/pounds
1.47	4ft 10ins	48–50	7st 7lb–7st 12lb
1.50	4ft 11ins	50–52	7st 12lb–8st 2lb
1.52	5ft	51–53	8st 1lb–8st 5lb
1.55	5ft 1in	53–55	8st 5lb–8st 8lb
1.57	5ft 2ins	54–57	8st 7lb–8st 13lb
1.60	5ft 3ins	56–59	8st 12lb–9st 4lb
1.63	5ft 4ins	58–61	9st 1lb–9st 9lb
1.65	5ft 5ins	60–63	9st 6lb–9st 13lb
1.68	5ft 6ins	62–65	9st 10lb–10st 3lb
1.70	5ft 7ins	64–67	10st–10st 7lb
1.73	5ft 8ins	66–69	10st 5lb–10st 11lb
1.75	5ft 9ins	67–70	10st 7lb–11st
1.78	5ft 10ins	70–73	11st–11st 7lb
1.80	5ft 11ins	71–75	11st 2lb–11st 10lb
1.83	6ft	74–77	11st 8lb–12st 1lb
1.85	6ft 1in	75–79	11st 10lb–12st 6lb
1.88	6ft 2ins	78–81	12st 4lb–12st 9lb
1.90	6ft 3ins	79–83	12st 6lb–13st 1lb
1.93	6ft 4ins	82–86	12st 12lb–13st 7lb

TABLE 5:
Fine Tuning Females – based on BMI of 21–22

HEIGHT		OPTIMUM BODY WEIGHT RANGE	
Metres	Feet/inches	Kilograms	Stones/pounds
1.47	4ft 10ins	45–48	7st 1lb–7st 7lb
1.50	4ft 11ins	47–50	7st 5lb–7st 12lb
1.52	5ft	49–51	7st 10lb–8st 1lb
1.55	5ft 1in	50–53	7st 12lb–8st 5lb
1.57	5ft 2ins	52–54	8st 2lb–8st 7lb
1.60	5ft 3ins	54–56	8st 7lb–8st 12lb
1.63	5ft 4ins	56–58	8st 12lb–9st 1lb
1.65	5ft 5ins	57–60	8st 13lb–9st 6lb
1.68	5ft 6ins	59–62	9st 4lb–9st 10lb
1.70	5ft 7ins	61–64	9st 8lb–10st 1lb
1.73	5ft 8ins	63–66	9st 13lb–10st 5lb
1.75	5ft 9ins	64–67	10st 1lb–10st 7lb
1.78	5ft 10ins	67–70	10st 7lb–11st
1.80	5ft 11ins	68–71	10st 9lb–11st 2lb
1.83	6ft	70–74	11st–11st 9lb

This immediately gives you a tighter, optimum weight range to aim for. Remember:
- Coarse tune your weight to achieve the healthiest weight for your body and especially your heart.
- You can then fine tune your weight according to how you feel about yourself and your shape. But don't overdo it. Most women don't need to go below a BMI of 21.

Write your fine tuning optimum weight range here ....

How Many Calories Do You Need?

The old-fashioned 'recommended daily amounts' for calories are now superseded by the Committee on Medical Aspects of Food Policy (COMA) report published in 1991.

TABLE 6: Estimated Energy Requirements For Adults (COMA)

AGE	kcal/day MEN	WOMEN
11–14	2220	1845
15–18	2755	2110
19–59	2550	1920
60–74	2355	1900
75 and over	2100	1810

These estimated calorie intakes are averages only. Half the population will need less calories than those quoted – and half will need more.

Your calorie intake also depends on your current weight. The heavier you are, the more calories you need to maintain this extra bulk.

An approximate idea of your calorie needs can be obtained by multiplying your weight in pounds by 15.

e.g. A person weighing 10st (140lb) needs:
$140 \times 15 = 2,100$ kcls per day.

A person weighing 11st (154lb) needs:
$154 \times 15 = 2,310$ kcals per day.

A person weighing 17st (238lb) needs:
$238 \times 15 = 3,570$ kcals per day.

And that's just to maintain your weight.

This is only a rough guide however, and as we shall see in the section on metabolism, every individual varies greatly.

A female eating 1,800 kcals per day may gain weight compared with another woman of exactly the same height, weight and age, who will lose weight. Unfortunately, life is never fair in the slimming stakes.

One kilogram of fat is roughly equivalent to 7,000 kcals energy. Therefore, if you are 5kg (11lb) overweight, in theory you need to increase your energy output over your energy input by 35,000 (11 × 7,000) kcals in order to metabolize this excess fat.

This is not the same as saying that by eating 35,000 kcals less than usual you will lose those 5kg of excess fat. The process is much more complicated than that.

Other factors such as a changing metabolic rate, the activity of brown fat cells and the amount of energy dissipated (wasted) as heat all play an important role (*see Appendix 2: Metabolism And Fat*).

How Good is Your Posture?

Correct posture and balance can make you look instantly slimmer.

By standing incorrectly and slouching, we look fatter, shorter and put unacceptable strains on muscles, joints and ligaments. Over long periods of time, this can lead to permanent changes in shape and exacerbate curvature of the spine.

It is accepted that bad posture can lead to ill-health. Several therapies have been developed which aim to rectify a faulty body alignment. These include the Alexander technique, osteopathy and chiropractic.

The Mirror Test

Stand barefoot in front of a full-length mirror, naked or wearing a leotard/bodysuit/swimsuit. If you have long hair, tie it out of the way so you can see the curve of your neck and shoulders.

Stand as you normally would, don't consciously straighten up at this stage. Examine yourself critically from both front and side views, then answer the following questions as honestly as you can:

- Does your head poke forwards?
- Does your neck seem shortened?
- Are your shoulders rounded?
- Do your breasts sag?
- Does your stomach protrude?
- Does your waist seem wide?
- Does your bottom poke out?
- Does your bottom sag?
- Is the curve of your spine exaggerated?
- Do your knees 'knock' inwards?

Now try standing properly, with your body's natural posture corrected and aligned. Draw your body upwards, as if trying to add an extra six inches to your height. Lift your head up high so it sits balanced above your spine, straightening and elongating your neck.

Draw your shoulders back and pull in your stomach muscles.

Tilt your pelvis by rolling your bottom forwards and down so your pubic bone lifts forwards and up.

These movements naturally lengthen and straighten the spine. This lifts the rib cage and breasts and allows the shoulders to drop into a relaxed position.

Now study your reflection in the mirror, from the front and side. See how:

- you look taller, with a longer neck
- your shoulders have a better, squarer shape
- your trunk has elongated

- your breasts have acquired a more attractive shape
- your waist looks narrower
- your legs look longer
- your knees are less knock-kneed

By being aware of your body and posture, you have instantly created a better shape. Try to master this new body alignment until it's second nature.

You may find this hard initially, but as your weight decreases and your body fitness and suppleness improve through exercise, your posture will improve by leaps and bounds too.

Every time you pass a shop window, *check*! Consciously re-adjust any poor alignment. Soon, you won't even need to think about it — it will happen automatically.

Do You Smoke?

There are 14 million cigarette smokers in the UK, of whom two-thirds want to give up. But 80 per cent of smokers who try to give up relapse within one year. Only 35 per cent of smokers succeed in stopping before the age of 60. And 300 new smokers are hooked every day — in the UK alone.

Unfortunately, quitting smoking is easier said than done. You've got to crack the habit — as well as your nicotine addiction. Every time you smoke a cigarette, you put your hand to your mouth at least 10 times.

If you're a twenty-a-day-er that's your hand-mouth habit reinforced 200 times a day, 1,400 times per week, 73,000 times per year. And that's a lot of habit to kick.

Within seven seconds of puffing your cigarette, a powerful mind-drug — nicotine — reaches your brain to act as a stimulant and, in larger doses, as a relaxant.

If you suddenly stop taking this drug, withdrawal symptoms of tension, aggression, depression, insomnia, loss of concentration, constipation, cravings and weight-gain can occur.

A study involving half-a-million smokers has proved conclusively that the risk of premature death in smokers is nearly double that of non-smokers. On average, non-smokers live six years longer than smokers.

Health Risks of Cigarette Smoking

- 4,000 chemicals have been isolated from tobacco smoke, many of which are known to trigger cancer.
- Up to a quarter of all cot deaths are associated with passive smoking.
- Passive smoking is implicated in 4,000 spontaneous abortions per year.
- Passive smoking causes asthma, eczema and glue ear in young children.
- Smokers have 2.4 times the risk of a major depressive illness.
- Smoking impairs the rigidity of penile erections with a clear dose-related effect.
- Sub-arachnoid brain haemorrhage is six times more likely in young smokers than in non-smokers.
- Infertility is more likely in smokers.
- Smoking-related diseases kill 40 per cent of smokers before they reach retirement.
- Smoking during pregnancy causes malfunction of the placenta, still-birth, growth-retarded babies and babies of lower intelligence.
- Smokers are five times more likely to have premature wrinkles on the face than non-smokers.
- There are 300 deaths per day in the UK from smoking – and doctors can now write 'smoking' as the cause of death on certificates.

If that hasn't convinced you that smoking is not worthy of a body aware person, cigarettes are also associated with the following diseases:

Diseases Associated with Smoking Tobacco

Coronary heart disease
- Angina
- Myocardial infarction (heart attack)
- Palpitations

Circulatory disease
- Thrombosis (blood clots)
- Embolus (clots travelling round the body)
- Aortic aneurysm
- Hypertension (high blood pressure)
- Stroke
- Poor blood flow to legs
- Impotence
- Senile dementia
- Blindness

Lung disease
- Chronic bronchitis
- Emphysema
- Lung cancer

Gastro-intestinal tract disease
- Gingivitis (inflamed gums)
- Halitosis (bad breath)
- Peptic ulcers

Cancers

- Lung
- Breast
- Mouth, lip, tongue, throat
- Stomach
- Pancreas
- Large bowel
- Penis
- Bladder
- Kidney
- Cervix

Every time you have a shot of nicotine, blood vessels in your body go into spasm. Clotting factors in your blood are raised so your risk of a serious thrombosis or embolus increases.

The good news is: within 48 hours of giving up smoking, the levels of clotting factors in your blood fall low enough to reduce your chance of a heart attack or stroke. Within one year, your risk of contracting other diseases will also have come down to a near normal level. It is therefore never too late to become body aware – and give up smoking to save your life.

The Body Awareness Quit Plan: The Easy Way to Stop Smoking

1. Name the day and get into the right frame of mind.
2. Find someone to give up with you. It's much easier to give up with a friend or relative.
3. Throw away all your smoking paraphernalia – papers, matches, lighters, ashtrays and spare packets.
4. Take it one day at a time. The thought of never smoking again is frightening – but all you have to do is get

through one day without smoking. The trick is to tell yourself the same thing every day.

5. Keep a 'star chart' and stick in a gold star for every successful cigarette-free day. Plan a reward for every week of success with all that 'ash cash' you haven't spent on the weed.

6. Find something to occupy your hands. Remember, they're used to doing something at least 10 times for every cigarette you smoked per day. Try: model building, origami, painting or drawing. The worst thing you can do is sit in front of the television. What are you going to do when your favourite star lights up?

7. Become more active. Exercise regularly and improve your overall fitness. Exercise releases a chemical in the brain (serotonin) which gives you a natural 'high' and curbs your craving for nicotine.

8. When you get that urge to put something in your mouth, suck on an artificial cigarette. You can buy these in chemist shops — but why not make your own out of celery or carrot sticks? Another tip is to clean your teeth. The strong, tingling taste of peppermint will help to beat the need for something in your mouth.

9. Avoid situations where you used to smoke or plan ahead to overcome them. Ask friends not to smoke around you. In your coffee break, go for a brisk walk round the block rather than smoke in the rest room with everyone else.

10. Practise saying 'No thanks — I've given up!'

If you find your craving for nicotine is driving you mad, try nicotine patches to see you through. Patches can double your chance of success. They are particularly good if you suffer withdrawal symptoms such as irritability, loss of concentration or problems sleeping.

Stick a patch on any hairless bit of skin, such as your upper arm. Change the patch every day and *don't* take it off at night. You can also swim, bathe or shower with it on. Don't smoke whilst wearing your patch – this can be dangerous.

Use nicotine patches for up to three months – a short time when you consider you've probably been smoking for most of your adult life.

The Body Awareness Alcohol Assessment Plan

Over a quarter of all hospital admissions in the UK can probably be blamed on alcohol. Make sure you don't join this statistic by answering these simple screening questions designed to warn you (or your partner) of possible problems.

The first test is nicknamed **CAGE**. Score one point for each **Yes** you answer. A total of two or more points means you might have an alcohol problem – see your doctor for advice as soon as possible.

CAGE

Do you ever feel you should **C**ut down on your drinking?
Are you ever **A**nnoyed by people criticizing your drinking?
Do you ever feel **G**uilty about your drinking?
Do you ever drink first thing in the morning – i.e. have an **E**ye-opener?

Another useful quiz helps to detect signs of alcoholism. It was devised in America and is short, simple and to the point.

Answer **Yes** or **No** to each of the following 10 questions and add up your scores in the columns.

Question	Yes	No
Do you feel you are a NORMAL drinker?	0	2
Do friends or relatives think you are a NORMAL drinker?	0	2
Have you ever been to Alcoholics Anonymous?	5	0
Have you ever lost friends because of your drinking?	2	0
Have you been in trouble at work/school through drink?	2	0
Have you ever neglected family, work or obligations for two or more days in a row through drink?	2	0
Have you ever had the shakes (DTs), heard voices or seen things that weren't there?	5	0
Have you ever sought help about your drinking?	5	0
Have you ever been to hospital because of drinking?	5	0
Have you ever been arrested for drink/driving or failed a breathalyser test?	2	0

A score of 6 or more points indicates you might suffer from alcoholism. Seek advice from your doctor straight away.

Units of alcohol
1 unit of alcohol = one glass (100ml) wine *or*
= one measure (50ml) sherry *or*
= one tot (25ml) spirits *or*
= half a pint (280ml) normal beer

Safe weekly alcohol limits
	Safe	Dangerous
Men	21 units	50 units
Non-pregnant women	14 units	35 units

It's easy to *underestimate* how much you drink, especially

with beer. Extra-strong beers or lagers will quickly put you over the top.

- A man drinking two pints of normal beer has had 4 units of alcohol.
- A woman drinking two glasses of wine and a double vodka has also had 4 units of alcohol.

CHAPTER 4

How You Are Going to Get There

The Diet Process

The term metabolism describes all the chemical changes in the body that convert food energy from our diet into energy the body can use. These processes are either:

- **efficient** so most food energy is converted into energy-rich storage molecules (including fat) and little energy is wasted as heat, *or*
- **inefficient** where certain chemical reactions are uncoupled and instead of making energy-rich storage molecules, more energy is dissipated as heat.

Yo-Yo Dieting

Many diets fight themselves by slowing down your metabolism and making it super efficient. Food energy is converted into energy storage molecules and little is wasted as heat. Every calorie sticks and this is one reason why many diets − especially crash diets − fail.

The ultimate nightmare scenario results: you starve yourself for several days or even weeks and lose relatively little weight. When you start eating normally again, your metabolism stays in super-efficient mode and the weight piles back on at frightening speed.

Even worse, it bounces right back up to where you started from and then – effortlessly – soars higher.

You now weigh more than when you first decided your weight was unacceptable. Many dieters oscillate between high and low weights, swinging between desperate, semi-starvation diets and the binges brought on by depression and low blood sugar levels.

It is not *you* that is at fault, however. The nature of the diet you have been following has set your metabolic alarm bells ringing and resulted in your body's extraordinary, protective mechanisms clicking on.

The Body Awareness Programme

The body awareness weight-loss programme harnesses your metabolism and works *with* it rather than against it. It encourages those uncoupled reactions so more of the calories you eat are expended as heat.

It will beneficially change the ratio of cholesterol molecules in your blood and begin reversing the hardening and furring up of your arteries which started in your teens. This will reduce your risk of developing coronary heart disease which is linked with our unhealthy Western diet and lifestyle.

The Body Awareness Programme is designed to provide:

• Enough calories per day to encourage the normal, energy-wasteful metabolic reactions to continue in your body and discourage the switch to super-efficient mode.
• A high carbohydrate intake which allows the body to burn fat stores more easily. Carbohydrate also has an effect on the

33

brain to keep you feeling fuller for longer and kick-starts your metabolic rate.

- Essential fatty acids your body requires to prevent the deficiencies which often occur in low-fat dieting regimes. These will also balance out the effects of harmful fatty acids released from your body fat stores.
- A high level of vitamins C, E and betacarotene to boost the metabolism, improve your skin and mop up the damaging free radicals formed during normal metabolic reactions.
- Regular meals throughout the day to boost your metabolic rate through the specific dynamic action of food. This will also stop you feeling hungry or craving sugar. With a little-and-often system you can lose weight faster than by eating the same quantity of food during three big meals.
- A back-to-nature, healthy-eating plan based on the Mediterranean diet: fresh fruits, vegetables, natural-source, unrefined complex carbohydrates, olive oil, garlic, herbs, fish and a little red wine.

It is the sort of diet our ancestors would have followed and is boosted with a few carefully chosen supplements that complement our current understanding of how the human physiology works. Combined with a regular exercise programme, your metabolic rate will work faster than it has ever worked before. You will lose weight safely, healthily and – best of all – easily.

If you want to know more about the principles used in the Body Awareness Programme, refer to the appendices at the back of this book. It is not essential to read this section, but if you are interested in how the body works, and why certain dietary nutrients have been selected, it will make fascinating reading.

In short, the Body Awareness Programme is a delicious, no-hunger plan using a high-carbohydrate, high-fibre, essential-fat, snacking system which harnesses your metabolism and physiology so they work for you rather than against you.

It combines a scientific eating programme with exercise, relaxation, pampering and motivational techniques, and unlike most diets which ban alcohol, or make you feel guilty if you indulge, it even incorporates a daily allowance of wine.

The Body Awareness Diet will work, but only if you are enthusiastic, motivated and stick to it.

If you are half-hearted and eat more than your daily allowance, you are unlikely to achieve optimum results. Whenever your resolve starts to flag, try re-reading the chapter on motivation.

Remember, dieting isn't just a temporary thing to see you through your current overweight phase. Healthy eating must permeate your life until it becomes second nature. Otherwise, as soon as you revert to the old eating and lifestyle habits that made you fat in the first place, the weight will pile back on.

Start now and become body aware for ever. You will probably live longer as a result.

The Benefits of the Body Awareness Programme

• You'll rapidly feel better
If you have been following a typical Western diet high in saturated fat and low in vitamins, minerals, fresh fruits and vegetables, you may have had niggling problems with your health for some time. Lethargy, sluggishness, indigestion, constipation and fluid retention are inevitably linked to diet. We are what we eat! The Body Awareness Programme will soon have you feeling more vital and energized.
• Your skin, hair, eyes and nails will improve
Substituting the correct dietary fats for harmful ones will overcome enzyme deficiencies in the skin and central nervous system. Your eyes will appear whiter and brighter;

35

your skin will be smoother, clearer and less oily. Spots will disappear. Flakiness and dingy tones will improve. In the long term, your hair and nails will grow stronger, glossier and less brittle.

• Your digestive system will improve

An increased intake of fibre and fluid will flush your system through. Constipation will be a thing of the past. Motions will become bulkier, easier to pass and regular. You may notice they become paler and smell less offensive.

• Gynaecological problems will improve

Dietary fats (lipids) are important building blocks for sex hormones such as oestrogen, progesterone and testosterone. Including the correct types of lipid in your diet will prevent the enzyme blockages that cause hormonal imbalances. If you suffer from cyclical breast pain or heavy, painful, irregular periods, you will find these improve with time.

By eating a higher proportion of carbohydrate in your diet – and by eating it little-and-often, research has shown that premenstrual syndrome will improve – and in many cases disappear.

• Blood cholesterol levels will fall

There are two main types of cholesterol circulating in the blood. Low density (LDL)-cholesterol is harmful. Its molecules are small enough to seep into artery walls and accumulate, causing narrowing in a process called atherosclerosis. This is linked with high levels of saturated fat in our diet.

High density (HDL)-cholesterol is beneficial and protective against coronary heart disease (CHD). These molecules are too large to seep into artery walls and remain in the blood to perform essential functions.

Blood Total Cholesterol Levels

Desirable	<5.2 mmol/l
Borderline	5.2–6.4 mmol/l
Abnormal	6.5–7.8 mmol/l
High risk	>7.8 mmol/l

LDL-cholesterol levels should not be greater than 4 mmol/l.

If the ratio of total blood cholesterol to HDL-cholesterol is:

<5.0	– low risk of CHD
5.0–6.5	– moderate risk of CHD
>6.5	– high risk of CHD

Several factors are working together in the Body Awareness Programme to lower your blood level of harmful LDL-cholesterol significantly and raise the level of protective HDL–cholesterol. These factors include:
- decreased saturated fat intake
- increased monounsaturated olive oil intake
- increased fish intake
- increased intakes of garlic, walnuts and fresh herbs
- the beneficial effects of exercise

In addition, the profound relaxation achieved by flotation therapy has been scientifically proven to lower high blood cholesterol levels.

• You will improve the health of your heart

Exercise, lowered blood cholesterol levels, weight loss and relaxation will significantly improve the health of your heart. Most importantly, your risk of coronary heart disease will reach an all-time low.

Once you've lost your excess weight, you will have no difficulty keeping it off. The transition to the Body Maintenance Plan involves principles you've already learned – and will want to follow for the rest of your life.

Prepare delicious meals for the family based on

traditional Mediterranean recipes and, as a bonus, their health will improve too.

How Quickly Will I Lose Weight?

The rate at which your excess weight comes off depends on a number of factors, including your current Body Mass Index (BMI), your personal metabolic rate, your level of activity, your age and your starting weight.

In general, the more fat you need to shed to reach your fine-tuning, optimum weight for health, the quicker your initial weight loss will be.

The first week of the diet will produce the most dramatic weight loss. This is because you are burning up glycogen stores found mainly in your muscles and liver.

Glycogen is bound to four times its weight in water and this will be lost in the first week too. It's not unusual to lose 2.5kg (5½lb) during the first seven days.

This fast-track weight loss will then slow to an ideal 0.5-1kg (1-2lb) per week. It may not seem very fast, but remember: the excess weight crept up over a long period of time.

If you try to lose weight too quickly a number of unwanted effects will occur:

- Your metabolism will revert to super-efficient mode. Less food energy will be dissipated as heat and every calorie you eat will stick.
- Lean body tissue will be burned rather than fat stores. Your ratio of body fat to lean tissue may go up.
- You will get bored and a snack-attack will occur. You are in danger of having a binge.

By losing weight slowly and safely, you are more likely to keep it off.

Accept That Your Weight Loss May Be Slow

You can't expect to lose in one month what it took you several months or even years to put on in the first place.

Unfortunately, one of the commonest reasons for giving up on a slimming diet is that the weight-loss process is too slow.

All that effort in counting calories, weighing food and sweating in the gym is translated into a minuscule downward blip on the scales. Is all that self-denial really worth it? The answer is YES, YES and YES again!

One of the main reasons for losing weight is to improve your overall health. This will decrease your risk of a serious, obesity-related disease.

Studies in overweight patients with late-onset diabetes have shown that each kilogram of fat lost is associated with an extended life expectancy of three to four months.

A successful weight loss that brings you down into the healthy BMI range is likely to prolong your life as well as improve your appearance and self-esteem. That's why it's worth persevering.

Let's take the worst likely scenario: a slow weight loss of only 0.5kg (1¼lb) per week. This slow weight loss will occur in someone with a naturally efficient metabolic rate. It is also likely to happen to someone who is over 50 years old, as the metabolic rate slows with age.

0.5kg per week may not seem like a lot of fat to lose but it all adds up. Over one month, that's 2kg (4½lb) lost. Big deal, you might think, but over three months you will have lost a total of 6kg (13½lb) – almost a stone.

In six months you will have shed a massive 12kg (27lb) excess body fat. Given that it probably went on over several years, six months is not really a lot of time to spend in slowly taking it off.

And that's just the worst possible scenario. Most people

following the Body Awareness Programme will find they shed excess fat safely, healthily and easily at least twice as quickly as this.

If you look at it another way, every month in which weight is lost is a month in which it hasn't been gained.

What would happen if you gave up the diet just because your weight loss was too slow? The weight that had taken all that effort to lose would just pile back on. The tight clothes would remain tight – or become even tighter. Your health would continue to be at risk from all that excess fat.

Your Weighing and Plotting Routine

It is important to weigh yourself regularly when losing weight – and to weigh yourself at the same time of the day – in the nude.

Weigh yourself first thing in the morning after getting out of bed – and after going to the loo. During the day, fluid slowly accumulates in the body due to a combination of gravity, hormones and various processes of metabolism.

Once we lie down and go to sleep, our fluid balance is corrected and we excrete any excess first thing in the morning. This is the time when we will weigh the least.

Most diets recommend that you only weigh yourself once a week. If you prefer to do this, fine, but it might not give you an accurate idea of how well you are doing.

Our body weight fluctuates naturally during the day. Sometimes we can retain a surprising amount of fluid. If your weekly weigh-in occurs on a fluid-retaining day, it may seem as if you've lost no weight at all. In reality you will have managed to lose several pounds of fat, but this is disguised by the retained fluid.

Daily weighings which show an upward swing on

occasion, even though you know you've stuck to the diet, are nothing to worry about. They represent fluid retention – perhaps just before a menstrual period – and you can recognize them as such.

Controlled trials in hospital have confirmed that fat losses equivalent to about 15,000 calories (around 2kg) can be completely masked by fluid retention, so patients can seem to put on weight whilst actually losing fat.

Try not to place too much importance on the daily fluctuations in your weight. It is the average, overall weight loss for any particular week which will guide you on how well you are doing.

Look at the following graph. This shows an average weekly weigh-in chart. Not terribly heartening, is it?

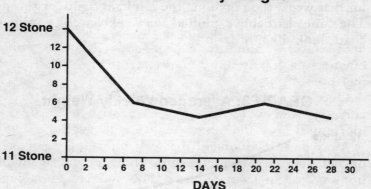

GRAPH 1: Weekly Weight

Now consider the same chart, but with daily weighings included. This provides a much more interesting and encouraging record of the dieter's progress.

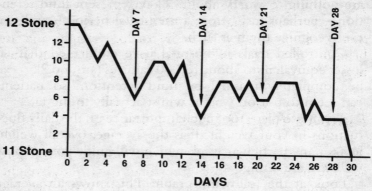

GRAPH 2: Daily Weight Chart

The best, most accurate way to record your weight is to plot your weekly average weight. This is obtained by adding together the seven daily weights you've recorded for that week, then dividing the resultant figure by seven. The same chart above, plotted as a weekly average weight chart, looks like this:

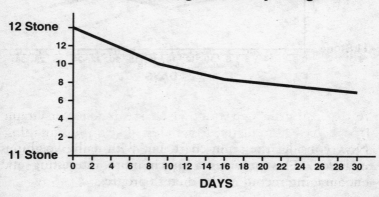

GRAPH 3: Averaged Weekly Weight

42

If you can find time to plot this average weekly weight, you will find it much more encouraging.

In addition, by weighing yourself every day, you are constantly re-affirming your desire to lose weight and are bringing that fact to the foremost part of your consciousness.

Plotting Weight Loss

Another favourite way to plot your progress is to record accumulative weight lost rather than total body weight. For example, on the following graph, Mrs W.M. managed to lose 2lb in the first week, 1lb in week two, 2lb in week three and 1lb in week four.

GRAPH 4: Accumulative Weekly Weight Loss

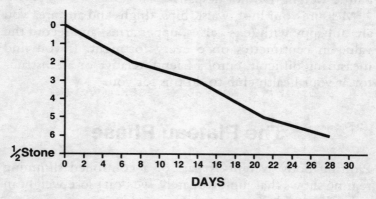

You can easily draw up your own chart (modelled on Graph 4) to record accumulative weight lost. The important thing is to try to ensure that the downward line you plot is not too steep (i.e. you are not losing weight too rapidly) and, furthermore, that your chart does not indicate an overall weight gain. If it does, you are beginning to slide off the tracks and need to review your weight loss strategy.

Using a Tape Measure

In some people, unflattering measurements and a bulging silhouette are as much due to poor muscle tone as to excess body fat.

You may find that your appearance improves dramatically from the exercise programme, even though your overall weight loss is small. For you, the tape measurements that you record on the Body Awareness Self-assessment Chart (*see Appendix 9*) are more important than what the scales say.

By toning up your body, you will lose inches without losing much in the way of pounds. In fact, as muscle is more dense than body fat, you may find you even put on a little weight. Do not despair.

Measure your bust, waist, hips, thighs and any area you are unhappy with (e.g. calves, upper arms) and record the value in centimetres once every fortnight. If you find measuring difficult, enrol a friend, relative or an instructor at your health club to do this for you.

The Plateau Phase

Plotting body weight as part of a controlled slimming regime shows that, unfortunately, we don't lose weight in a simple straight line. If only we could.

Sooner or later – probably sooner – we're going to run into the dieter's brick wall, the plateau phase.

Look at the following weight-loss chart.

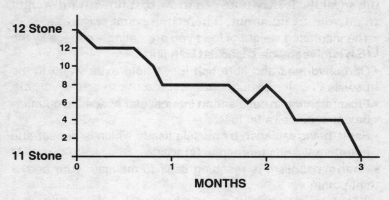

GRAPH 5: Plateau Phases

12 Stone

12

10

8

6

4

2

11 Stone

0   1   2   3

MONTHS

This dieter has had to suffer three weight plateaux. This is not an unusual number over a three-month diet. The more weight you have to lose, the more plateaux you will endure.

Body Set-points

The latest evidence suggests that we each have a series of body set-points. These are weights which our body will try to maintain – either by altering our metabolic rate or by manipulating our fluid balance.

These physiologically ideal weights occur over a wide range and some are well outside what we would think of as a healthy weight.

From Day 1 of following the Body Awareness Food Exchange or Mediterranean Slim diets, you will lose excess fat. You are eating less calories than your body needs, you are boosting your metabolism by eating regular quantities of complex carbohydrates and you have increased the amount of energy you burn by starting a regular exercise programme. However, your body is quite capable of acting sneakily. It may refuse to show that downward weight trend you dream about. There are several reasons:

- The increased weight of food you are eating – especially the fruit and vegetables, packed with fibre.
- Carbohydrates and fibre-rich foods hold extra water in the bowels.
- Fluid retention in cellular and intercellular spaces to counterbalance the cell's fat loss.
- Fat is being replaced by muscle tissue which is denser and therefore weighs more than fat tissue.
- Your metabolism is resetting itself to maintain your body's set-points.

These factors together account for the plateau phase – where your weight sticks maddeningly at one point and refuses to budge downwards, even though you know intuitively that your diet is working.

Do not get disillusioned, and do not give up. In a perverse sort of way, that is exactly what your body wants you to do. This is a survival mechanism.

Some of us, more than others, have predetermined body weights which the body fights to maintain. A few people only seem to lose weight in 1kg (2¼lb), 2kg (4½lb) or even 3kg (6¾lb) jumps.

In my diet and healthy-eating clinics I hear stories like this all the time:

Case 1

'When I first started losing weight, I was disheartened and disillusioned. For days, no weight loss would appear on the scales, despite sticking to my diet avidly. I changed the battery in the bathroom scales – and in desperation even bought some expensive new ones. All to no avail. The maddening thing was I *knew* I was losing weight. I could see a slimmer me in the mirror. I felt lighter and definitely firmer, but my weight seemed to be going up. Then, one week later, just when I was about to give up and fling away my dieting ideas for ever, it happened. I sat on the loo and released what seemed like 10 gallons of water. The result? On stepping on the scales I was 4lb lighter.'

Case 2

'When losing weight, no matter what I do, my scales steadfastly refuse to record certain body weights. This month, I hovered between 10st 11lb, 10st 9lb and 10st 7lb. To my knowledge, I have never weighed 10st 10lb or 10 8lb.'

Case 3

'Whenever I've dieted in the past, I only ever lose weight in blocks of 4lb. Last week I stuck at 13st 7lb, then plummeted to 13st 3lb. When I was heavier, weighing around 17st, I noticed the same thing. I'd stick at a weight, then spend a day in the bathroom and emerge 4lb lighter.'

Case 4

'My weight jumps around by 2kg even when I'm sticking to a strict diet. I yo-yo between 75kg and 73kg but never seem to lose or gain less than this. I even changed my electronic scales, thinking they were inaccurate, but the same thing keeps occurring.'

Case 5

'I find it relatively difficult to lose the last few pounds in any one stone. I went from 11st 10lb to 11st 5lb very easily. Then I stuck and had to really struggle to get down to 11st. The same thing happened again. From 11st down to 10st 5lb was simple. But could I get down to 10st? I'm now stuck at 10st 5lb despite eating 1,000 kcals per day.'

Case 6

'I used to suffer from anorexia nervosa. I now know when

my weight is getting too low. Whenever I go below 8 stone, my periods stop automatically.'

Body Set-point Theory

The body set-point theory is partly explained by how our metabolism varies according to the amount of dietary energy available.

In times of plenty, our metabolism is inefficient. It hasn't got to worry about where the next meal is coming from and energy is wasted as body heat generated in brown fat cells (*see Appendix 2: Metabolism and Fat*).

We can eat many more calories per day than we need and yet not put on any weight. We stick around one body set-point.

When times are hard and meals are scarce (slimming diets), the metabolism recognizes the threat and switches to super-efficient mode. Every calorie eaten is processed and few are wasted. Again, we remain around the same body weight we stuck to in times of plenty – even though our calorie intake is restricted. From this set-point, two scenarios can develop:

1. Returning to normal calorie intake
If we go back to eating a high-calorie diet, our metabolism stays in super-efficient mode. A high percentage of the extra daily calories is converted to body energy stores – fat! We will put on weight until we reach equilibrium – our next body set-point, which is higher than the one we were on before.

Slowly, the metabolism will settle down into wasteful mode once more. However, we now have more fat on board – and weigh more.

2. Maintaining a reduced calorie intake

If we stick to our diet, the body goes on to a form of red alert. Hormonal and metabolic changes occur that try to maintain the status quo. Glycogen and fat stores are mobilized to maintain blood sugar levels and we start to lose fat volume.

However, as we are on alert for possible impending starvation, many physiological changes occur, including the release of a hormone called ADH (anti-diuretic hormone) from the pituitary gland. ADH acts on the kidneys so that fluid filtered from the blood is re-absorbed and not passed into the urine. In other words, ADH causes fluid retention.

Retained fluid masks the fat loss achieved by dieting and our weight remains at our predetermined set-point. This fluid retention cannot go on indefinitely. Once our blood becomes too dilute, powerful control mechanisms take over and switch off ADH secretion. We then experience a massive diuresis and end up taking frequent trips to the loo, with the result that our body weight suddenly drops.

We are now at a new body set-point and the process may start all over again.

Not everyone will experience these set-point sticking places. They are more likely in smokers, women who experience bloating just before a period or who are taking hormonal treatments such as the oral contraceptive pill.

Some drugs used to treat conditions such as diabetes, epilepsy, high blood pressure, pain or high cholesterol levels can also increase ADH secretion.

Alcohol actually switches off ADH secretion, so our daily glass of red wine on the Body Awareness Diet will help to counteract the fluid-retaining effect and plateau phase.

Changing Our Body Set-points

Each of us has many body set-points. They are mostly inherited but can be modified by our diet and lifestyle.

Regular exercise will induce metabolic changes which favour a lower body set-point. This is in addition to any downward weight loss brought about by burning up excess calories.

Low-fat, low-sugar wholefoods encourage us to maintain a lower set-point body weight than a high-saturated fat, high-sugar diet. As dietary fat is so easily converted into body fat, it makes sense that the body should adjust physiologically to accommodate the storage of all this dietary energy.

Increasing age generally results in increasing body set-points too; another reason why middle-aged spread creeps up on some of us so insidiously. Ectomorphs tend to gain very little weight with age, while mesomorphs and endomorphs have to struggle to maintain their youthful shapes.

Body Awareness Goals

By eating a low-saturated fat, low-sugar diet, body awareness encourages the attainment of a lower body set-point. This is reinforced by exercise and by relaxation therapy – such as flotation.

After a float, a marked diuresis (voiding of body fluid) occurs. This is a result of the profound relaxation and the lowered levels of stress hormones. Decreased secretion of ADH is probably involved too.

CHAPTER 5

Motivation

How Motivated Are You?

- How many times have you tried to lose weight?
- How many times have you got so far, then stuck at a stubborn weight?
- How many times have you rebounded right back to where you started from?
- How many times, misery of miseries, have you suddenly discovered you're even heavier than when you started to lose weight?
- Unless you are totally motivated and determined to win at slimming, you will fail.

Having read this book so far, you have proved you have that inner spark, that determination to succeed in achieving health and fitness.

Successful slimming requires a lot of effort over a long period of time. Your weight probably crept on over many months or years and it's best to let it creep off the same way.

If you are too hard on yourself and try to lose weight too quickly, you are doomed to fail. Boredom, hunger, impatience and appetite will be your undoing.

For pure, intense, unwavering motivation, you need a

firm mental grip on where you are going, why, and how long it is likely to take.

Why Do You Want to Slim?

Write down your 10 main reasons for wanting to lose weight, in order of priority. They may look something like this:

1. To look more attractive
2. To have more energy and zest for life
3. To improve my health and live longer
4. To get into fashionable clothes
5. To improve my confidence and self-esteem
6. To improve my career prospects
7. To look good sun-bathing nude on holiday
8. To make love with the light on
9. Because my partner wants me to
10. Because I owe it to myself

These are all important reasons to lose weight, but primarily you must tackle the job because *you* want to. If you're doing it for someone else, half your motivation is lacking. Don't do it to please a partner, do it for *you*. Because *you* deserve it.

When you have decided which reasons for losing weight are the most important for you, you need to fix them in your mind.

Buy some thin card in your favourite colour. Cut it into credit card sized pieces. With a silver or gold felt pen, write down on each card a reason for losing weight in best copper script.

Place one of these cards wherever temptation lurks and where you are likely to see them regularly:

- in the fridge
- in the store cupboard

- in your purse
- in the car
- in your cheque book
- in your make-up bag

Now you know exactly why you want to lose weight. Now you have to focus on what it will be like to achieve your goal.

Be Brutal with Yourself

Here's an exercise in total honesty. Take all your clothes off in a warm room in front of a full–length mirror (it's best to lock the door and ensure there's no window cleaner about). Some gentle relaxing music will help as this exercise takes a little time if done properly.

Study your face
- Are your cheeks on the chubby side?
- Do you have a double chin?
- Are the shapes of your eyes compromised by sagging, excess flesh?
- Is your skin pale, sallow, spotty, blotchy, lined, greasy, dry, patchy or scaly?
- Do your make-up skills leave a lot to be desired?
- Are your lips too big? Too small?
- What about your eyes?
- Analyse your hairstyle. Does it suit you? Is the colour flattering? Is your hair lank? Greasy? Going grey? Showing signs of a perm or tint growing out?
- Is your neck thicker than you would like?
- Is it lined?

If you feel negative about aspects of your appearance, your self-esteem is suffering.

Now go back and re-analyse the parts of your face you

don't like. Some can be improved – facials may help the texture and glow of your skin. Hairstyles can be changed; contact lenses bought in place of glasses; make-up skills learned.

Make a list of areas where positive action will produce results. Make a list of problem areas that will improve by losing weight.

Now study the rest of you – your breasts, waist, hips, thighs and ankles in the same critical manner. Turn sideways to the mirror and study your profile and rear view too. A triple mirror, or another long mirror placed at an angle makes this easier.

Don't be afraid to be honest. It's the only way you will galvanize yourself into making improvements.

What part of your body do you like the most? Which do you like least? Work out the bits you can definitely change, which you can improve a little, and which you are stuck with.

Write these lists down and use them to reinforce your aims and goals in losing weight and getting slim.

Now go back and apologize to all those bits of your body that you decided you could do nothing about – the jutting chin, the long nose, the small breasts, etc.

They are part of you. You may not be able to change them but you must learn to like and live with them, because if you don't love all of you, other people will find this difficult too. Only when you have learned to accept all of you, the way it is, can your self-esteem improve enough to assist your weight-loss goals. You want to lose weight because you deserve it. You owe it to yourself.

A Peek Into the Future

Now, put your clothes back on. Lie down, close your eyes

and concentrate on forming an image of what you have just seen. Picture every excess roll of fat, every area of cellulite and every sprig of excess hair.

Then, work at imagining what you will look like when you have reached your ideal weight.

Melt away those bulging contours. Sketch in your mind the sort of curves you covet. Picture the clothes you will wear; how you will look in a bikini. Imagine the admiring looks from colleagues, family and friends. Nice, huh?

And if that isn't enough to get you raring to go, picture a struggling heart pumping away. It is trembling with flabby, unhealthy muscles, clogged up arteries and an outer coating of excess fat. It's not difficult to see why it's going to struggle to pump for those three score years and ten.

Now picture a lean, fit heart with plump, healthy muscles, sparkling arteries and no excess layers of fat. This is the heart that will let you enjoy life to the full, which will carry on pumping past its biblically allotted span. That heart can be your heart if you stay within your ideal BMI range, exercise regularly, and eat a healthy diet.

Visualization is a powerful mental tool. If you say things like:

- I can't see myself losing weight
- I can't picture myself in a size 12 dress

then you can guarantee you will never achieve these goals. If you can picture them in your mind's eye however, you have reinforced where you want to be – and will subconsciously find it easier to get there.

Practising this positive thought exercise in a flotation tank will imprint your aims even more firmly in your mind.

Think Positive

Good motivation entails positive thought. It IS possible to

diet. You CAN lose those excess pounds, however many you need to shift.

The human who can photosynthesize (make solid matter out of water, air and sunlight like plants) hasn't yet been genetically engineered. Excess weight comes off when:

ENERGY IN (calories) is less than ENERGY OUT
(metabolism + level of activity + heat)

This is a sound equation with a scientific basis. You WILL lose weight by cutting down the number of calories you eat and increasing your level of activity. You can't fail – as long as you persevere and don't give up at the first hurdle.

Rapid Health Benefits

There are immediate health benefits from losing weight. These will also help to motivate you if you suffer from certain illnesses. Losing weight will:
- significantly decrease a high blood cholesterol level
- improve the way your body handles sugar
- reduce the frequency of angina
- significantly reduce high blood pressure
- relieve the discomfort of varicose veins
- reduce the incidence of heart-burn and indigestion
- reduce breathlessness
- reduce backache
- improve gout
- improve joint pain and mobility
- improve self-confidence
- reduce anxiety, stress and depression
- improve fertility
- improve energy levels and zest for life

The Body Awareness Diet will show you how.

Setting an End-point Target

Targets are important motivators that focus your mind and give you a goal to achieve. We all need a challenge in life – make yours the attainment of life-long fitness and slimness, with all the health benefits that these entail. It will help you exert the self-discipline you're going to need.

Set yourself a target and picture it several times a day. Make sure it's:

- realistic
- achievable
- something you *really* want

It may be getting into a size 12 dress for a wedding, looking good in a holiday bikini, or improving some aspect of your health.

Whatever your goal is, fix it firmly in your mind. If you really believe you can do it – you will. It's only you that has the power to achieve your target – and the self-destructive ability to fail if you aren't properly motivated.

Setting Smaller Targets

If you only aim for your end-point target, it will seem daunting and very far away. You need to set yourself little targets, ones that are easily met and frequently achieved.

The best targets are small, weekly ones like losing 0.5–1kg (1-2lb) a week. This may seem nothing compared to how much you have to lose, but week-by-week, these little achievements will add up to a significant weight loss.

Most importantly, the weight will be lost easily, without undue hardship or suffering – and without fail. Remember that. Losing weight is a scientific process which *is* possible if you tackle it in the right frame of mind. Your weight built up slowly and in small amounts. You must lose it in the same way or your metabolism will rebel.

If you try to lose weight any faster than 0.5–1kg (1–2lb) a week, your body will readjust its metabolic pathways. It will shift from processes that are wasteful of calories to super-efficient reactions where every calorie sticks. You will start to burn up body protein (lean tissues) rather than body fat (adipose tissues). This is discussed further in Appendix 2: Metabolism and Fat.

Secondary Motivators

In order to reinforce your motivation, you need to reward yourself frequently. Rewards are wonderful motivators, but they must be things you *really* want and otherwise wouldn't have.

It is important that the reward isn't food. Ever since childhood, you have probably been rewarded for good behaviour with chocolate or sweets. That's one of the reasons you are overweight now.

Your rewards should be aimed at improving you further: upgrading your appearance, knowledge or wardrobe to complement your slowly improving shape. Depending on how much motivational reinforcement you need – and depending on your pocket – for every 1–3kg (2–7lb) lost, reward yourself with a treat. Draw up a reward chart such as the following:

Weight Loss	Reward
1kg	A good book; a CD; new lipstick
2kg	A painting trip to the country
3kg	A trip to the theatre or seaside
4kg	An aromatherapy massage
5kg	A sauna or jacuzzi
6kg	A professional make-up
7kg	A new hair-do
8kg	An item of clothing or jewellery
9kg	A visit to an opera or concert
10kg	A session in a flotation tank
11kg	Being colour-printed
12kg	A new track suit or swimsuit
Target weight:	A parachute jump
	A hot-air balloon trip
	A mountain bike

Alternatively, a course of evening classes – pottery, wine-tasting, flower-arrangement, creative writing, business studies – anything that will improve your knowledge base and improve your self-confidence and self-esteem should be considered worthwhile.

Be adventurous and daring as more weight comes off. A slimmer, fitter you can expand your horizons and turn into reality what before were only dreams.

If money is a problem, don't feel daunted. Make your targets cheap ones, like an evening spent pampering yourself in the bath; give yourself a home-made face-mask; allocate time to go round an art gallery or museum. Trace your family tree, do something different that ordinarily you wouldn't think to find time for: have a low-calorie picnic in the country with the family or a good friend; go for a paddle in the sea; fly a home-made kite; borrow a boat and have fun getting wet on the river; pick sloes and make sloe gin – by the time it's mature you'll be slim enough to enjoy it without feeling guilty.

Collecting Stars

As well as rewarding yourself for losing weight, give rewards for willpower and self-control too.

Buy packets of silver and gold stars. Draw up a star chart and reward yourself with a gold star for every day you stick to your diet.

Stick on a silver star every time you resist a particular food temptation e.g. going shopping and not buying some desperately wanted white chocolate, or a beckoning cream doughnut.

When you've collected 10 silver or 10 gold stars, award yourself a non-food luxury from your reward chart, such as a facial.

The Body Awareness Programme is all about new experiences, new skills, new aspirations and a new you. As you lose weight you will gain confidence and learn to become more creative. You will get more out of life.

By adopting a healthier eating plan for weight loss and weight maintenance you will have a healthy body at your disposal. Skin will be clear, eyes bright, brain refreshed and your metabolic reactions occur at the right rate.

Slim Together

It's always easier to share a difficult task with someone else. Recruit a friend or relative to help, so when you start to flag they can listen, sympathize – and keep you on the straight and narrow. Enrol:

- A friend who needs to lose weight too. Set targets and rewards together. Even if she/he has less weight to lose –

don't be discouraged. Share their triumphs or sticking-point blues and they will share yours too.

- A relative. Does your husband, wife, child, mother, father, sister, brother need to lose weight? Work together to achieve your goals.
- Don't know anyone? Too embarrassed to ask? Join a slimming club. Most areas have at least one. Here, you will meet similarly motivated people with similar hopes and fears. In addition, you will gain the experience of a team-leader who will point out where you are going wrong or be quick to praise when you're knocking off those targets.
- Take part in a sponsored slim. By losing weight you will be helping a charity as well as helping yourself. There's also the extra motivation which comes from others knowing how successful you've been.
- Enrol an item of clothing to help. Hang a sexy piece of under-wear, or a slinky dress two sizes too small where you will see if frequently. Every time you pass it, think positive. Think: I'm going to get into you soon. I'm going to achieve my weight-loss goals.

Coping with Failure

If, despite all your best efforts, you don't seem to be getting anywhere, there are two things you can do:

1. Analyse what has gone wrong and plan determinedly to overcome the hurdle.

2. Accept the status quo and allow the pounds to creep back on.

The first response is the correct, motivated, survival response. The second is no longer worthy of you. Write down what has gone wrong:

Have you stuck at a particular weight?

Have you regained weight?

Have you had a binge–out and now feel guilty?

Is the waistband of that new dress feeling tight?
Have you lost weight but still feel fat and horrible?

POSITIVE ACTIONS you can take to beat this temporary set back:

Read about the plateau phase in Chapter 4. You may be at a body set-point and have started to retain fluid – even though you are continuing to burn up excess fat.

Plan a week of hard physical exercise and a strict dieting regime.

Do some spot exercises to tone up stubborn areas of fat.

Go for a brisk, invigorating walk.

Relax in a luxury bubble bath, followed by a rigorous oil and salt scrub down.

Write down 10 things you *like* about yourself. Start seeing yourself as a worthwhile person again.

Make an appointment to get your hair done, have a facial, anything that will raise your self-confidence and elevate the self-esteem that just acquired a dent.

Think positive. This is the first day of your adventure to find the new you. Make getting slim your absolute top priority. Remember, you're doing it for yourself – and not for anyone else.

Keep battling on. Fix your goals firmly in mind. Peek into the future once more. Re-write your motivating cards. Get out that slinky dress or sexy underwear and imagine yourself wearing it. Re-formulate your targets. Re-invent your reward chart. This time, include on it something you *really* want and can realistically budget to achieve. How about a dream holiday in the sun?

Some days are bound to be difficult. You may be feeling low because of something that's happened or something someone has said. You may be due a period and be feeling bloated stodgy and irritable. If you feel an irresistible urge to nibble, try any – or all – of the following:

Get out of the house. Take some fresh air and exercise. Go for a brisk, rousing walk – even if it's raining.

If you are feeling low, it's often due to a mild, chemical imbalance in the brain. Exercise will help to redress this. One of the reasons we crave food when feeling low or depressed is because carbohydrate triggers the release of a brain chemical called serotonin which makes us feel better. Exercise also induces the release of brain chemicals that have euphoric effects, plus it dampens the appetite and improves our level of fitness.

Have a low-calorie, healthy snack. Eat a juicy apple; chop some fresh fruit and vegetables into some natural yogurt and wash this down with a glass of sparkling mineral water.

Clean your teeth. You may be experiencing 'appetite' rather than hunger. Your tastebuds are on the prowl. Try cleaning your teeth vigorously for five minutes, using plenty of strongly flavoured toothpaste. Follow up with a glass of sparkling mineral water into which you have squeezed the juice of half a lemon. That should help kill your appetite.

Work up a sweat. You may be feeling bored. Boredom often leads to nibbling. Put on some loud, disco music with a good beat. Start with some simple stretch exercises to warm up, then dance or run on the spot. Keep this up for at least 15 to 20 minutes. Speed up and slow down depending on how breathless you feel. Take your pulse and make sure it is in the fat-burner range (*see Chapter 6*).

Temptation at Work

Several aspects of work may revolve around food: the tea-trolley, the canteen, pub meetings at lunchtime, birthday cakes, chocolate/soft drinks machines. Plan ahead. Take a lunch box in every day, filled with interesting salads, low-calorie drinks, yogurts and fresh fruit. Keep crisp-breads, low-calorie spreads, low-cal drinks and fruit at work.

Try not to eat in the pub. If you have to, choose the lowest calorie food available. Go for a baked potato and salad – ask them not to add butter or mayonnaise. Avoid stodgy pies and puddings. Drink sparkling mineral water mixed half-and-half with wine to make a spritzer. Low-cal tonic water with angostura bitters will satisfy tingling tastebuds.

When birthday cakes are flourished, try popping out to the loo in order to avoid one. Claim you have indigestion – or, if forced, take the smallest, least fattening slice and count this into your daily calorie allowance.

Temptation in the Supermarket

Plan ahead. Always shop after a meal, when you are no longer hungry. Take a list and promise yourself that you will stick to it. If you know your willpower will let you down, get a relative or friend to shop for you. Don't take too much spare cash which will burn a hole in your pocket.

Shop so that your family eats more healthily too. Cut out fattening, stodgy foods such as pork pies, cakes and biscuits. Re-train your family to appreciate fresh fruit, yogurts, vegetables and herbs. Buy fish and white meat rather than red meat.

Buy foods for vegetarian days and Mediterranean-style meals. Buy low-calorie, low-fat versions of salad dressings, milk, drinks, etc. Replace saturated fats (e.g. butter) with monounsaturated fats such as olive oil and olive oil-based spreads.

Temptation at Home

If you have a family

Learn to throw excess food away. A leftover piece of cake or nugget of cheese will do your health and weight targets more good in the bin than on your hips.

Try getting your family to eat more healthily with you. Cook tempting Mediterranean-style meals for them. Help yourself to smaller portions, or eat separately until you are on the Body Awareness Maintenance Plan.

Whilst actively dieting, eat before your family. You won't need superhuman control when serving them if you are no longer hungry.

Or, try feeding the kids separately. Then have a romantic meal for two with your partner. Light candles, use the best dinner service and cutlery. Drink plenty of mineral water with your meal. Serve yourself plenty of vegetables and a small portion of the main dish. Chew slowly and aim to leave some food on your plate. Enrol your husband into helping you.

If you live alone

Make your slimming campaign a full-time, absorbing project around which the rest of your life rotates.

Keep a strict food diary, plan meals ahead and keep active. You are lucky as in your spare time you can go to the gym, or for a brisk walk. You need only buy food for yourself with no-one else's requirements to distract you.

Evenings are probably your worst time for temptation. Save a treat for the evening – a glass of wine or a low-calorie, hot chocolate drink. Try to avoid socializing in restaurants and pubs if possible.

When eating out, choose low-calorie foods and drink lots of mineral water or tonic with angostura bitters.

Self-esteem

A positive self-esteem is essential for successful weight loss.

Only one in three normal-weight people have good self-esteem. That means two out of three don't.

Ninety-nine per cent of people on a diet – whether or not they are significantly overweight – also have a low self-esteem which reduces their chances of success.

When you feel negative about yourself, you end up feeling low, eating too much, drinking too much, not bothering with exercise, achieving low productivity in the rest of your life – and failing to lose weight.

Self-esteem provides you with the internal strength to succeed. Winners are those people who make a habit of doing the things that losers are uncomfortable to try. Winners take risks. Winners can visualize where they're going and how they're going to get there.

Imagine yourself losing weight. Imagine yourself thin. Cut out a picture of your head, put it on top of a slim body and stick it onto your fridge. This will reinforce your self-image of becoming thin. Don't stick a picture of yourself in which you look fat, or a picture of a pig onto your fridge. That will just reinforce the thought: Hey, I'm fat or I'm a pig.

When your self-esteem is low – write down 10 things you are good at and 10 things you think you are bad at. Then work out how you can gain more recognition for your skills – and how you can improve the things you know you can do better at.

Don't blame other people for your being overweight – or your inability to diet. Too often it is easy to fall into the trap of thinking . . . if only I didn't have to cook for the family, I could lose weight. That's why I'm fat. If only . . . I had more money, I could buy diet foods and lose weight. I'm fat because I don't have enough money. If only . . . I had more energy, I could exercise and lose weight. That's why I'm overweight.

Instead, think about how you are responsible for your situation. Only you can change it.

Think positive: Up until now, I haven't been able to lose weight. Now I'm going to.

Focus on your successes – if you lose a pound in weight – focus on it, remind yourself of your success. Feel good about it and go for it again.

CHAPTER 6

Exercise

Inactivity is a major feature of the Western lifestyle. Although we evolved to cope with a high level of activity that would enable us to survive in the wild, we've become 'couch potatoes', skulking on the sofa in front of the TV – often in a back-straining posture screaming for correction.

Inactivity has a detrimental effect on our health. It encourages sluggish metabolism, weight gain, high blood pressure, high blood cholesterol levels and poor handling of body glucose.

Muscles – including the heart – become flabby, joints seize up and ligaments stiffen. We become lethargic, tired all the time and have a tendency towards depression. Worst of all, our sex-drive can slink off the lower end of the register.

In contrast, regular physical exercise has a positive effect on our health. It curbs our appetite, boosts our metabolic rate and makes us feel energized. Furthermore, it:

- improves strength, stamina and suppleness
- reduces blood cholesterol levels
- reduces blood pressure
- reduces the waist/hip ratio
- speeds up the metabolism and burns fat
- tones up muscles and firms the silhouette
- improves the efficiency of the heart

- strengthens bones and decreases the risk of osteoporosis
- relieves depression
- generates feelings of euphoria
- improves self-esteem

People who are physically inactive tend to eat more saturated fat than those who are fit. They are also more prone to overweight.

A sedentary lifestyle is linked with high blood pressure and high blood lipids (fats), both of which hasten hardening and furring of the arteries (atherosclerosis). Regular physical activity can help to reverse both these coronary heart-risk factors and most importantly, it increases your aerobic capacity.

Aerobic Capacity

Our heart pumps blood around the body to provide cells with essential nutrients such as oxygen and to remove waste products such as carbon dioxide gas.

Blood passes through the lungs, where it becomes saturated with oxygen and off-loads carbon dioxide for excretion.

Together, our heart, blood vessels and lungs make up the cardio-respiratory system. The efficiency of our cardio-respiratory system determines how much oxygen our body receives. During vigorous exercise, muscles use increased amounts of oxygen and produce increased amounts of waste carbon dioxide.

The largest amount of oxygen your body can consume per minute is called your aerobic capacity. This capacity is the most sensitive indicator of both the fitness and efficiency of your heart and lungs.

The amount of oxygen your body uses is calculated by measuring how much your pulse rate increases during a known amount of energy expenditure (exercise).

Aerobic capacity is measured in units of millilitres of oxygen per minute per kilogram of body weight e.g. my reading after eight weeks of a prescribed exercise programme was 44.63ml/kg/min.

I started off with an aerobic capacity of 33.11ml/kg/min, so my cardio-respiratory system improved rapidly and significantly with proper, enjoyable exercise.

Getting Assessed Before You Start

If you can afford to, join a professional gym, such as Holmes Place of London, where your fitness level can be properly assessed both before and during your weight-loss, get-fit programme. Most importantly, you will be guided at every step of the way and assigned a fitness training programme specially tailored to your needs.

Your progress should be reassessed every two to three months so you can see how your body is responding to your personal training programme.

The sort of things that need assessing include your:
- height
- weight
- skin fold thickness
- body dimensions
- waist to hip ratio
- percentage body fat
- blood pressure
- pulse at rest
- pulse after exercise
- aerobic capacity
- lung function
- strength
- stamina
- suppleness

Fitness Index

A good gym will calculate your fitness index regularly during your fitness programme. This is determined by computer from your aerobic capacity and your percentage body fat – the two most important indicators of health and fitness. A fitness level of:

      8–10 is below average
      11–13 is average
      14–16 is above average
      17–20 is excellent

If you haven't exercised enough to raise your pulse rate for 20 minutes continuously, at least twice a week during the last six months, your fitness level is probably below average – or average.

Don't forget that average fitness is pretty poor and means an average (i.e. high) risk of a poorly conditioned heart and coronary heart disease too.

Your goals in joining the health club will also be assessed, e.g. do you want to:

- lose fat weight?
- gain lean weight?
- firm, tighten, tone?
- fill out?
- reshape your body?
- reproportion your body?
- improve the condition of your heart?
- improve your overall health?
- increase your energy levels and vitality?
- reduce stress and relieve tension?
- increase your self-confidence?
- improve your flexibility, co-ordination or balance?
- improve your metabolism?
- improve your reflexes?
- improve your sleep pattern?

All these things can be achieved by the use of a correctly

prescribed exercise programme. That's where your personal trainer comes in.

Personal Trainers

A personal trainer will assess you at least every two or three months to analyse your progress, identify where you are not achieving as much as you might – and where you are taking it too easy.

People who have achieved optimum looks and health – e.g. Princess Diana – can probably thank their personal trainer for providing:

- achievable goals
- motivation
- encouragement
- mental pushing
- sympathy
- understanding
- results
- a proper stretch programme
- a suggested maintenance programme

Your trainer will give you an individual explanation of what you can expect; how your body is likely to change; what expectations are unreasonable, e.g. you can't change your basic body type from endomorph or mesomorph to ectomorph. They will also advise on what limitations you should accept due to your medical history, and any drugs you are taking.

Furthermore, your trainer can prescribe a training programme to help tone up muscle in problem areas. Then, as you slowly lose fat through your combined eating and exercise programme, the musculature revealed underneath will be more attractive.

Stamina, Strength and Suppleness

Exercise improves three major parameters: *stamina* – by making the heart fitter and increasing muscle energy stores; *strength* – by building up muscle bulk; *suppleness* – by improving our ability to stretch and our range of joint movements. These three factors – stamina, suppleness and strength – are known as the three Ss.

Different sports help to improve our fitness in different ways. They should be done regularly and with a certain amount of effort to provide maximum benefit. Always start a new sport gently and work up to higher effort levels using your pulse as a guide – *see* p.91. Sports such as squash should not be attempted until you are fairly fit.

The following table gives you an idea of the benefits gained from different activities:

THE SSS GUIDE TO DIFFERENT SPORTS

ACTIVITY	STAMINA	SUPPLENESS	STRENGTH
Aerobics	★★★	★★★	★★
Athletics	★★★	★★	★★★
Badminton	★★	★★★	★★
Circuit training	★★★	★★★	★★★
Cricket	★	★★	★
Cycling	★★★★	★★	★★★
Football	★★★	★★★	★★★
Golf	★	★★	★
Jogging	★★★★	★★	★★
Karate/judo	★	★★	★
Rounders	★★	★	★★
Rowing	★★★	★	★★
Skiing (downhill)	★★	★★	★★
Skipping	★★★	★★	★★
Squash	★★★	★★★	★★

ACTIVITY	STAMINA	SUPPLENESS	STRENGTH
Swimming (hard)	★★★★	★★★★	★★★★
Tennis	★★	★★★	★★
Walking (ramble)	★★	★	★
(brisk/hill)	★★★	★	★★
Weight training	★	★★	★★★★
Yoga	★	★★★	★

★ = slight effect   ★★ = beneficial effect

★★★ = very good effect   ★★★★ = excellent effect

How Supple are You?

Try the following tests to see how supple you are. Give yourself points for each one you can do easily, without excess straining.

Shoulder Shuttles

Stand comfortably, with your feet apart. Bend your left arm up behind you to touch your right shoulder blade. Now, raise your right arm and place your right hand down behind your right shoulder, trying to touch the fingers of both hands behind your shoulder blade.

If you can do this easily, award yourself 1 point. Repeat on the opposite side for another 1 point.

Toe Touchers

Stand comfortably, with your feet 6 inches apart. Bend forwards keeping your legs straight and try to touch your toes. If you can do this, award yourself 2 points.

Can you place your palms flat on the ground? If so, you are especially supple. Award yourself 2 extra points.

Hamstrings

Sit on the floor with your back straight and your arms by your sides. Stretch your legs out in front of you, flat on the floor without bending your knees or curving your spine. Can the backs of both knees touch the floor? If so, award yourself 2 points.

Now, bend forwards, so the backs of your knees stay touching the ground.

Can you touch your toes? If so, award yourself 2 points.

Can you comfortably grasp your toes, keeping your legs flat on the floor as before? If so, award yourself 2 points.

Knee Knockers

Stand comfortably with your feet 12 inches apart and your hands by your sides. Keeping your back and legs straight, bend down to one side so your hand runs down your leg.

Can you comfortably grasp your leg just below your knee joint? If you can do this on both sides, award yourself 2 points.

Lumber Looseness

Lie on the floor and bend up both knees. With both hands behind your knees, bring them in to touch your chest. Can you comfortably grasp your hands behind your knees and keep them close to your chest? If so, award yourself 2 points.

Now, keeping one knee grasped to your chest,

straighten out the other until it lies on the floor, with the back of your knee touching the ground. If you can do this on both sides, award yourself 2 points.

Pelvic Roll

Lie flat on the floor with your arms by your sides. Bend up your knees but keep your feet flat on the floor. Your pelvis should tilt so that your lower spinal curve is flattened and your lumbar area touches the floor. Hold this for a count of 10 for 2 points.

Add up all the points scored and write them here:

My suppleness score is..........out of a possible 20.

Assessment Results

If you scored below 10
You are not very supple. Your muscles and ligaments need gentle stretching and your joint mobility needs improving. You need to concentrate on fitness stretches.

It is especially important for you to warm up properly before doing any form of exercise (*see* p.79). Your muscles are tight and will tear easily if strained. Your ligaments are prone to painful spraining. You may well find your joints click and creak quite noticeably. These noises are due to tight ligaments.

Try the Walking Regime (*see* p.86) to begin with. Start off gently and slowly speed up until you are walking briskly every day.

If you enjoy swimming, try gentle aquarobics too.

If you scored 10–15

You are reasonably supple but there's room for improvement. Always warm up properly before exercise as your muscles and ligaments are not as supple as they could be and will easily be strained or sprained.

Start walking regularly and briskly.

Swim briskly using breast stroke.

Cycle to improve the suppleness of your lower joints.

You can start a supervised cardiovascular programme at a gymnasium, concentrating on the exercise bike, the treadmill for brisk uphill walking, the Cybex machine to exercise your arms and the step machine. As you begin to feel more fit and supple, introduce a gentle weight-training programme too. Aerobics and step classes will also improve your stamina and fitness.

If you scored 16–20

You are supple enough to enjoy most activities without undue strain on your muscles, ligaments or joints. Warming up is important because, although you are supple, sudden bursts of activity can still cause damage.

Concentrate on a cardiovascular programme at a gymnasium and start a weights programme to build up your strength. Aerobics and step classes will greatly improve your fitness.

You can also consider increasing your efforts by wearing wrist and ankle weights as you get fitter and stronger.

Repeat the suppleness assessment tests in this book as you work through an exercise training programme. If you are not doing warm-ups and stretch exercises properly, you may find that your suppleness score decreases. This is because toned muscles and ligaments become tighter – you need to stretch before and after every exercise period to maintain and improve your suppleness.

Is Exercise Safe?

All activities carry some risk; nothing is ever completely safe. If, after 20 years of inactivity, you suddenly take up jogging or squash, you will put your heart under un-necessary – and dangerous – strain.

People starting an exercise programme too vigorously are likely to tear muscles or ligaments, damage joints and end up stiff, sore and demotivated. You need to start slowly and increase your exercise levels gently and sensibly as your fitness level improves.

If you are over 50 years of age, and haven't exercised regularly, ask your doctor for an initial check-up and advice before you start. If you have already had a heart attack, consult your specialist first.

The evidence suggests that gentle exercise will signifi-cantly improve your life expectancy, but you must tackle it the right way – and if you have a medical condition, with your doctor's blessing. The safety rules to follow are:

- Don't eat a heavy meal less than two hours before you exercise.
- Don't drink any alcohol in the six hours prior to exercise.
- Warm up properly.
- Start off slowly.
- Cool down correctly.
- Stop if you feel dizzy, very short of breath, break into a cold sweat or experience any pain.
- Wear recommended clothes and shoes.
- If out at night, make sure you are fully visible when near traffic.

How Much Exercise Should You Take?

To achieve fitness, you should take regular exercise which

lasts at least 20 minutes, and is done a _minimum_ of three times per week. Note that little word minimum. Once you have achieved a reasonable level of fitness, you should do more.

Non-weight-bearing exercise, e.g. cycling or swimming, is excellent for those in poor health or with joint problems – but start slowly.

If you haven't taken much exercise during the last six months, start your fitness programme with a brisk, walking regime. Make sure you warm up before exercising and cool down afterwards.

Why Stretch and Warm-up?

Warming up before exercise is important to:
- literally warm your body – cold muscles can seize up
- raise your pulse rate
- increase your suppleness and joint mobility
- increase blood flow to your muscles in preparation for exertion
- stretch your limbs and decrease your risk of tearing a muscle or spraining a ligament
- allow mental preparation and concentration

On joining a fitness club, you will be taught how to stretch and warm up both before and after exercise.

Stretching

The Holmes Place Method

Stretching is easy but there's a right and wrong way of doing it. A stretch should be relaxed, sustained and with your attention focused on the muscles being stretched. Don't bounce up and down and don't stretch to the point of pain.

Remember to stretch after your exercise period is over too, otherwise your muscles will become tight and you will lose flexibility.

Chest Stretch

Interlock your hands behind your back with your palms facing inwards. Raise your hands as high behind your back as possible. Hold for 10 seconds.

Triceps Stretch

Raise your right arm above your head. Bend the elbow so your right hand comes down behind your left shoulder. Place your left hand on your raised right elbow and gently push that elbow down — so your right hand is pushed a few inches further down your back. Hold for a count of 10. Repeat with the left arm.

Upper Back

Raise both arms above your head. Clasp your hands together and turn your palms so they face upwards. Push up towards the ceiling as far as you can. Hold for 10 seconds.

Calf Stretch

Stand two to three feet away from a wall. Take one step forward with your right leg, so this is bent and the left is stretched behind you.

Rest your forearms against the wall at the level of your

head. Clasp your hands together. Rest your head against your hands on the wall. Press both heels into the ground and try to push the hip of your straightened left leg into the wall. You should feel a stretch in the left calf. Hold for 10 seconds. Repeat with the other leg.

Quadriceps

Stand about two feet away from a wall. Raise your right arm and rest it against the wall to steady you. Bend up your right foot behind you and clasp it with your left hand. Pull your heel as tightly into your bottom as you can. You should feel a pull at the front of your thigh. Hold for 10 seconds. Repeat with the other leg.

Bottom

Sit on the floor with both legs stretched in front of you. Bend up your right leg and cross it over your left leg. Place your right foot flat on the floor to the side of your left knee.

The next bit can be difficult. Balance yourself by placing your right hand on the floor 12–18 inches to the side of your body. Cross your left elbow over to the outside of your right knee and use the elbow to push the right knee down towards your left. At the same time, swivel your head around as far as you can to the right. You should feel a pull in your right bottom and hip. Hold for 10 seconds. Repeat with the other leg.

Hamstring Stretch 1

Sit on the floor with both legs straight out in front of you.

Bend up your right leg and place the sole of your right foot as far up against the inside of your left thigh as possible. Your right knee should be on the floor and your right heel up against your crotch. Lean forwards and, using both hands, grasp your left leg as far down towards the ankle as you can. Stretch forwards as far as possible. Hold for a count of 20–30 seconds as there is room for significant improvement in flexibility here. Repeat with the other leg.

Hamstring Stretch 2

Lie on your back. Keeping your bottom on the ground, bend up one knee and clasp both hands behind your thigh. Hug this leg as close to your chest as possible, allowing your other leg to bend too. Hold this position for a slow count of 10, then repeat with the other leg.

Groin Stretch

Sit on the floor. Pull up both feet and place both heels as close to your groin as possible. Keeping the soles of your feet together, let your knees flop out towards the sides. Lean forwards and grasp your feet with both hands. Using your elbows, push your knees as close to the ground as you can. Hold for 20–30 seconds as there is room for improvement here.

Lower Back Stretch

Don't do this exercise if you have had problems with your lower back. Lie on the floor on your back with both legs stretched loosely out in front of you. Stretch out your left

arm so it lies on the ground at a right angle to your body.
Bend up your left leg so your left knee comes up towards
your chest. Grasp your left knee with your right hand and
pull it over so your hips swivel and your left knee comes
down to touch the ground to the side of your right hip.

You may feel and hear creaks and cracks in your lower
spine. Hold for 20–30 seconds. Repeat with the other leg.

Suggested Warm-up Exercises

Neck Rolls

Stand comfortably with your feet apart. Place your hands
on your hips. Drop your chin to your chest and gently
rotate your head side-to-side 10 times. If this hurts, or if
you feel dizzy, stop.

Shoulder Shrugs

Stand comfortably with your feet apart and arms by your
sides. Lift your shoulders as high as you can and keep them
there for a count of 3. Then relax. Repeat these shrugs 10
times.

Shoulder Circles

Stand comfortably with your feet apart. Let both arms
hang by your sides. Slowly circle one shoulder forwards,
upwards, then backwards and downwards. Do this 10
times with each shoulder, speeding up as you go.

Arm Swings

Stand comfortably with your feet apart and arms by your sides. Lift one arm forwards and up, keeping it straight, until it is high above your head. Then spread your arm out sideways and down, completing the circle. Repeat this 5–10 times.

Do the same with the other arm and then with both arms together. Repeat both these movements 5–10 times.

Do the reverse, with arms initially going backwards and up. Repeat 5–10 times.

Side Curls

Stand comfortably with your feet apart and hands by your sides. Flex slowly and smoothly sideways to the left, so your left hand travels down the side of your leg. Then slowly straighten and repeat on the right-hand side. Do not lean forwards or backwards, but sideways only. Repeat these sideways curls, left then right, 10 times.

Waist Twists

Stand comfortably with your feet slightly apart. Link your hands together with your arms straight out in front of you. Without moving your hips, swivel smoothly to the left, twisting your waist. When you have twisted as far as you can, hold your position for a count of 3. Then return to the starting position and repeat the twist to the right. Repeat to left then right, 5–10 times.

Knee Bends

Stand comfortably, feet slightly apart, by the side of a chair.
Rest one hand lightly on the chair back. Slowly bend your
knees and squat. Slowly stand up again. Repeat 5–10
times.

Touch Toes

Stand comfortably, feet slightly apart, arms by your sides.
Bend forwards keeping your legs straight and try to
touch your toes. Slowly stand up again. Repeat 5–10
times. If you feel dizzy, stop.

Sit Stretches

Sit on the floor with your legs together and stretched out
in front of you. Reach forwards and try to touch your toes.
Hold as far forwards as you can stretch for a count of 10.

Steps

Jog lightly up and down the stairs (beware of loose carpet,
etc.) for one minute. Or, march on the spot, lifting your
knees up as high as they will go, and marching as fast as
you can.

Power Marching

March up and down on the spot, bringing your knees up
so your thighs are at right angles to your body. Do this as
fast as you can. At the same time, punch the air with your

fists. Either punch the air in front of you, or if you are feeling adventurous, punch above your head. You will soon work up a warm glow.

How to Walk Yourself Fit

Walking is an excellent, low-impact exercise for building up fitness, especially if you've been relatively inactive during the past year. Brisk walking will burn up over 350 calories an hour, more if you swing your arms and put extra effort into it.

Walking for fitness is a major pastime in the USA, with over 77 million participants. This makes it the most popular participatory sport in the nation. In one American study, a group of women followed a two-month walking programme, building up from two 15-minute sessions a week to a total of two hours. They all continued their usual eating habits, yet each lost a total of four inches from their waists, hips and thighs.

In the UK, the 1992 National Fitness Survey also found that walking was our most popular recreational activity. Using a scientific programme, walking can bring health and fitness benefits. By starting with three walks a week and building up regularly, you should notice a firming of your silhouette in four to six weeks. If you follow a sensible reducing diet at the same time, results will show even faster.

A walking for fitness programme involves brisk, regular walks, not infrequent leisurely strolls. Make sure you have recommended footwear with cushioned soles and some ankle support. Warm up first with a few simple stretch exercises. Begin slowly and lengthen your strides gradually. You should soon start to feel warm and generate a light sweat, but you should not feel out of breath to the extent that you can't walk and talk. After your brisk walk, stroll gently for a few minutes to cool down, then do some simple stretch exercises to maintain muscle suppleness.

Avoid isolated areas and, if walking at night, wear reflective clothing. If possible, walk with a companion for additional safety.

Perhaps the easiest way of walking yourself fit is using a treadmill. These machines tell you how fast you are walking, how far you have managed and how many calories you have burned.

Suggested Walking Regime

Obviously you don't need to stick to the days of the week suggested, but try to spread your activity evenly throughout the week.

WEEK	MONDAY	WEDNESDAY	FRIDAY	SUNDAY
1	10 mins	10 mins	15 mins	
2	10 mins	10 mins	15 mins	
3	15 mins	15 mins	15 mins	
4	20 mins	15 mins	20 mins	10 mins
5	20 mins	20 mins	20 mins	15 mins
6	20 mins	25 mins	30 mins	20 mins
7	20 mins	25 mins	30 mins	30 mins
8	30 mins	35 mins	35 mins	40 mins
9	35 mins	45 mins	35 mins	45 mins
10	45 mins	45 mins	45 mins	45 mins
11	45 mins	45 mins	45 mins	60 mins
12	45 mins	60 mins	45 mins	60 mins

To maintain your new fitness level, continue walking three or four times a week. Try to average at least three hours of brisk exercise spread out over each seven-day period.

How to Cycle Yourself Fit

There are now over 15 million regular cyclists in the UK, with over two million new bikes sold each year. Cycling is definitely in fashion. With the development of the all-terrain and mountain bikes, we can now literally cycle where we please, up hill, down dale or even splash through riverbeds.

Cycling is one of the best all-round exercises you can indulge in, improving your stamina, strength and suppleness. It is a low-impact, non-weight-bearing, aerobic activity which, like swimming, doesn't put your muscles, ligaments or joints under excessive strain. This makes cycling particularly beneficial to the overweight.

Cycling exercises your legs, bottom, heart, stomach, lower back, arms and chest and rapidly burns up calories at a rate of up to 650 kcals per hour.

If you haven't learned to cycle, obtain the benefits on an exercise bike at a gym. But why not make learning to ride one of your body awareness self-improvement goals?

Suggested Cycling Regimes

In the gym:

The average, non-fit person should start off with the following regime: Hill Profile.

		BEGINNERS		
WEEK	**DIFFICULTY LEVEL**	**VISIT 1**	**VISIT 2**	**VISIT 3**
1	Two	6 mins	6 mins	6 mins
2	Three	6 mins	12 mins	12 mins
3	Three	12 mins	12 mins	12 mins
4	Three	12 mins	12 mins	12 mins
5	Four	12 mins	12 mins	18 mins
6	Four	12 mins	12 mins	18 mins
7	Five	12 mins	12 mins	18 mins
8	Five	12 mins	18 mins	18 mins

If you can manage a fourth gym visit per week, do the same as for visit three. Most gyms provide music or television for entertainment, or you can take a portable cassette-player with you to while away the time.

You can then move on to further cardiovascular training programmes or do some weight training.

Out and about

If you own your own bike, it is important to be aware of cycling safety:

• Use lights at dusk.
• Fit a red reflector to the rear and amber reflectors to your pedals.
• Maintain and oil your bike regularly.
• Wear reflective clothing at night.
• Avoid roads where there is fast or heavy traffic.

- Consider taking a cycling proficiency test as one of your body awareness self-improvement goals.
- Always wear a safety helmet to BSI 6863 (not for speed cycling or racing) or to American Snell or ANSI standards.

Initially, cycle during the day on a route you know well. Keep to level ground for the first few weeks, then slowly tackle gentle hills, and steeper ones too if you feel up to it.

Beginner's Outdoor Cycling Regime

WEEK	MONDAY	WEDNESDAY	FRIDAY	SUNDAY
1	15 mins	15 mins	15 mins	
2	15 mins	20 mins	20 mins	
3	20 mins	20 mins	20 mins	
4	20 mins	15 mins	20 mins	15 mins
5	20 mins	20 mins	20 mins	20 mins
6	20 mins	25 mins	20 mins	25 mins
7	25 mins	25 mins	25 mins	30 mins
8	30 mins	30 mins	30 mins	35 mins
9	30 mins	35 mins	35 mins	40 mins
10	35 mins	40 mins	35 mins	45 mins
11	35 mins	40 mins	45 mins	60 mins
12	45 mins	60 mins	45 mins	60 mins

To maintain your new fitness level, continue cycling three or four times a week. Try to average at least three hours of brisk exercise spread out over each seven-day period.

Using Your Pulse Rate

You don't have to measure your pulse to exercise effectively but if you do, you'll be adding a scientific dimension to your work-out.

Moderate, low-intensity exercise will help you lose weight, build up fitness and improve your overall health; but you may not be pushing yourself enough to burn excess fat and strengthen your cardiovascular system most efficiently.

You can use your pulse rate throughout your walk or exercise period to obtain the maximum benefit for your cardiovascular system. Your pulse rate will also tell you the safe limits within which you can exercise your heart.

Your heart is a muscle of similar size to your fist. At rest, it beats approximately 70 times per minute in men, and 70–80 times per minute in women. Try clenching your fist at this rate. You'll be surprised at how difficult it is.

Your pulse is caused by the heart pumping a volume of blood into the circulation. This surges forwards, stretching arterial walls in a wave-like motion. Your pulse is most easily felt in three places:
- On the inner side of your wrist on the same side as your thumb (radial pulse).
- On the outer side of the front of your neck, under the jaw (carotid pulse).
- Centrally, at the top of the thigh, where your leg joins your abdomen.

With practice, these pulses are easily detected. Your pulse becomes more pronounced after exercise, when you are stressed or nervous, and with stimulant drugs such as nicotine, alcohol or caffeine. Certain prescribed drugs will slow the pulse rate down to make less work for your heart. If you have any medical condition (especially a heart problem) or are on any medication, always consult your doctor before embarking on an exercise regime.

Feel for your pulse on the right wrist with your left

hand's middle three fingers. It's best not to use your thumb, as this has a strong pulse of its own which may cause confusion. Count your resting pulse after sitting quietly for 15 minutes.

Resting Pulse Rate
(beats per minute)

Level of Fitness

Resting Pulse Rate (beats per minute)	Level of Fitness
50–59	Excellent (trained athletes)
60–69	Good
70–79	Fair
80 or over	Poor

NB: Your pulse rate is affected by some drugs and some heart conditions. If your resting pulse rate is below 60 or above 80 beats per minute and you know you are unfit, consult your doctor for a check-up.

Now, calculate your maximum pulse rate. This is done by subtracting your age from 220.

Activity levels need to raise your heart rate to between 60–80 per cent of this estimated maximum. This ensures that you will be burning fat rather than muscle energy stores (glycogen) during aerobic activity.

Monitoring your pulse should also enable you to exercise for 20 minutes feeling invigorated rather than exhausted.

Within the 60–80 per cent pulse range, a variety of fitness levels are catered for. Beginners, who haven't exercised for at least six months, should initially work at up to 65 per cent of maximum pulse rate. This can be calculated as follows:

$$\frac{(220 \text{ minus age}) \times 65}{100} \quad OR \quad \frac{(220 \text{ minus age}) \times 13}{20}$$

The table below has worked this out for you. It is easiest to count your pulse over a 10-second period and memorize the 10-second pulse range which corresponds to your age.

Exercise Pulse Rates to Aim for Versus Age

AGE	Estimated Max Pulse Rate (220 minus age)	60% Max Pulse Rate	65% Max Pulse Rate	80% Max Pulse Rate	10-Second Pulse Range
15	205	123	133	164	21–27
20	200	120	130	160	20–27
25	195	117	127	156	20–26
30	190	114	124	152	19–25
35	185	111	120	148	19–25
40	180	108	117	144	18–24
45	175	105	114	140	18–23
50	170	102	111	136	17–23
55	165	99	107	132	17–22
60	160	96	104	128	16–21
65	155	93	101	124	16–21
70	150	90	98	120	15–20
75	145	87	94	116	15–19
80	140	84	91	112	14–19

To start with, make sure your pulse stays at the lower end of the 10-second pulse training range (equivalent to 60–65 per cent maximum pulse).

If your pulse rate is below this range, perform your exercises more vigorously next time. If it is above this range, stop immediately and rest. Next time, you MUST take things at a slower pace, otherwise you risk damaging your health.

Take Your Pulse

• several times during exercise – every 10 minutes.
This will enable you to tailor your efforts and keep within the fat-burning, fitness range;

• immediately after finishing your exercise period.
This will confirm that you have been working at the correct level of effort and not over- or under-exercising;

• one minute after exercising, while resting.
The difference between your post-exercise pulse and your one-minute resting pulse is important. This tells you how quickly your heart is recovering from its exertion. The quicker your pulse drops, the fitter you are. After 10 minutes' rest, your heart rate should fall to below 100 beats per minute. If you are very fit, your pulse will drop by up to 70 beats in one minute.

Take Things Slowly

It's important to build up your activity and fitness levels gradually. It can be dangerous to launch straight into a training programme if you are unfit or in poor health.

Once you are relatively fit, you can increase your pulse rate to 70–75 per cent of your target range. When you reach super-fitness, you will be able to exercise comfortably at 75–80 per cent of your target range. Once you go above this level, you are in the athlete training zone and may risk endangering your health. You will also be burning lean tissue, such as muscle, rather than metabolizing the optimum amount of fat.

Chart Your Progress

Fitness can be gained at a significant rate by exercising for at least 20 minutes, three times a week. Draw up a chart like the one below. Fill it in at the beginning of each week to monitor your progress. This will help reinforce your motivation and give you a fitness goal to aim for.

This is a chart suitable for a 35-year-old woman, initially exercising at 65 per cent maximum pulse rate, increasing to 70 per cent maximum and 75 per cent maximum over a three-month period. Maximum pulse = 220 minus age = 185.

TARGET PULSE RANGE (60–80 per cent maximum pulse) = 111–148
10-second pulse range (for quick assessment) = 19–25

WEEK	% MAX PULSE	TARGET PULSE PER MINUTE	10-SECOND PULSE	PULSES RECORDED DURING EXERCISE	PULSE AT END OF EXERCISE	PULSE 1 MINUTE AFTER EXERCISE
0	65%	120	20	24, 22, 20	20 × 6 = 120	100
1	65%	120	20			
2	65%	120	20			
3	65%	120	20			
4	65%	120	20			
5	65%	120	20			
6	70%	130	22			
7	70%	130	22			
8	70%	130	22			
9	70%	130	22			
10	70%	130	22			
11	70%	130	22			
12	75%	139	23			

Burning Fat

As well as improving strength, suppleness and stamina and having beneficial effects on your health, exercise burns up fat. This fat-burning process is at its most efficient when your pulse is at the lower end of the training range – i.e. around 65 per cent of maximum pulse for your age.

The following table gives an idea of the number of calories burned during several activities by a person of average fitness. If you are signficantly overweight, the good news is that you will actually burn up more.

Only about 25 per cent of this energy is used by muscle activity – the rest is given out as heat. Our body temperature rises and we start to sweat. As sweat evaporates off our skin, this excess heat is removed.

Calorie-burning Values of Different Exercises

ACTIVITY	CALORIES BURNED PER HOUR
Sitting	90
Standing	100
Driving a car	140
Walk (stroll)	180
Washing and dressing	220
Bowling	250
Gardening	250
Swimming	300
Golf	300 plus
Walk (brisk)	350
Dancing	350 plus
Jogging	500 plus
Tennis	500 plus
Cycling	650 plus

Resistance Training

An exercise programme that incorporates both aerobic activity (e.g. walking, cycling, aerobic classes) and resistance training (free weights, weight–resistance machines; callisthenics, training rubber bands) is the best combination for getting in shape.

Aerobic exercise burns calories, promotes fat loss and strengthens the cardiovascular system. Resistance training complements aerobic processes by toning muscles and strengthening them.

It encourages increased muscle metabolism which, in turn, burns calories more efficiently. In addition, when you add resistance training to a weight-loss and aerobics regime, you ensure that you preserve muscle bulk – and only metabolize excess fat.

Using Weight-resistance Machines

When you join a health club, you will be given a weights programme to follow in the gym if this is suitable for your long-term aims. The weights programme will be individually tailored and based on your current level of fitness, your strength and your ultimate goals.

If you want to lose weight, your programme will entail repetitive muscle movements using low weights to tone muscle and burn fat.

If you want to put on muscle bulk and body-build, you will lift heavier weights fewer times.

A suggested beginner's regime follows. The resistance weights used, and their calibration, will depend on the make of machine. The number of repetitions and the number of sets repeated will stay constant until strength is built up and the trainee reassessed.

MACHINE	SET NUMBER OF REPETITIONS	NUMBER OF SETS
Leg extension	12	2
Leg curl	12	2
Calf raise	12	3
Leg abduction	12	2
Leg adduction	12	2
Chest press	12	1
Fly (peck deck)	12	1
Shoulder press	12	2
Lat pulldown	12	2
Arm curl	12	2
Triceps press	12	2

Muscular strength is the ability of a group of muscles to overcome a resistance. By gradually increasing the amount of resistance a muscle must overcome (adding on more weights to the machine) you will slowly increase muscular bulk, strength and the energy stores (glycogen) within.

Muscular endurance is the ability of a muscle to exert force to overcome a resistance over a long period of time. Endurance is improved by increasing the number of exercise repetitions whilst keeping the resistance relatively low. This improves stamina and tightens the silhouette, but will not bulk up your muscles in the typical, body-builder way.

Another way to add resistance training to your regime is to use an exercise elastic band (e.g. Flex-a-band, Dynaband) made from latex rubber. These increase the strength and endurance of muscle groups, especially those in problem areas such as stomach, bottom, hips and thighs. It can also firm up flabby areas around the upper arms, pectoral muscles and breasts. Your current fitness level will determine the strength of band you should use.

CHAPTER 7

Stress and the Importance of Relaxation

Stress and Disease

Relaxation is a powerful, stress-relieving tool. Stress is increasingly recognized as a major contributor to disease, but unfortunately most of us have lost the art of relaxing correctly.

When we feel pressurized, our body secretes powerful hormones such as adrenaline and we go on red alert. This reaction evolved to help primitive man survive by fighting or fleeing dangerous animals. We now rarely resort to actual fight or flight and stress hormones build up to cause harm.

Some stress is good for us and allows us to meet life's challenges. Too much results in unpleasant symptoms such as sweating, dizziness, palpitations, and even chest pain. Our bowels start to work overtime and we may hyperventilate and panic. In short, we experience dis-stress.

Distress can reduce us to gibbering wrecks, raise blood pressure dangerously high and cause spasm of our coronary artery walls. This leads to angina and, in some cases, a heart attack.

A mind-over-matter connection has long been suspected as patients who are pessimistic, lonely or under stress become markedly sicker than those who are optimistic, sociable and relaxed.

Many diseases worsen under stress, including skin disorders such as eczema or psoriasis.

It is now known that nerves in the skin's upper layer produce a substance that transmits signals between nerves and regulates the function and activity of surrounding immune cells.

This substance, called calcitonin gene-related peptide (CGRP) is a protein supplied directly to immune cells through a nerve. CGRP is an exciting discovery as it shows how central nervous activity (e.g. stress) can affect the body's immunity.

People under stress are classically more likely to suffer serious disease linked with a faulty immune system – such as cancer.

Most symptoms of stress are due to hyperventilation and the physiological effects of adrenaline hormone.

Symptoms of Stress

Physical
- Tiredness
- Sweating
- Flushing
- Insomnia
- Palpitations
- Extra heart beats (extra systole)
- Rapid pulse
- Dizziness
- Faintness
- Trembling of muscles
- Restless legs (von Ekbom's syndrome)
- Pins and needles (paraesthesiae)
- Numbness

- Headache
- Chest pain
- Stomach pain
- Nausea
- Diarrhoea
- Premenstrual syndrome
- Irregular, heavy periods
- Absent periods
- Excessive appetite
- Obesity

Mental
- Overwhelming feelings of anxiety and panic
- Fear of rejection
- Fear of failure
- Loss of ability to concentrate
- Increased risk of accidents
- Loss of sex drive
- Premature ejaculation
- Impotence
- Reliance on alcohol, smoking or drugs
- Obsessive behaviour
- Compulsive behaviour
- Bulimia nervosa
- Anorexia nervosa
- Feelings of isolation from friends/relatives
- A feeling of impending doom
- Suicide or para-suicide

When stress reaches our threshold for coping, disease and death can occur. Stressed people die young from coronary heart disease, accidents and suicide. They also have a tendency toward serious disease such as diabetes and cancer.

Stressed people lose their sense of judgment and jeopardize the stability of relationships. Friendships and marriages break up, alcohol becomes a major crutch and a potential new source of problems.

Internal Versus External Stress

Stress comes from two main sources:
- within an individual (internal)
- from the environment (external)

Most stress is self-generated for, although external factors are the stimuli, it's how we react to these factors that's important.

Internal Causes of Stress

- Tiredness
- Physical unfitness and lack of exercise
- Physical disease
- Disruption of bio-rhythms, e.g. late nights, crying babies
- Uncertainty of goals in life
- Negative self-image, e.g. overweight
- Personality type

Type A personality

Certain personality characteristics are associated with high levels of internal stress, the type As.

These people are excessively competitive, always setting deadlines and striving ahead at work. They have difficulty relaxing and become frustrated and impatient with delays. Type As need constant reassurance of their worth and may become hostile when thwarted. They tend to dominate conversation and are always finishing other people's sentences.

Type B personality

Type B personalities may be equally ambitious, and achieve just as many goals, but lack the big sense of time-urgency and panic.

They are self-confident and don't seek approval so

avidly. They get on with the job and complete it to everyone's satisfaction. They are calm, easy-going and pleasant to be with.

Do you think you are a type A or a type B personality?

External Causes of Stress

Sources of external stress are mainly related to change. Change causes uncertainty, uncertainty induces anxiety and anxiety leads to stress.

You may experience changes in relationships, in the family or at work. Your boss or you yourself may set unrealistic goals. Make sure your weight-loss targets are achievable, so they don't induce feelings of frustration, inadequacy, not being in control, failure and stress.

Coping Mechanisms

There are two ways of reacting to stress:
- the subconscious, defensive approach
- the conscious, adaptive approach

The adaptive approach usually works, while the defensive approach usually fails.

Defensive Mechanisms

These are subconscious ways of distorting reality; the ostrich head-in-the-sand approach: pretend it isn't there ('My weight isn't really affecting my health') and eventually it will go away. Unfortunately it never does and even if it seems to, anxiety still lurks to provoke feelings of inadequacy and doom.

Problems can be projected onto others and we lose responsibility for them ('It's my glands making me fat').

We rationalize and find acceptable excuses for things that are really quite unacceptable.

Problems are isolated and talked about clinically. We regress to earlier stages of development and sulk and eat more when depressed.

Sleeping postures become more foetal. Stressful concepts are conveniently forgotten, but often revealed in so-called Freudian slips.

Adaptive Mechanisms

These are deliberate means of adjusting to stress in a positive, constructive way. Thoughts are isolated from feelings and situations seen in perspective. Problems are analysed logically and plans made to resolve them. The very fact that you are reading this book shows that you are applying an adaptive approach to your dietary problems and have a good chance of succeeding at your weight-loss goals.

How to Beat Stress

Psychologists advise the following:
- Work out what situations and people cause you stress, and why. Often only a few sources are involved.
- Change those things that can be changed, then accept it is normal to operate as an imperfect person in an imperfect world.
- Identify and respect your good points. Improve your shortcomings as much as possible, then accept them as part of you.
- Don't compare yourself unfavourably with others.

- Don't expect others to change before you are prepared to change yourself.
- Set realistic goals – tackle big problems, such as being overweight, one step at a time.
- Expect to make mistakes. Apologize, then learn from them. Don't give up when the going gets tough – this is a waste of valuable life experience.
- Learn to be patient. Let the pushy so-and-so with a Porsche into the queue in front of you; stop at amber lights instead of racing through just-red ones.
- Talk more slowly and listen without interrupting.
- Formulate decisions in unhurried circumstances, rather than under deadline pressures.
- Be assertive. Say 'No' and mean it. This will help prevent you being put upon and overloaded with tasks.

Finally, try injecting a 'Meichenbaum' as an antidote to stressful situations, i.e. substitute a positive, calming thought for a stressful, negative one, e.g.:

I do this as well as anyone.

I am enough.

Up until now, I haven't managed to lose weight. Now I'm going to.

This is the first day of the rest of my life.

Every day, in every way, I get better and better.

Diet and Stress

Caffeine and nicotine mimic the stress response, so limit your tea and coffee intake to three cups per day. Better still, switch to decaffeinated brands or try the many fruit and herbal teas available.

Vitamin C and the vitamin B complexes are depleted under stress as they are utilized in the fight–or–flight response. Vitamin B is further depleted by the metabolism of alcohol and sugary foods, often resorted to in excess in times of stress.

Vitamin B deficiency leads to symptoms of anxiety and irritability – a vicious circle is propagated.

- Eat high-fibre wholefoods.
- Decrease dietary sugar, salt and saturated fat.
- Eat little and often to prevent hypoglycaemia.
- Stop smoking and keep alcohol intake to a minimum.

In other words, follow the Body Awareness Diet.

There are a number of exercises and techniques you can use to reduce stress and keep it within safe limits.

Basic Relaxation Exercise

When stressed, we breathe rapidly and shallowly. This leads to headaches and dizziness. Learn to breathe abdominally so the inspiration moves the abdomen and not the chest.

Find somewhere quiet and warm to practise. Remove your shoes and loosen tight clothing, especially around the waist.

Close your eyes. You are going to work round your body, tensing and relaxing different muscle groups to relieve tension.

Lift your **forearms**, bending at the elbow and clenching your **fists** hard. Lift your arms into the air and feel the tension in your forearms and upper arm muscles. Be aware of the tightness in your hands and any discomfort in your arms. Keep your eyes closed and concentrate only on your arms.

As you breathe out, slowly start to relax and let the tension go. Release the fingers and fists and lower your arms gently until they are at rest. Imagine the tension flowing down your arms and away through your fingers. Let your arms become heavier and more and more relaxed. Feel the tension flow out of you until your fingers start to tingle. Your arms may feel like they don't belong to you. Each time you breathe out gently, say the word 'relax'.

Now tense your **shoulders** and **neck**. Shrug your shoulders up as high as you can and tense them. Feel the tension in your head, shoulders, neck and chest. Hold it for a moment. Then slowly lower your shoulders and let the tension flow away. Relax your chest and breathe gently and slowly. As you breathe out, say the word 'relax'.

Now tighten your **head** muscles by lifting your head up and pushing it forwards. Feel the tension in your neck. Tighten all your facial muscles. Clench your teeth, frown and screw up your eyes. Feel the tension on your face, the tightness in your skin and jaw, the wrinkles on your brow. Hold it for a few seconds, then start to relax. Let go gradually so you become aware of all your muscles as they relax. A feeling of warmth will spread across your head as the tension is released. Release your eye muscles, your jaw, your tongue, your nose. Your head will feel very heavy and very relaxed. Breathe slowly and every time you breathe out, say 'relax' to yourself.

As long as you have no back problems, concentrate now on the tension in your **back** muscles. Tense them by pulling your shoulders and head backwards and arching your back slightly. Hold this for a few moments. Then start to relax completely. Allow your back to sink comfortably down. Feel the weight sinking down as you relax. Check your arms, head and neck are still relaxed too.

Now tense your **abdomen** by pulling it in as tightly as you can. Feel the tightness so you have to breathe in your chest area. Then, as you breathe out, slowly release and feel the tension drain away. Now blow out the stomach as if tensing against a blow. Hold this tension for a few moments, then slowly relax and feel the tension flow away. Make sure the tension has not crept back into parts of your body you have already relaxed.

As you breathe out, make sure you feel your whole

upper body feels heavy, calm and relaxed.

Now concentrate on your **legs**. Pull your toes up towards you and feel the tightness down the front of your legs. Then push your toes away from you and feel the tightness spread up your legs. Hold this for a few moments, then lift your legs into the air, either together or one at a time. Feel your buttocks, thighs and stomach tense. Hold this for a few moments and then lower your legs until they are at rest.

Relax your thighs, buttocks, calves and feet. Let them flop under their own weight and relax. Feel the tension flow down your legs and out through your toes. Feel your legs become heavy and relaxed. Your toes may tingle.

Now, your whole body should feel very, very heavy and very relaxed. Breathe calmly and slowly. All the tension has drained from your body.

Place one hand on your abdomen and check that your tummy rises and falls slightly as you breathe. Your breathing should lift your abdomen, not your chest. Slowly and evenly breathe in and out. You should now be fully relaxed.

Constantly check and re-check your body to make sure it's relaxed and tension has not crept back in.

Imagine you are lying on a warm, sunny beach and relaxing in the sun. Constantly check your body for tension. Relax . . . relax . . . relax.

Aromatherapy

We know that smell has a powerful effect on our emotions. The olfactory nerves from the nose connect with the limbic system of the brain, where our emotional response is centred. Just think about the powerful effects of sex pheromones – or the startling feelings accompanying certain evocative smells.

It should come as no surprise that pungent smells derived from plant essential oils can strongly affect our emotions and mood. Some aromatherapy oils are stimulating and invigorating, others soothing and relaxing. When diluted oils are rubbed onto the skin, their effects are even more potent.

Many modern drugs are derived from plants. We also know that drugs can be absorbed through the skin – several drug patches are prescribable by doctors.

Aromatherapy oils are widely available. Buy a selection with relaxant and anti-stress properties.

- Dilute 2–3 drops in one tablespoon of carrier oil and rub into your skin.
- Place a drop on a tissue and breathe in the vapour.
- Put oil drops in a diffuser – either one which is heated by a candle or placed over a light bulb or radiator – to scent the air.
- Run a hot bath and add a few drops as directed. Then lie back, wallow and relax for at least half an hour.

Oils with relaxant or anti-stress properties include:
- ★★ Basil
- ★ Bergamot
- ★ Cardamom
- ★ Camomile Roman
- ★ Clary-sage
- ★ Coriander
- ★★ Fennel
- ★ Geranium
- ★★ Grapefruit
- ★ Jonquil
- ★★ Lavender
- ★★ Lemon
- ★★ Lemongrass
- ★ Marjoram
- ★ Melissa
- ★ Narcissus

- ★ Neroli
- ★ Nutmeg
- ★★ Orange
- ★ Osmanthus
- ★ Patchouli
- ★ Rose
- ★★ Rosemary
- ★ Sandalwood
- ★★ Thyme
- ★ Vetiver
- ★ Ylang-ylang

NB: oils marked with a double asterisk are also said to tone the muscles and aid the slimming process.

Flotation Therapy

Flotation therapy takes place in a light-proof, sound-insulated tank in which you float on a pool of water more buoyant than the Dead Sea. The water is at skin temperature, light, sound and other external stimuli are removed, and you relax for at least 50 minutes in silence. If you wish, gentle music can be piped in.

During a float, high blood pressure falls significantly. Levels of stress hormones go down and with a series of floats, cholesterol readings improve. The brain starts to generate theta waves, the mystical state sought through meditation.

When external stimuli such as sound, vision and temperature are taken away, the brain, which is divided into dominant and non-dominant halves, is suddenly cut off from the thousands of stimuli it has to filter every second.

The non-dominant side of the brain is then free to do what it is best at – produce creative thoughts and bursts of insight. Problems become crystal clear as we literally experience a brain wave.

Some floaters experience feelings of euphoria due to the release of brain chemicals similar in effect to heroin. This is useful for patients with chronic pain (e.g. arthritis) and their need for pain-killers can go down.

Some floaters focus in on themselves so well that they can speed up or decrease their heart rate at will. Others listen to language tapes and can learn a foreign language in a fraction of the usual time.

Flotation therapy can help you relax, help you become more creative and empathic – and can also help you to lose weight.

Whilst you are lying in the tank:

- Imagine yourself slim, fit and healthy.
- Let that excess flab peel away in your mind.
- Picture your fat cells slowly letting go of their fat stores as fat is burned for energy.
- Imagine your metabolism clicking up into high speed.
- Imagine the calories you eat being converted into energy and wasted as heat – not deposited on your hips.
- Imagine a healthy meal full of ACE vitamins, fish, olive oil, garlic, grapes, red wine and unrefined carbohydrates. Feel good about that meal. Imagine how delicious it is.

During flotation therapy, your brain has time to concentrate on your goals. You can reinforce your willpower, visualize your target weight – and aim straight for it. Do not underestimate the power of positive thought.

Give flotation therapy a go at least once during your weight-loss or healthy-eating programme. It will expand your horizons and I can guarantee you will feel a different person on coming out. You will obtain most benefit by floating every 7–10 days.

If you would like to know more about flotation therapy, refer to the appendices at the back of this book.

CHAPTER 8

Body Awareness Foods

Certain foods are more healthy than others. If they're eaten in the right quantities, they lower our risk of heart disease and certain cancers. These foods, used extensively in the Body Awareness Programme, tend to be high in vitamins, essential fatty acids, antioxidants or unrefined carbohydrate. These nutrient–rich foods are:

- olive oil
- fish
- garlic
- fresh herbs
- grapes – especially red ones
- red wine
- walnuts
- oil of evening primrose
- yogurt
- pasta
- bread
- fresh fruit and vegetables

The ACE Vitamins

The Health Benefits of Vitamins

It used to be fashionable to dismiss the need for vitamin supplements. It was declared they were literally money down the drain in the form of expensive urine. We now know that this expensive urine protects against cancer of the bladder.

Until recently, it was thought that we could obtain adequate vitamins from a proper diet full of fresh fruits and vegetables. However, this is no longer thought to be the case for the ACE or 'super' vitamins A (betacarotene), C and E.

I would also add gammalinolenic acid (evening primrose oil) to that list and, for people who don't like eating fish, would strongly recommend the use of a fish oil supplement (high in eicosapentanoic acid), such as Maxepa. Oil of evening primrose and fish oil are available in one pack as Efamol Marine.

Our diet should always come first. In addition to eating as many antioxidant-rich foods as possible, our dietary intake of ACE vitamins is boosted to optimal limits by the use of supplements. Most experts agree that diet alone cannot supply the necessary levels.

- 98 per cent of the population do not achieve European recommendations of 10mg of vitamin E per day;
- 60 per cent don't achieve European recommendations of 60mg vitamin C per day;
- 90 per cent of the population only obtain 2mg betacarotene per day. The National Cancer Institute recommends at least 6mg betacarotene per day to reduce the risk of cancer.

An adequate intake of vitamins is particularly important for smokers. Extra vitamins A, C and E are needed to mop up damaging free radicals produced by smoking cigarettes.

The elderly population is especially vulnerable to low blood vitamin levels. An American study of 96 independent elderly individuals showed that those who took multivitamins for one year had significantly improved levels of immunity and a decreased risk of infection. Immune T-cell subsets and natural killer cells were increased in number and were more active. In addition, they mounted a significantly more effective antibody response to influenza vaccine.

Overall, those who took supplements only had infections for an average of 23 days in the year, compared with an average of 48 days for those not taking multivitamin supplements, i.e. infection-related illness was halved.

It is now accepted that vitamins not only reduce the incidence of chronic, debilitating diseases, they also have a profound effect on the incidence of age-related conditions such as cataracts and arthritis.

Nutritional status is important in determining the function of our body. We are what we eat. If we provide our body with inadequate materials and nutrients, our metabolism simply goes wrong. We need an optimum intake of micro-nutrients to enhance our immunity (especially in old age) and to protect us against free-radical attack.

Vitamins A, C and E are antioxidants. Antioxidants neutralize free radicals produced by our metabolic pathways, chemical pollutants, cigarette smoke and radiation.

Free radicals only exist momentarily but are powerful enough to set up chain reactions that can damage our genetic material and oxidize fats in our body. Oxidized cholesterol in the blood is more likely to get absorbed into artery walls, resulting in atherosclerosis – hardening and furring up of the arteries – which in turn leads to coronary heart disease.

A trial involving 6,000 middle-aged males has shown that the risk of developing angina was three times higher in men with low levels of vitamins E, C and betacarotene.

The vitamins seem to work together for a maximal

114

antioxidant effect. It's known, for example, that when vitamin E exerts its protective function it becomes a free radical itself before rapidly being regenerated by vitamin C. It is important therefore to have adequate blood levels of all vitamins. It is less effective taking vitamin C supplements if your intake of vitamin E is inadequate.

Certain trace minerals (selenium, manganese, copper and zinc) are also thought important in scavenging free radicals. They combine with proteins to form intracellular antioxidant enzymes.

Vitamin E

Vitamin E is increasingly recognized as an important constituent of health. It can help prevent a wide range of problems including cataracts, cancer, rheumatoid arthritis and coronary heart disease. Although the latter is the only disease so far in which vitamin E has proven benefits, independent prospective studies have linked low blood vitamin E levels with an increased risk of developing cancer.

Vitamin E is shown experimentally to inhibit oxidation of low density LDL-cholesterol. In two recent trials, involving 87,000 female nurses and 40,000 male doctors, the risk of major cardiovascular disease was reduced by one-third in women taking vitamin E supplements for up to two years, and by up to 50 per cent in those who took it for longer.

Those taking vitamin E in multivitamin preparations had a 12 per cent reduction in coronary heart disease.

The risk of major coronary heart disease in men was reduced by 25 per cent in those taking vitamin E for more than two years.

It is now accepted that vitamin E, together with other antioxidants, reduces the risk of heart disease. It is especially helpful for people who are overweight, who smoke and who have high blood LDL-cholesterol levels.

Most experts believe it is essential to both increase vitamin E levels in our diet *and* to take vitamin E supplements.

A diet rich in vitamin E will only provide around 20mg per day. A daily intake of at least 40mg to 50mg is needed to provide adequate protection against free-radical damage causing coronary heart disease.

The Vital 3 supplements recommended in the Mediterranean Slim Diet contain 134mg of vitamin E per capsule. The increased intake is essential to mop up free radicals released from body fat stores during the weight-loss process.

The good news is there are no known toxic side effects from taking too much vitamin E. The only people for whom it is not recommended are those with blood-clotting disorders or those known to have a vitamin K deficiency.

Vitamin E is found in vegetable oils, seeds, avocado, wheatgerm, nuts and seafood.

Vitamin E content of various oils

OIL	LEVEL OF VITAMIN E (mg/100g)
Wheatgerm	136
Sunflower	49
Safflower	40
Palm	33
Rape seed	22
Cod-liver	20
Corn	17
Peanut	15
Olive	5

Vitamin C

There is now strong evidence that vitamin C supplements lengthen our lifespan. A 10-year study, involving 11,000 men and women, undertaken by the University of California has shown that a high intake of vitamin C (including the use of supplements) lowers the risk of heart disease in males by a dramatic 40 per cent – the risk of dying is reduced by 35 per cent.

The women in the survey enjoyed a reduced coronary heart disease risk of 25 per cent compared to the normal population.

The authors felt there was possibly a decreased risk of cancer of the oesophagus and stomach in males as well, but this requires further investigation.

Dietary vitamin C is obtained from liver, fruit and vegetables. Citrus fruits, guava, peppers, paw-paw, broccoli, mangoes, berries and kiwi fruit are especially vitamin C-rich.

Lack of vitamin C causes scurvy. Until recently, this was a relatively rare disease in the UK but is now becoming more common – particularly amongst teenagers and the elderly following an inadequate diet.

Many teenagers eat no fresh fruit or vegetables at all. In one recent case, a girl living on a diet of crisps, hamburgers, chocolate, and cola developed bleeding gums, broken thread veins in her skin and dry, fissured lips. She was only obtaining 8.5mg of vitamin C per day. The minimum daily requirement to prevent scurvy is 10mg. Interestingly, the girl was overweight and not anorectic.

The other group of teenagers at high risk of developing this disease are those with eating disorders. Symptoms of scurvy also include weakness, tiredness, shortness of breath and aching limbs.

Diabetics have a marked reduction in blood vitamin C levels compared with non-diabetics – despite no obvious difference in dietary intake. Some experts recommend that diabetics, especially if they smoke, should take vitamin C supplements – perhaps in dosages as high as 200mg per day.

Experiments have shown that vitamin C applied topically to the skin reduces the number of sunburn cells after exposure to ultraviolet radiation. This is probably because it mops up free radicals produced by ultraviolet radiation.

The reference nutrient intake for vitamin C remains behind the times at 40–60mg per day. Most experts now believe that around 500mg per day is required to give protection against free-radical attack, coronary heart disease and other age-related diseases such as cancer.

The Vital 3 supplement recommended in the Mediterranean Slim Diet contains 150mg of vitamin C. In addition, the typical dietary intake per day from the eating programme provides around 350mg vitamin C to take you into the 500mg per day range.

Betacarotene

Betacarotene is converted in the body to vitamin A (a powerful antioxidant) when vitamin A stores are low. Otherwise, it is retained as the pro-vitamin, a powerful antioxidant in its own right.

Betacarotene is found in dark green leaves (e.g. spinach, broccoli) and yellow/orange fruit and vegetables such as carrots, apricots, mangoes and red/yellow peppers.

Research in the USA on 87,000 female nurses and 22,000 male doctors showed that those with the highest intake of the pro-vitamin betacarotene reduced their risk of coronary heart disease by 22 per cent in females and 25 per cent in males. Research with 13,000 elderly people in Massachusetts showed that those with a high intake of betacarotene were less likely to develop cancers of the mouth, throat, larynx, oesophagus, stomach, large bowel and bladder. Several studies have also found a link between low levels of betacarotene and cancer of the lung and cervix.

The average British adult obtains 2mg of betacarotene per day from their diet. This is below the National Cancer Institute recommendation of at least 6mg per day.

The Vital 3 supplement recommend in the Mediterranean Slim Diet provides 15mg of betacarotene per day. Betacarotene may reduce the risk of:

- breast cancer
- lung cancer
- cervical cancer
- heart disease
- stroke
- macular degeneration in the eye – a common cause of blindness in the elderly

Vitamin A

Vitamin A supplements are not recommended. Unlike vitamins C and E, too much vitamin A is dangerous. Side effects include hair loss, blurred vision, headaches, liver damage and even death. In pregnancy, excess vitamin A can lead to foetal damage and even miscarriage.

Vitamin A itself is only found in foods derived from an animal source such as liver, seafood, egg yolk and dairy products. Liver and liver products are not recommended during pregnancy. Betacarotene is a safe alternative.

Olive Oil

Olive oil is one of nature's finest products which has many desirable effects on the body's biochemistry. It is adopted as a body awareness food for its positive effects on choles-terol, skin and hair.

It is derived from the fruit of the olive tree (*Olea europaea*) and is native to the Mediterranean region – an area with a low incidence of coronary heart disease.

All olives start off green. These are the unripened fruit with firm skin and a slightly bitter taste. As the olive ripens, it goes through various shades of purple to black and the flesh becomes increasingly wrinkly. Flavour mellows as the percentage of oil increases.

Olives intended for producing oil are picked when unripe. They taste bitter and are totally inedible. Unripened green olives have a low acid content which is crucial; the lower the acidity, the better the oil.

Extra virgin olive oil is the best quality and has not been purified. It has a distinctive green hue and often hazes at room temperature. Its flavour is superb as it comes from the first pressing of the fruit and retains the fresh, olive aroma. It contains less than 1 per cent acidity.

Fine virgin olive oil comes next in quality with between 1–1.5 per cent acidity.

Virgin olive oil is slightly more piquant in taste and con-tains 2–3 per cent acidity.

Pure olive oil is a blend of refined oils mixed with extra virgin oil to provide a quality suitable for cooking. Acidity averages 1.5 per cent, but the flavour is less pleasing. It's best not to use cheaper versions for salad dressings as the bitter flavours will come through.

The major problem with olive oil is ageing. As the oil matures, extra acidity is gained which detracts from the original flavour. Most oils are best used within one year of pressing. If left longer than this, stale or even rancid flavours can develop – so don't lay down olive oil along-side your clarets.

All olive oils contain vitamin E and are rich in mono-unsaturated fat. The principal component – oleic acid – is processed in the body to lower blood cholesterol.

Significantly, it only lowers the harmful low density cholesterol (LDL) without modifying desirable high density cholesterol (HDL). As a result, in Mediterranean regions where olive oil is used liberally for culinary and medicinal purposes, the incidence of coronary heart disease and other cholesterol-related illnesses is low.

Many studies have confirmed that olive oil is good for the heart. We now, therefore, have an almost bewildering choice of different olive oils on the shelves of our supermarkets.

Each country and region yields its own style of oil with its own unique flavour. Just as with wine, flavour depends on factors such as mineral content of the soil, the climate, how the olives are cultivated and the way the final product is blended.

Occasionally, leaves are added when the oil is pressed from the fruit. This adds an attractive green colour to the final product, but is really a bit misleading because it emulates the green of extra virgin, first-pressed oil and allows the price to rise.

Connoisseurs look for flavour and aroma in their olive oil and maintain that colour is of secondary importance.

Words used by professional tasters to describe olive oil flavours include: grassy; lemony; spicy; peppery; dark brazil-nut chocolate; leafy; fruity; nutty; bitter; almondy; tangy; limey; buttery; bacony; like fresh green pears; appley; earthy; heavy; thyme; and even pure vanilla – so clearly there's a wide variety available.

As with wine, a little practice is needed to become familiar with the olive in all its glory. My personal favourites are oils from Tuscany and Crete.

Whichever oils you choose, keep them somewhere cool and dark and use them as soon as possible. Avoid buying from small shops where turnover is likely to be low and the oils on display correspondingly old.

Olive Aperitif

This makes an attractive aperitif or hors d'oeuvre when served with a pile of cocktail sticks for guests to pick away at the jar.

enough black or green olives to fill a glass jar
sprig of fresh rosemary
sprig of fresh thyme
sprig of fresh oregano or marjoram
stalk of lemon grass
1 small dried chilli
2.5cm peeled ginger root, heavily scored with a knife
zest of 1–2 lemons
2 cloves garlic, crushed
extra virgin olive oil to cover

Pack the ingredients loosely in a glass jar. Cover with olive oil and seal. Leave the olives to marinade for at least a week – they will continue to improve in flavour over several months. Any herbs and flavourings can be used – whatever is to hand.

Herb Oils

If you have olive oil that needs using up, try concocting your own herbal infusions. These are simple to make and look and smell as delicious as they taste.

Herbed oils add an extra dimension to cooking and salad dressings. I've found the best oils are made using mint, basil, rosemary, oregano, fennel, marjoram, thyme, savory or tarragon. For some reason, parsley doesn't work.

Sweet oils made with clove pinks, lavender, lemon verbena, lemon thyme and rose petals are also useful.

Herb Oil

300ml olive oil (any quality)
2–4 tbsp crushed herb leaves
1 tbsp wine vinegar

All you have to do is select fresh, dry leaves and crush them in a pestle and mortar. Alternatively, chop them roughly with a little added oil.

Add 2–4 tablespoons of crushed leaves to each 300ml of olive oil and pour into a corked, clear bottle, leaving plenty of room at the top.

Add 1 tablespoon of wine vinegar and cork the bottle. Shake vigorously.

Place the bottle where it will receive direct sunlight for several hours a day. This brings out the flavour of the herbs. Leave for two or three weeks, shaking twice a day.

Then, strain off the oil and extract as much of it as possible from the strained herbs. Taste the oil and see if it's flavoured strongly enough for your taste. If not, repeat the process using fresh crushed herbs.

When the oil is finally to your liking, re-bottle and add a decorative sprig of fresh herbs.

You can make herbed wine vinegars in a similar way, although a larger quantity of leaves is required and hot rather than cold vinegar is poured over the crushed herbs.

Herbs to add to wine vinegars include: basil, bay, chervil, dill, fennel, lemon balm, marjoram, mint, rosemary, savory, tarragon and thyme.

Garlic Oil

Peel three or four cloves of garlic and score the flesh heavily. I cut each clove into thin slices that are still attached at one side, though you could crush the cloves if you wish.

Don't put the cloves into the oil whole without cutting the flesh in some way – the pungent flavour of allicin is only released when the cell walls are disrupted. Intact, whole cloves have no aroma.

Cover the chopped or crushed garlic with oil (or vinegar) and leave in a jar or bottle for at least two weeks, shaking twice a day.

A blend of herbs and garlic produces a fragrant Mediterranean-style oil which is excellent when mixed with lemon juice and freshly ground black pepper for basting grilled fish or meat.

Chilli Oil

When making chilli oil, add as many chillies as you wish. If you cut the chillies open to release the seeds, the hotter the oil becomes.

Fish Oils

Fish oils have proved valuable in many areas of medicine.
- Research has shown that a modest increase in dietary fish can help prevent death due to coronary thrombosis (heart attack).
- In those who have had a heart attack, eating fish significantly reduces the possibility of a second heart attack occurring. If one does occur, the chances of dying from the second thrombosis are decreased.
- Dutch doctors have shown that people who eat fish once or twice a week cut their risk of dying from a stroke.

- Cod-liver oil is valuable for easing pain and stiffness in people suffering from arthritis.
- Seven years worth of research in Israel has pinpointed a substance present in fish which helps repair damaged nerves. This could lead to future treatment for victims of paralysis.
- Danish research suggests that fish oil may help avoid premature births, as pregnant women on fish-rich diets have longer pregnancies and heavier babies than average.
- Fish oil greatly improves the health of people with ulcerative colitis. A four-month study has confirmed that taking fish oil supplements resulted in weight gain and decreased colonic inflammation. In addition, patients who required oral steroids could halve their intake of these drugs.
- Other chronic, inflammatory diseases such as rheumatoid arthritis and psoriasis are associated with excessive production of immunologically active chemicals in the body. Many of these are derived from the metabolism of non-fish oils (e.g. arachidonic acid). By eating more fish, especially oily fish, molecules which neutralize the harmful effects of these undesirable, immunologically active chemicals are produced. This explains the beneficial effects of fish oil in the conditions mentioned above.
- Most exciting of all, new research suggests a substance found in fish oil may have a role in beating cancer. Researchers have found a fish oil derivative which halts the growth of tumours and reverses the weight loss associated with cancer in animals. Studies are now taking place with humans and look equally promising.

Eicosapentanoic Acid

The magic substance found in fish which imparts all these beneficial effects is EPA – eicosapentanoic acid. EPA can shrink solid tumours and halt the dramatic weight loss (cachexia) associated with cancers. It appears to work by altering hormone-like proteins synthesized by abnormal cells in some tumours.

In one study, pre-cancerous polyps of the colon responded dramatically to treatment with fish oils and reduced in frequency by 50 per cent.

Preliminary studies suggest that a daily dose of 5–8g of pure eicosapentanoic acid is ideal. Most importantly, EPA has none of the side effects associated with traditional, cytotoxic drugs.

EPA may well prove to be the wonder drug we've all been seeking – a prototype elixir of life.

The fish classed as oily which have an especially high content of EPA are: mackerel, herring, pilchards, sardines, salmon and trout.

Glycoproteins found in green-lipped mussels also have a medical benefit. They display proven anti-inflammatory activity and relieve the pain of arthritis. They work by preventing inflammatory cells (neutrophils) from crossing the endothelium of blood vessels to the sites of inflammation. Once there, these cells would release potent chemicals which contribute to pain and swelling.

The green-lipped mussel found in New Zealand is the only mollusc with this property. Scallops, blue mussels and oysters have been tested but were found to be inactive.

Seafood

Fish is a major component of the Mediterranean and Eskimo diets. It is eaten regularly by the healthiest peoples in the world – those with little risk of coronary heart disease.

Over 50 varieties of seafood can be bought in Great Britain, yet most of us seem rather reluctant to try this delicious and nutritious source of protein. The most adventurous we get is a boned trout fillet or a breaded piece of hake.

To many people, the word fish conjures up visions of bland-tasting dishes, but it's possible to feast on fish every day – and never repeat the same dish or the same exquisite combination of flavours.

For a long while, fresh fish was difficult to buy in many parts of Great Britain. It's now more widely available thanks to the efforts of various famous chefs. The ebullient Keith Floyd probably did more for our ailing hearts than any health-food messages from the Department of Health.

Selecting really fresh fish

Never be afraid to ask your fishmonger if you can inspect the fish. After all, you're the one who's going to eat it – and suffer in the bathroom if it's off. If he doesn't want to play ball, the simplest thing is to vote with your feet. However, I haven't yet met a fishmonger who doesn't leap proudly to display his wares when a customer expresses interest and a desire to experiment.

Fresh fish should smell of seawater – salty, with a tang of ozone and sometimes slightly sweet. It should not smell of fish. This characteristic smell comes from the breakdown of chemicals, so if your fish smells fishy it's not fresh.

The eyes of fresh fish are clear, bright, shiny and gleaming, but as the fish deteriorates, the eyes become shrunken and cloudy – compare the eyes of a fresh trout to that of its frozen brother.

Inspect the gills of your potential purchase too. They should be a healthy pink or bright red – not a dingy brown.

Fresh fish skin should gleam like expensive shot silk and feel young and firm to the touch.

When you push a finger into the fish body, the flesh should spring back with elasticity and not remain collapsed and dented. This is the prod test. Even fresh fish can be flabby and in poor condition after spawning, so prodding as well as sniffing is important. Scales (if any) should be tight rather than loose.

On cutting, the flesh should feel firm and tight – not flabby, water-logged or flaky.

It's always best to buy fish whole as that way you can assess the above features more easily. If you only want fillets or steaks, choose your fish then ask the fishmonger to cut the amount you require.

Shellfish (lobsters, crabs, mussels, scallops, oysters etc.) should be bought alive and kicking. Pick them up and assess their weight. They should always seem heavy for their size.

It's important that the shells of bivalved molluscs (i.e. those with two shells: mussels, oysters etc.) should shut firmly on tapping and not be coated with decaying weeds, barnacles or mud.

How much fish to buy

The wastage with fish (through discarding skin, heads, bones, shells) varies from around a third with monkfish to over two-thirds with lobster. As a rule of thumb, flat or round fish have as much skin and bone as edible flesh – so buy double the amount you actually want to eat.

With fish that have exceptionally large heads (e.g. John Dory, gurnard) you need to buy more generously, as two-thirds of the fish is inedible.

The discarded parts aren't really wasted however – most (except oily fish) can be boiled up with herbs and vegetables to make wonderful stocks, soups or sauces to enhance any meal.

To whet your appetite for wet fish, I've included a description of the more common creatures you're likely to find at your fishmonger's. I've grouped them according to families so you can get an idea of which fish look and taste fairly similar.

Please ignore the temptation to batter your fillets and deep-fry them before serving with chips. They'll all taste the same if you do – and pile on extra calories.

The best way to appreciate the wide variety of flavours is by experimenting with simple recipes. Try poaching fillets in a court-bouillon – or wrapping them in grease-proof paper or foil with fresh herbs, spring onions and wine, and baking en papillote.

Recipes for different types of fish can be found in Chapter 10 of this book.

The Salmon Family

Atlantic salmon; Pacific salmon; Arctic char.

Salmon is classed as an oily fish. It was the fish of paupers in medieval times due to its abundance. It then became the fish of kings as pollution flushed them out of the rivers. The advent of salmon farms has now brought this magnificent beast back into the the realm of affordability.

Wild salmon has flesh which is paler and stronger tasting than farmed salmon – but it is often twice as expensive.

Salmon flesh tends to flakiness and is best undercooked so the flesh has just set. Otherwise, it can be gritty and dry. I prefer salmon fillets to steaks. These cook more evenly and the bones are more easily removed.

Salmon needs to be poached or covered with a light sauce for moistness. If baking with herbs and a dash of wine, always wrap salmon in foil to retain the juices.

Both smoked salmon and gravadlax – raw salmon mari-naded with citrus juices, vinegar or alcohol, plus dill weed – extend the culinary range of this fine fish and allow increased opportunity to enjoy its health-giving oils.

If you can find fresh, whole Arctic **char** – go for it. The delicate, sweet flesh melts in the mouth and is as good for the palate as it is for the heart.

The Herring Family

Sardines; anchovies; herring; shad.

The herring family is oily and rich in EPA.

Fresh sardines – of which there are several species – are quite different from those encountered crushed in a tin. Fresh sardines are best grilled, which has the advantage of draining away some of the natural oil if you're watching calories.

A sardine is nothing more than a young pilchard – and a pilchard a mature sardine.

Anchovies are renowned for their pungent, salty flavour which adds a distinctive tang to classic Mediterranean dishes. The practice of eating fresh, unsalted anchovies is uncommon in the UK, but it is worth trying. The anchovies are split open raw, cleaned and marinaded in lemon juice for 24 hours. They can be served as an antipasto with drinks – rather like an Italian gravadlax.

Herrings are one of our finest and best known fish. They are sold fresh, salted, smoked or pickled. The Scots cook herrings by rolling them in coarse-cut oatmeal and frying – though grilling is healthier.

Shad are marred by their numerous small bones. According to legend, they represent a discontented porcupine turned inside out by a mean-minded spirit. The best time to eat shad is in May as they start swarming up river to spawn.

The Cod Family

Cod; hake; haddock.

Cod is the fish which comes closest to being a staple in our diet. Specimens weighing over 90kg have been recorded – but the usual market weight is around 4.5kg.

The flesh is white with big, chunky flakes and a mild, slightly sweet but bland flavour. Cod cries out for a robust, strongly flavoured sauce. Using red wine as a base is ideal.

Cod is also popular salted. When soaked in cold water it becomes stronger flavoured – but if dried it stinks.

Hake must be eaten very fresh. Its flesh is denser than cod and quickly becomes insipid and watery. The whole fish then looks washed out and squashy and falls apart when filleted. Hake is popular poached, steamed or baked and is also used to make fish balls.

Haddock has a distinctive black smudge behind each gill which are said to be the thumb prints left by St Peter when picking up the fish on Christ's instructions. In its mouth he found the silver to pay a tribute. The story is spoiled by the fact that haddock is not found in the Mediterranean or the Sea of Galilee.

Haddock has a stronger flavour and a greyer flesh than cod. It also needs a robustly flavoured sauce or plenty of fresh herbs and garlic. Haddock can be bought fresh, dried or smoked.

The Perch-like Fish

Barracuda; sea bass; sea bream; grouper; red and grey mullet; wrasse; parrotfish.

Having watched a large **barracuda** lunge at me as I stood on the deck of a banana boat in the Caribbean, I sometimes get the shivers when eating this fierce fish with its devastating array of teeth. (Revenge was obtained at the barbecue later that evening.) However, char-grilled with garlic, rosemary and marjoram, I can think of nothing better to eat on a romantic, warm and starry night. Barracuda has a reputation as an aphrodisiac – probably because of its outrageous aggression and virility.

Sea bass has a soft, dense flesh of delicate flavour. The texture is firm, it is relatively free of bones and retains its shape well during cooking.

Bass is often difficult to obtain as, in parts of the country sales are forbidden in order to conserve natural stocks. When bass is available, it is snapped up by Oriental chefs who prize it highly.

Sea bass is a round fish whose skin gleams like beaten silver. Unfortunately it's almost as expensive.

Be careful of the spikes on the fins and around the gills. Always gut whole bass as soon as possible. It has innards that ferment and burst quickly – tainting the delicate flesh.

Never serve a strongly flavoured sauce with bass or you will drown the gourmet flavour of the flesh.

Sea bream are attractively coloured – black or red with distinctive orange stripes. They are almost too beautiful to eat. Bream can be grilled, baked whole or filleted. They benefit from being marinaded in fresh herbs and wine prior to cooking.

Grouper has firm, flaky meat of good flavour. It is a popular fish in the Mediterranean and is now more widely available in the UK.

Red mullet is a glorious crimson colour tinged with yellow. The flesh is delicately flavoured with a hint of lobster and comes apart in thick, firm flakes. Red mullet is a Mediterranean staple, where it is grilled, fried or baked. It is often cooked and eaten whole and uncleaned – the liver is considered a delicacy. It lacks the gall bladder and bile which make so many fish livers bitter.

Grey mullet can be finely flavoured but, as they are bottom feeders, often taste of mud. For this reason I poach grey mullet in a strong stock, then sprinkle them liberally with garlic, thyme and cheese (Cheddar and Parmesan) before flash-grilling to release the flavours of toasted cheese.

Wrasse are an interesting fish in that when sleeping, they experience periods of rapid eye movement (REM). In humans this is associated with dreaming – so what do wrasse have to dream about? Holidays in warmer climes?

Wrasse are added to stews and soups as their flesh has a yellow colour which is off-putting when served alone. Along with their cousin, weaver fish, wrasse are a basic component of bouillabaisse.

Parrotfish are named after their mouth which is beaked like a parrot. The fish gnaws and crunches coral for a pastime – when not sleeping like the wrasse. It is a spectacular fish, rich in reds, pinks, greens and blues, with splashes of yellow. Steaming is the recommended method of cooking.

The Mackerel Family

Mackerel; tuna; swordfish.

I grew up on fresh **mackerel** caught round the coast of Padstow in Cornwall. It is a handsome fish, iridescent with greens, blues and blacks, with a silver-white belly, and is well named – the French word *maquereau* means pimp or dandy.

The cooked flesh is greyish with bands of brown meat near the skin. The flavour is strong and reminiscent of sardines.

Mackerel goes off quickly because of its high oil content. Since the 17th century there has accordingly been a special dispensation to sell mackerel in England on Sundays.

In Cornwall, mackerel fillets are grilled with a liberal spattering of flour to absorb the healthy oils and form a delicious, crispy topping. I then douse the grilled fish with lemon juice and parsley and eat them with salad and minty, boiled new potatoes.

Because of mackerel's oiliness, acidic sauces (e.g. gooseberry, cranberry, rhubarb) or sousing (the Cornish term for pickling) in balsamic vinegar complement it best of all.

Tuna also glories under the name of tunny. Thanks to an increased interest in fresh tuna steaks, it's now less likely to be eaten out of a tin. Tuna are an unusual fish in that they are warm-blooded and have a greater need for oxygen. In order to obtain this, they must swim constantly at high speed to drive water over their gills. They can never slow down – hence their musculature is highly developed with a distinctive flavour. Tuna flesh is a firm, heavy meat that flakes easily. In Japan, it is highly prized raw as a component of sashimi.

Tuna steaks (skipjack and yellowfin are the most common) are delicious grilled, but care must be taken that they don't dry out. They are not classed as oily.

Tinned tuna preserved in brine or olive oil is very different from the fresh meat. It is excellent for slimmers and extremely tasty when part of a salad niçoise.

The **swordfish** is a magnificent creature. Its meat is compact with a flavour reminiscent of chicken. It is delicious char-grilled and drizzled with olive oil, lemon juice, fresh herbs and lashings of black pepper. Make sure the meat is fresh. Frozen swordfish steaks hold all the attraction of eating leather.

The Gurnard Family

Gurnard; redfish; rockfish; scorpion fish.

The fish of this family (other than gurnard) are only

suitable for fish stews and soups, and they are essential in classic bouillabaisse. Most are small with dry flesh.

The **gurnard** grows larger and has firm, white flesh capable of being filleted, although it is usually cooked whole, stuffed with herbs, or with a sweet nutty sauce.

The Thin/Flat Fish Family

Brill; halibut; John Dory; plaice; sole; turbot.

Brill is similar to turbot, but lacks the bony lumps which feel like baby limpets when you run your fingers over the skin. The taste and texture are similar with sweet, white meat that is nicely moist.

Halibut can easily weigh over 227kg – as much as three average human males. The meat is not surprisingly cut into chunks before it reaches the fishmonger's. In the 19th century, halibut was seasoned with freshly grated nutmeg, salt and pepper and baked in the oven. It can be cooked in any of the ways described for firm, white fleshed fish and is lovely poached with mushrooms and dill.

John Dory is a remarkable-looking fish – thin-bodied rather than flat, with vicious spines and gills. Its profile head-on is razor thin so it can creep up on its prey without being seen. One dark, black spot adorns each side of the fish rather like a malevolent eye. These marks are also claimed to be St Peter's thumb prints (*see* **haddock**) as he apparently threw one back into the sea because of the distressed noises it made.

John Dory belongs to the genus *Zeus* named after the Greek god. It is very much the deity of fish – one of my favourites if I can find one big enough to deliver fair-sized fillets. Its large head and gut account for 60 per cent of its weight and, because it's so thin, meat is scarce on smaller fish. You need to allow 720g of John Dory to obtain 240g of usable flesh.

John Dory has a lovely firm texture and is delicately flavoured – hence its French name of *poule de mer* – sea chicken. Each fillet divides into three natural sections that are easily separated if larger fish are used. It is excellent in an orange sauce flavoured with Cointreau.

Plaice is a familiar flat fish, popular and abundant. It has a shiny brown skin with hints of British racing green, plus fluorescent blood-orange spots. Plaice is similar in appearance to flounder, but has bony nodules on its head which flounder doesn't.

When fresh, plaice is delicate but wishy-washy in flavour and rapidly stales. Some gourmets say they are best eaten in the spring, whilst others shun them at this time of year as they are spawning.

Plaice feeds on bivalves such as cockles and mussels and also forages on the sea floor. The flavour is therefore preferable if they live over sandy bottoms. Gravel and mud tend to dull the flavour and eradicate all traces of sweetness.

Plaice can be poached, grilled or fried – the latter being more common in British eating establishments.

Sole is so-named because the Greeks considered the fish would make an ideal slipper for ocean nymphs. Dover sole is considered the king of sole as the fish is well suited to cooking on the bone. The meat remains firm and the skeleton intact, allowing for easy removal on the plate. Lemon sole does not have this attribute and belongs to a different family.

Despite its name, Dover sole is found all the way from the Mediterranean to southern Norway. Dover had the distinction of being the best market from which the fish was sent to London.

The eye side of Dover sole is a pinky-brown similar to the sepia of faded photographs. As it ages, dark smudges appear. During daylight, Dover sole burrows under the sea floor so only its eyes and gills are exposed. The best catches are therefore made at night. Sandy bottoms make for firmer, sweeter flesh than mud or gravel sea floors.

Slip soles are small Dover sole weighing up to 240g each. Those caught around Plymouth are endearingly known as Plymsoles. You would need two per person for a decent-sized meal.

Interestingly, some gourmets claim the flesh of Dover sole tastes best several days after death – though other flat fish rapidly deteriorate.

Fresh **turbot** is difficult to surpass and often honoured with intricate, exquisite sauces marketed as chef's specials. It even has a cooking pot – the *turbotière* – especially designed for it.

Turbot is an unremarkable-looking, oval fish which resembles nothing so much as a marine cowpat, with a speckled grey/dung/black back. Bony protuberances are palpable on its skin – hence its nickname of nail-head.

The flesh is firm and a lovely clear white which is moist and succulent. The skin is edible and delicious. It is in the same class as lobster – a treat for that special occasion.

My favourite accompanying sauce is a beurre blanc – made with Greek strained yogurt rather than cream, olive oil rather than butter, plus balsamic vinegar.

Turbot can be steamed, poached, fried, grilled or baked en papillote. The head and bones make one of the finest fish stocks.

Fish Without True Bones

Monkfish; dogfish; shark; ray; skate.

Monkfish is in a class of its own, but I include it here with the cartilaginous fish as a near relative. Monkfish is more properly called angler fish.

Only the tail of the monkfish is edible. This flesh is firm, pearly white and slightly gelatinous. After spawning, the meat is similar to a tasteless milk jelly (known as 'slink-fish') – so don't forget the prod test.

Lovers of monkfish claim it resembles lobster meat. It is used commercially to simulate crab sticks, lobster claws and scampi. Its major advantage is the lack of bones there are to negotiate.

Monkfish must be eaten fresh and only lightly cooked. If stale or overdone, it rapidly resembles latex rubber. The meat can be poached, steamed, grilled, fried or even roasted like a leg of lamb. The head, though difficult to obtain, makes an excellent stock.

A tough membrane accompanies the tail meat and is best removed before cooking.

Dogfish (or rock salmon/huss) is merely another name for smaller members of the shark family.

The skin resembles sandpaper and dogfish possess large, volatile intestines which need removing immediately if you are buying the fish intact.

Dogfish has a robust flavour and texture. It is well suited to soup or a strongly flavoured sauce.

I first ate **shark** on PeePee Island in Thailand, having watched the contestants of a game-fishing competition limp home with a spectacular catch of shark, marlin and swordfish.

I was struck by how fresh shark meat resembled chicken in flavour and texture, whilst marlin was a dead ringer for pork.

Forget all you ever learned about sharks perfusing their flesh with urea to offset the osmotic effects of seawater. You honestly wouldn't know – until the meat starts to go stale. Then an ammoniacal smell reminiscent of pungent latrines will take your breath away.

Shark eaten in England is usually frozen and disappointing. It needs to be fresh as it's blackened on the char-grill, with fresh herbs and lime to extract the most succulent flavour.

I also believe that **skate** and **ray** should be eaten fresh

– never old or frozen. If you don't believe me, try freezing a piece of wing. You will remove flesh smelling so strongly of ammonia it knocks you over from five paces. I am told this signals the departure of urea and should be welcomed. Experts state that skate and ray are best eaten a couple of days after death. Rather them than me.

When fresh, the white meat peels off the wings in sweet-tasting strips. The classic sauce to accompany these fish is a beurre noir flavoured with ghee and capers. I, however, prefer a sauce made from white wine, Greek yogurt, nutmeg, rosemary and thyme.

Shellfish

Crustaceans

Crayfish; langoustine; lobster; prawn; shrimp; common brown (edible) crab; spider crab.

Crayfish is similar to lobster but lacks claws, lives in warmer waters and grows to a larger size. Its carapace is dark wine-red before cooking, in contrast to the lobster's blue or green. Crayfish meat is coarser and less sweetly flavoured. It must be cooked and eaten absolutely fresh as the flavour disappears on chilling in the fridge.

Langoustines are also known as Dublin Bay prawns or in their breaded, deep-fried form as scampi. They are small lobsters growing no more than 25cm long. Their carapace is orange-red or pinky-rose though some are a pale salmon bisque. The French serve their langoustines whole, so you have to suck the sauce off the carapace before shelling to get at the meat. Real audience-participation food.

Lobster is the king of the sea. It varies in colour from blue to green and on cooking the carapace turns a bright vermilion red. Lobster meat is sweet and intense and comes out in satisfying, large chunks which are easy to slice. The green mush (fatty liver) found in the body cavity is known as tomalley. This is a great delicacy in New England but most inhabitants of 'old England' leave it on the side of their plate.

Lobster meat should not be drowned with strongly flavoured, rich sauces. You might as well use monkfish instead and save money.

Due to over-fishing, lobsters rarely grow large these days. Monsters over a metre long, weighing 20kg used to be commonplace. A lobster weighing 1kg is ideal for two people.

Do cook a fresh lobster for yourself. You never know how long a cooked lobster has hung around and the flavour deteriorates markedly after just one day. Bought lobster tends to be overcooked and can be dry and disappointing.

Lobster must be cooked alive. After death the flesh rapidly becomes soft and mushy. A lobster suffering from shock also has mushy flesh, so some gourmets recommend resting live lobster overnight, wrapped in a damp cloth at the bottom of the fridge. This allows it to recover from the trauma of being moved.

The smallest species of **prawn** are no larger than the biggest shrimps – but some king prawns reach an impressive 23cm in length. Giant tiger prawns can reach 33cm long.

Too many people only eat prawns stuffed into an avocado or placed on lettuce and smothered in pink sauce. Although these creations are delicious, it's worth experimenting a bit further. Tiger prawns lightly cooked with garlic, ginger and spring onions are gorgeous – as are tomato, garlic and herb creations from the Mediterranean.

When buying fresh prawns, their aroma should be reminiscent of fresh seawater. Avoid any that smell of iodine or ammonia. Ensure their bodies are firm-fleshed and the shell adheres tightly to the body. Discard prawns with loose heads and blackened bodies or legs.

Quick-frozen prawns are usually cooked. They must be defrosted slowly to preserve their flavour.

When you buy cooked, shell-on prawns, try making a prawn bisque using the shells with added vegetables.

The term **shrimp** designates both brown shrimps and prawns in the USA. Large prawns are known as jumbo shrimps.

Live shrimps are transparent as anyone owning a shrimping net as a child will know. On briefly dunking in boiling water, shrimps turn a pinky-brown and on shelling, only a tiny morsel of meat comes forth.

The French and Japanese often eat their shrimps and prawns whole – a taste-texture which has to be acquired. As a nation, we can cope with prawn-flavoured crisps – but crisp-flavoured prawns are another matter.

Potted shrimp, shrimp pastes and shrimp soups are the most accessible ways of eating this labour-intensive crustacean.

The **common brown crab** is the one most often found at the fishmonger's. They weigh up to 2.7kg though specimens twice this size have been recorded. The meat tastes similar to lobster but is less sweet.

Crab bodies yield mainly brown, creamy flesh, while the claws and legs produce white, firm flesh. This comes out in fibrous bits rather than chunks and is awkward to remove from the shell. Large crabs are less fiddly than small ones and are just as well-flavoured. Crab-picks and claw-crushers make cleaning the legs simpler, but a professional crab-cleaner can dress a crab in seconds.

On average, you will obtain one-third the weight of your crab as meat – of which only one-third will be white meat.

When buying crab, make sure it's alive and choose one which feels heavy for its size. If it feels light, it contains too much water. Always pick up the crab and shake it (assuming its claws are bound) and discard any that slosh with fluid. A healthy crab keeps its claws tucked up close to its body. If they hang loose and the crab is sluggish, it's not a well animal.

If you buy crab ready cooked, check it has just come out of the steamer.

Spider crab is my favourite delicacy, despite my crippling arachnophobia. Unfortunately, spider crabs are difficult to obtain; the ones caught off our coasts are instantly transported to France where they are held in high esteem.

Uncooked, the carapace is an exotic cardinal red and covered with spines, encrusted weed and barnacles which provide excellent camouflage.

Spider crab has a distinctly sweet flavour – far superior to that of the common crab. However, they are also more fiddly to dress and yield less meat.

Cephalopod Molluscs

Cuttlefish; squid.

Cuttlefish are mid-way between squid and octopus as regards appearance, texture and flavour.

All cephalopods possess ink sacs from which a dark cloud is ejected to hide them from predators. Many cooks regard the ink as a delicacy in itself and make inky sauces. It is also possible to buy black pasta flavoured and coloured with squid ink.

Cuttlefish and squid have ten tentacles whereas the octopus has eight.

Smaller cuttlefish are less tough and rubbery than larger specimens, but to many they are an acquired taste. Sliced into rings, dredged in tempura batter and fried in olive oil, they make a tasty hors d'oeuvre.

Squid are found throughout the world except the Black Sea. They are ideal for stuffing and easy to prepare. All you have to do is pull off the head and de-glove the thin skin from the body. This peels away easily. Insert your fingers into the body and pull out the single transparent bone and the intestines. Chop up the tentacles and use them to stuff the body, with rice, vegetables or herbs. Alternatively, slice the cleaned squid into rings and deep-fry in olive oil as calamari – a Mediterranean staple.

Bivalved Molluscs

Oysters; mussels; scallops.

Oysters are the most prized marine mollusc. At one time they were a staple food of the poor, but over-harvesting has depleted natural beds. They are now a luxury, often cultivated, food.

Mature oysters are trained to survive up to 10 days out of water for transportation to the world's markets. This process is known as *expédition*.

Most people prefer their oysters raw, when they smell and taste of the sea. I like mine topped with herbs, black pepper, yogurt and breadcrumbs and flashed under the grill until the flesh has just set.

Oysters have a surprisingly high-fat and cholesterol content.

Mussels are increasingly popular and are now available all the year round from a newly evolved industry known as myticulture. Traditionally, mussels were only eaten when there was an 'r' in the month. The risks of food poisoning and flabbiness due to spawning made them bad news during the summer months until professional farming took off.

Because of the indiscriminate way mussels filter sea water it is unwise to pick them yourself unless local fishermen inform you they are safe. Sewage outlets, polluted seas and a particular type of poisonous plankton pose risks if concentrated in fresh mussels. Those purchased are subject to strict controls and usually safe if fresh. Occasional rogue mussels contain enough toxins to keep you in the bathroom all night. Mussels are also peculiar in that they can induce allergy in many people.

Fresh, properly cooked plump mussels have a flavour reminiscent of the sea, with a touch of beef thrown in. They should not be gritty, shrivelled or still attached to their beards. If anything crunches in your mouth it's best to investigate. I've often found little white pearls and even baby crabs or lobster only half an inch long. These seem especially prevalent in the Cornish giants that have such a wonderful flavour.

The classic moules marinière is still the best way of cooking mussels.

The succulent, green-lipped mussels from the Orient and New Zealand (*Perna canaliculus*) have a glorious, turquoise-green-tinged shell, which turns yellow on exposure to sunlight. They can grow up to 20cm long, though exported specimens are usually half this size.

When cooked, the flesh colours are an attractive combination reminiscent of peaches and cream. I eat them straight from the shell, dipped in lemon juice or olivey mayonnaise.

Scallops are increasingly easy to buy. Try, however, to obtain them in their shells. Those that are cleaned are usually soaked to plump them up – and you are paying for added water. Leave frozen scallops well alone unless you've prepared them yourself straight from the shell. The flavour of cooked, water-soaked, frozen scallops is negligible.

Most scallops propel themselves through water by opening and closing their shells rapidly. They skip around in a bizarre sort of dance, though some remain sedentary, clinging to the same rock throughout life.

Scallops are true hermaphrodites and possess a pink coral (ovary) plus a creamy testis to one side. In the UK, these titbits are often discarded, though in North America the genitals are revered.

The large, chunky white flesh that characterizes scallops is the well-developed adductor muscle used to open and close the shell. This meat has a sweet flavour and silken texture when cooked so that the flesh has just clouded and set. Overcooking, a common failing, will reduce this delicacy to unattractive rubber.

ANALYSIS OF FISH
per 100g raw fish

	TOTAL			
	PROTEIN	FAT	KCALS	
Cod	17g	0.7g	76	
Haddock	17g	0.6g	73	
Halibut	15g	0.6g	66	
Plaice	18g	2.2g	91	
Sole	17g	1.4g	81	
Tuna	24g	0.6g	99	In brine, drained
Anchovy	25g	19.9g	280	In oil, drained
Herring	17g	18.5g	234	
Mackerel	19g	16.3g	223	
Salmon	18g	12.0g	182	
Smoked				
salmon	25g	4.5g	142	
Trout	24g	4.5g	135	
Tuna	27g	9.0g	189	In oil, drained
Crab	20g	5.2g	127	Boiled
Lobster	22g	3.4g	119	Boiled
Prawn	23g	1.8g	107	Boiled
Shrimp	17g	0.8g	73	Shelled
Mussels	17g	2.0g	87	Boiled, shelled
Squid	13g	1.5g	66	

NB: Carbohydrate content of raw fish is zero.

Introducing Fish Into Your Diet

- Eat two or three portions of oily fish (mackerel, herring, pilchard, sardines, salmon or trout) per week. Tuna belongs to the mackerel family and contains useful oils, but is not classed as oily.
- Cod, haddock, plaice and other white fish are not classified as oily. They contain less EPA than the oily fish, but are still excellent for the blood, heart and overall health. They are a good source of protein and are low in calories.
- In Denmark, healthy bread containing refined fish oil is on sale.
- New Zealand adds fish oil to milk for health reasons.
- Switzerland have just reached a consensus making it likely that fish oil will be added to common foods as a healthy supplement.
- The British Nutrition Foundation recommends that the average Brit increases consumption of oily fish by a factor of 10 – to an equivalent of 300g mackerel per week.
- Fish oil capsules are sold in health food shops for those who do not want to add this amount of fish to their diet.

Garlic

The health benefits of garlic (*Allium sativum*) are extolled in many old wives' tales. Garlic has been cultivated for many millennia and even merits a mention in the Bible.

The garlic with the highest concentration of active ingredients comes from China where the plant has been revered for its life-enhancing qualities for over 4,000 years.

Experts in heart disease and lipids (fats) have now set their scepticism aside and are gathering evidence that confirms traditional herbalists' claims. The evidence that garlic lowers blood cholesterol levels and blood pressure is

146

overwhelming. Research also shows that garlic can boost the immune system and prevent stomach cancers.

Garlic tablets containing the equivalent of 4g of fresh cloves are available on prescription in Germany, as well as over the counter, for treating raised cholesterol levels and hardening of the arteries.

A scientific monograph on the use of garlic is being drawn up for the EC and, if adopted, garlic preparations may become available on prescription in the UK as well.

In patients taking 800mg of dried garlic powder a day, serum cholesterol levels fall by an average of 11–12 per cent after four months' therapy. Triglycerides (another form of fatty acid found in the blood) fall by up to 16 per cent.

Large doses of fresh garlic (7–28 cloves per day) would have a similar effect.

Compared with conventional cholesterol-lowering agents, which possess several side effects, the only known unwanted effect of garlic is the classic smell – noticed by 20 per cent of recipients or their contacts. Garlic on the breath can be freshened by chewing parsley, cumin or green beans, or drinking red wine.

Garlic was probably originally native to Asia, but is now grown throughout temperate climes. It is especially popular in Italy and France and is an essential ingredient of the Mediterranean diet.

Garlic bulbs are divided into 10–20 cloves, each encased in a brittle, parchment-like skin. This is usually white, but can be tinged with pink or purple. Cloves should be tightly packed; looseness is a sign of deterioration or inferior quality.

Elephant garlic, which as the name suggests comes in giant bulbs, is a cross between garlic and onion. This results in large, mild-flavoured cloves with a spongy, fibrous texture.

The active ingredient of garlic is allicin, a chemical

formed from the interaction of an enzyme, alliinase, on a precursor, alliin. This reaction only occurs when garlic cells are disrupted through cutting or crushing.

Garlic prepared for medicinal purposes is grown organically, cut into thick slices, dried slowly and powdered to remove water without disrupting too many cells. The dried and ground product then contains enough precursor chemicals to allow the active ingredient, allicin, to be released on dissolution in the stomach.

Garlic oil products are usually formed by boiling fresh garlic. As a result, the allicin content can be low. The same problem occurs with preparations made by steam distillation and solvent extraction.

Research suggests that allicin prevents human cells from taking up cholesterol and reduces cholesterol production in the liver.

Sulphur compounds, formed by the degradation of allicin, also contribute to the beneficial effects as they are incorporated into long-chain fatty acids, which prevent fat oxidation. This mechanism is particularly important in preventing coronary heart disease.

The blood-pressure-lowering properties of garlic are also thought to be due to allicin and ajoune, another garlic chemical. Garlic therapy reduces average blood pressures by 8 per cent (systolic) and 12 per cent (diastolic) over a three-month course. It's thought to work by dilating blood vessels and affecting the passage of sodium and potassium salts across cell membranes.

The latest research suggests that garlic can:

- boost the immune system by increasing the activity of immune cells (phagocytes);
- prevent stomach cancer. A substance in garlic – diallylsulfide – appears to prevent the genetic material of cells from mutating, thereby decreasing the occurrence of malignant tumours. Fresh garlic contains more of these organosulphides weight for weight than even the most expensive medicinal extracts.

The Japanese use garlic to treat arthritis and back pain and it may also have antibiotic, laxative and diuretic properties.

Herbs

The herbs commonly found in the Mediterranean diet have medicinal properties as well as providing important minerals, vitamins and trace elements. When added in relatively small amounts, they transform a dish from the mediocre to the sublime.

Do not allow dried herbs into your kitchen – unless you want to produce dish after dish tasting of dried hay. The majority of dried-herb flavourings are difficult to distinguish after cooking.

Basil (*Ocimum basilicum*)

Basil is the major component of pesto sauce – that exotic, aromatic mix of herb, garlic, Parmesan, olive oil and pine nuts which is so irresistible.

Basil is usually pigeonholed by cookery writers as 'good with tomatoes', but this bland description does the herb a grave injustice. Basil will boost any savoury dish into the realms of magnificence. The fresh flavour is warm and spicy with undertones of clove, aniseed and liquorice.

Basil comes in many varieties, including purple, lemon-scented and bushy forms. Its flowers are small and scented, with creamy white or pale pink petals appearing in late summer. Basil is not an easy plant to grow. It's a tender annual, easily damaged by wind, rain and hot sunshine. It is prone to mould, wilts soon after picking and will bruise almost instantly with rough handling.

Traditional remedies include steeping crushed basil

leaves in wine for several hours to prepare a tonic. Basil tea aids digestion, stimulates the appetite and acts as an anti-spasmodic, making it useful for irritable bowel syndrome. Basil allays fatigue, stress, depression and anxiety and combats insomnia. It is also reputed to be a useful treatment for snake bites.

Basil oil is an excellent starter oil for aromatherapy baths and massages.

Bay Leaf (*Laurus nobilis*)

Bay trees are magnificent specimens that can be trained into many attractive shapes. Left to the wild, multiple stems and branches will appear to form a dense, bushy thicket up to 7.5m tall. Sweet bay has the distinction of being the only member of the laurel family which isn't poisonous.

Bay leaves are pointed, glossy and leathery in various shades of green from light to dark olive. A yellow variety also exists. All types of leaf are easily scorched brown by cold winds.

Bay leaves are best fresh and used within a few days of picking. Otherwise, much of the pungent, aromatic, slightly bitter flavour evaporates.

Bay is a major flavouring agent around the Mediterranean. It is added by the handful to braised dishes of fish and meat, along with sweet peppers, tomatoes, lemon and garlic.

We tend to be less adventurous with it and add one or two leaves per dish. Try grinding fresh bay leaves into home-made curry powders as they add a subliminal warmth that enhances the flavour.

Remove bay leaves before serving. Because of their sharp, serrated edges, several cases of injury resulting from swallowing the leaves have occurred. These range from tears in the gullet to chest abscesses and even death through perforation of internal organs.

Bay is traditionally said to aid digestion and stimulate the appetite. It also eases the pain of rheumatism and muscle/joint sprains when bay leaf oil is massaged in locally.

Coriander (*Coriandrum sativum*)

Coriander is a herb you either love or hate. Once the flavour of its pungent green leaves has grown on you, it proves almost as addictive as chocolate. In the Bible it is compared to manna.

Coriander leaves and seeds enhance many dishes, especially those containing fish. Both are excellent in curries.

The Chinese were convinced coriander conferred immortality, and more recently, it was acclaimed as an aphrodisiac. As a 100 per cent convert to this delectable herb, I can understand why.

Coriander provides both spice and herb in the same plant. It is a hardy annual belonging to the parsley family and has attractive, emerald-coloured leaves divided into three, feathery lobes. The flowers are small and may be pink, blue or white. The plant is an important dietary ingredient in the Middle East, Southern Europe, Asia, South America and North Africa.

The small, spherical seeds are sweet and aromatic, with warm overtones of orange when ripe. They contain an essential oil which, when steam-distilled, is used commercially in liqueurs, gins and medicines. It has anti-bacterial and anti-colic properties. Furthermore, it aids digestion, eases flatulence and adds an unusual taste to food.

Dill (*Anethum graveolens*)

Dill weed is closely related to fennel and looks remarkably similar. Dill and fennel are capable of cross–pollination, but produce bland offspring lacking the character of either parent. If you grow both herbs in your garden, do not cherish the little weedlings that arise between the two.

The leaves are feathery and green with an unusual flavour. It is an essential ingredient of gravadlax – Norwegian cured salmon – though dill weed enhances any fish dish. Try adding a generous quantity of chopped leaves to tuna, cottage cheese and tomato salad.

The seeds are liked by some, though I have never really found a use for them. I am not fond of their caraway-like flavour. Dill seeds are added to pickled gherkins and cucumber to make . . . dill cucumbers.

Infused dill seed cures flatulence and stimulates the let down of milk in nursing mothers. Dill water has also been used to treat indigestion, hiccups, colic and insomnia.

Fennel (*Foeniculum vulgare*)

Fennel leaves are fine, feathery and green, with rich copper and bronze overtones. The flowers are small, aromatic and yellow, bearing brown, curved and ribbed seeds. These are well flavoured and complement mushrooms and garlic.

Fennel is excellent for counteracting the richness of oily fish such as herrings and mackerel. Only a few sprigs are needed – stuffed into the fish cavity or added to marinades or sauces.

Florence fennel develops a succulent bulbous rootstalk which is edible raw or cooked. Unfortunately, the plant runs to seed when cultivated in cooler climes such as our own.

Fennel aids the digestion and eases wind, colic and constipation. It is used to flavour cough remedies as it has expectorant properties. Fennel also helps to reduce the toxic effects of alcohol – an excellent remedy for hangovers.

Lemon Balm (*Melissa officinalis*)

Lemon balm has been used medicinally for over 2,000 years. When drunk daily as a herbal tea mixed with honey, it is said to promote longevity and dispel melancholia.

Lemon balm leaves are strongly scented with lemon and rather coarse and hairy in texture. Plants grown in sunlit soils tend to have a harsh flavour – overpowering, soapy and unpleasant. Those cultivated in a moist soil, shaded from sunlight during the hottest part of the day, are totally different: fresh, green foliage with a true lemony fragrance.

Use only the small young leaves in the kitchen. As the leaves mature, they become more harsh and soapy. Try chopping a few small leaves with mint and chives and sprinkling over a crisp, green salad.

Lemon balm may be added to fruit salads – everywhere in fact that real lemons are required.

Traditional herbalists use lemon balm as a poultice and rub for insect bites and sores. Infused as a tea, it relieves catarrh, colds, fevers, headaches and tension due to stress. Perhaps its most compelling use in aromatherapy is as a treatment for depression.

Mint (*Mentha* spp.)

Many varieties of mint are available, including those with

153

aromas such as lemon, ginger, bergamot, pineapple, apple, eau de Cologne, spearmint and peppermint.

The dried herb retains its flavour relatively well and a delicious herbal tea can be made combining the flavour of spearmint with that of camomile.

Fresh mint tips chopped with lemon balm, chives and yogurt make a delicious, low-calorie addition to summer salads.

Traditionally, mint is used to treat colds, indigestion, wind, colic, intestinal infections, migraine and rheumatic pains. It assists the digestion of fat by encouraging the flow of bile.

When peppermint is rubbed onto the skin, it is initially cooling as it constricts blood vessels. Then the vessels dilate, encouraging blood circulation in the area.

Peppermint oil is also used as an insect repellent, for scabies and as a fungicide for ringworm. Mint massages of the feet are soothing and relaxing after long periods of standing or exercise.

Oregano (*Origanum* spp.)

Oregano and marjoram are closely related.

Oregano is the wild herb growing unfettered round the Mediterranean. Marjoram is the cultivated variety.

Oregano is a vigorous, sturdy perennial. It varies from a mild-flavoured, tiny-leaved plant to an aromatic species which dominates a dish with just a few crushed leaves.

My favourite variety has golden leaves and gives an authentic, pizza-tang to garlicky tomato sauces and soups.

Sweet marjoram is used to treat colds and headaches and is recommended for nervous ailments, rheumatic pains, bruises, sprains, high blood pressure, poor circulation, stomach and gall-bladder problems amongst others. Marjoram is especially soothing drunk as an infusion to treat menstrual pains. The leaves are traditionally chewed to cure toothache.

Parsley (*Petroselinum crispum*)

Parsley is one of the most universally known and probably the most widely used herb.

It is rich in minerals and vitamins – especially vitamin C – and comes in two main forms: curled and flat-leaved. A version with edible roots, similar to parsnip, is popular on the Continent.

It is best to add parsley at the end of cooking, just before serving, as its flavour rapidly diminishes with prolonged heating. Flat-leaved parsley is excellent for adding to salads.

Do not bother with dried parsley. Its flavour is indistinguishable from that of hay.

Parsley is traditionally used to freshen the breath, as a tonic, to aid digestion and as a mild laxative. It is said to stimulate menstruation and to ease flatulence and colic.

It also has mild diuretic properties and has been used as an aphrodisiac.

Rosemary (*Rosmarinus officinalis*)

Rosemary is one of the herbs most strongly associated with the Mediterranean. Its leaves are a resinous, spiky, dark green with a silver patina. The herb becomes woody with age and can grow into a sizable hedgerow bush. The flowers are a pretty, pale lilac blue, pink or white.

Due to the strong resinous aroma, rosemary makes an excellent addition to barbecues and bonfires. The fumes contain camphor and purify the air.

Rosemary leaves retain their flavour well when dried.

When cooking, sprigs of rosemary are ideal for adding to all sorts of dishes. One of my favourite recipes uses large sprigs of rosemary threaded through a joint of lamb. When garlic slices are pushed into pockets in the meat, the resultant infusion of flavours during roasting is mouth-watering.

The medicinal uses of rosemary are as an anti-spasmodic, a digestive aid, an anti-depressant, antiseptic, a nerve stimulant and an anti-stress agent. Massaging with rosemary oil also eases rheumatic aches and pains.

Sage (*Salvia officinalis*)

Sage is closely connected with healing and longevity. In the UK, however, we only tend to use it mixed with onion and stuffed into roasting meats.

The leaves are a grey-green, thick and downy, with a strong aroma when crushed. Many variegated types are available, of which purple sage is the most attractive.

When suffering in Turkey from the most vicious attack of food poisoning I've ever experienced, my delightful landlady insisted on giving me an infusion of sage, which is imbued with anti-diarrhoea properties and eased my condition.

Sage is also used to combat fever, soothe colds and treat menopausal symptoms. Interestingly, the leaves contain oestrogen – a natural source of HRT (hormone replace-ment therapy).

Tarragon (*Artemisia dracunculus*)

Tarragon, the dragon herb, was probably named after its serpentine roots, though its flavour is said by some to be fiery.

This is the classic herb to accompany chicken dishes. The leaves are glossy, long and narrow, with a bluish-green tinge. Oil glands on the underside secrete the peppery, aromatic oil which makes the tongue tingle. Tarragon vinegar is widely available commercially.

There are two varieties of tarragon: French – which has the lovely, tangy, bitter-sweet, liquorice flavour; Russian – which is coarser in flavour and often bland.

Unfortunately, French tarragon is difficult to grow and perishes in the slightest frost. The Russian variety is hardier but less exciting to the palate. Like a fine claret, however, its flavour does improve with maturity.

Tarragon leaves are rich in iodine and vitamins A and C. It is used by herbalists to stimulate appetite, as a general tonic and as a cure for scurvy.

Thyme (*Thymus* spp.)

The fragrance of thyme in warm, summer air is the smell of the Mediterranean. Thyme is a powerful antiseptic and preservative and was used in the mummy business by embalmers in ancient Egypt.

Many different thymes are available, all with sharp, fresh acidic tangs. Lemon thyme is strongly scented with the aroma of fresh lemons and makes a wonderful addition to grilled fish.

Thyme flowers range from white, through yellow and pink to purple.

Thyme can be used medicinally to treat hangovers, coughs, colds, sore throats, headaches and insomnia. It is also used as a digestive aid and a tonic.

Walnuts

Walnuts (*Juglans regia*) feature frequently in the Mediterranean and Body Awareness diets. They contain beneficial (Omega-3) oils and can lower high cholesterol levels and reduce the risk of coronary heart disease.

Nine healthy men who added 84g (60g = 578kcals) of walnuts to their daily diet for four weeks reduced their total blood cholesterol by a massive 12 per cent more than a control group not eating walnuts. Even more importantly, harmful blood LDL-cholesterol levels were reduced by 16 per cent. However, these results need further investigation as participants may have altered their diet in other ways as well.

Studies using almonds and hazelnuts have also revealed beneficial effects on blood lipoprotein profiles.

Walnuts contain a high ratio of monounsaturated and polyunsaturated to saturated fat. Twelve per cent of the total fat content is essential linolenic acid which our bodies cannot synthesize. They also contain useful amounts of the vitamin B complex and vitamin E.

It is best to buy walnuts in shells or vacuum packs as exposure to air rapidly reduces their nutrient values.

Most of us eat less than 4g of walnuts per week. Increasing our intake to 28g (25g = 190kcals) per day is expected to decrease our blood LDL-cholesterol level by 6 per cent.

Pasta

Until relatively recently, all dieters threw their hands up in horror at the very word pasta, assuming it was dripping in calories and all things sinful.

The good news is it isn't. The only potentially bad thing about pasta is the butter- and cream-laden sauces often slapped on like camouflage. If your sauces are made with garlic, olive oil, tomatoes, vegetables, herbs and fish, pasta is an ideal food for a healthy diet.

Whenever you would normally serve chips or roast potatoes at home, try a helping of wholemeal pasta flavoured with freshly chopped herbs and black pepper instead.

Pasta is literally the Italian word for paste. Two versions are available – dough made with or without egg.

Dried pasta is usually made without egg from a variety of flours. The commonest is ground hard wheat or durum flour.

Many types of pasta are available, of which the most familiar are spaghetti, noodles and lasagna, and shapes such as conchiglie (shells), fusilli (spirals), tagliatelle (thin ribbons), fettuccine (fat ribbons), macaroni (thin tubes), ravioli (stuffed squares), cannelloni (large tubes) and penne (small tubes).

Fresh pasta is made from durum wheat semolina, flour and eggs. Home-made pasta is often said to be the best – lighter and better flavoured.

If you are feeling adventurous, try making pasta at least once. Inexpensive machines are available for rolling out the dough.

Pasta should be cooked in a large pot with plenty of boiling water so strands do not stick. Add a tablespoon of olive oil to the water to provide additional non-stick lubrication.

Dried pasta should be cooked until it is *al dente* – literally, 'to the tooth' – meaning it should be firm rather than mushy to bite. This takes anything from 1–9 minutes depending on the thickness and shape of the pasta.

Fresh pasta takes between 15 seconds and 5 minutes to cook and puff up depending on thickness and variety.

A cooked portion of 85g–100g is ample per person.

Yogurt

Yogurt most probably originated in the Balkans where milk carried in animal bladders rapidly fermented – leaving a white, sweet-sour substance for which miraculous properties are claimed. These include:

- encouraging long life
- boosting the immune system
- aiding digestion
- decreasing the risk of stomach cancer
- lowering blood cholesterol
- curing recurrent vaginal thrush

Even Mechnikov, the Russian immunologist and Nobel prize-winner (physiology/medicine) labelled yogurt a wonder food. He ascribed the longevity of Bulgarian mountain tribes and their lack of disease to their well-known love of yogurt.

Yogurt is produced by the bacterial fermentation of milk (whole, semi-skimmed or skimmed). The bacteria used commercially vary, but usually consist of a strain of *Lactobacillus* (*bulgaricus; bifidis; acidophilus*) or *Bifidobacterium* (*bifidum; longum*).

The fermentation process produces lactic acid from milk sugar (lactose) which results in curdling and the distinctive, tangy taste.

In most cases, bacteria remain alive after fermenting all the available lactose.

Yogurts labelled 'live' are heated to a low temperature which kills off pathogens (disease-forming bacteria) but allows fermenting bacteria to survive.

If pasteurization (prolonged, medium-high heat treatment) occurs to produce a longer shelf-life, all bacteria are killed. Sterile, long-life yogurts can be sold from supermarket shelves rather than fridges.

If live yogurt cultures are contaminated with other bacteria (e.g. in yak bladders) fermentation may produce other substances including toxins and alcohols. This results in an unpleasant smell and causes diarrhoea or vomiting.

Bio-yogurts are now popular in the Western world. They contain *Lactobacillus acidophilus* or *Bifidobacterium (bifidum* or *longum)*. These names are often abbreviated to acidophilus or bifidus – or even BA – on labels. Bio-yogurts taste mild and less acidic. In addition, acidophilus colonizes the bowel and vagina and lives in harmony with our own bacterial flora.

Although manufacturers are not allowed to make specific medical claims about live yogurt, it is widely believed to benefit the digestive system. Marketing phrases such as 'believed to aid digestion and dietary balance', or 'permit natural healthy digestion and metabolism' are common-place.

Certainly, the breakdown of milk sugar and lactose makes milk more easily digestible by those with lactose intolerance.

There is evidence that bacteria in live yogurt are able to stimulate other bacteria normally present in our intestines. Acidophilus and bifidobacteria are naturally present in the gut and help suppress pathogens such as salmonella and thrush.

To colonize the bowel however, bio-yogurt bacteria would have to survive the journey through acidic stomach juices designed to prevent this very thing happening. It's now thought that acidophilus and bifidobacteria are capable of doing this.

As a result, eating live bio-yogurt may be beneficial to people with naturally or artificially depleted levels of their own gut bacteria. This includes people who have recently:

- taken antibiotics
- had diarrhoea
- drunk a lot of alcohol
- suffered poor immunity to disease
- suffered serious disease
- undergone radiotherapy or chemotherapy

Most experts believe the minimum acceptable level for both Bifidobacterium and acidophilus bacteria is one million live bacteria per gram of yogurt. That's a minimum of two million live bacteria per gram.

Some believe levels of up to 100 million live bacteria per gram are preferable for maximum health benefits.

Bio-yogurts available commercially vary in their live bacterial content from a few hundred thousand to 300 million live bacteria per gram.

If you are healthy, your own intestinal bacteria are probably robust and present in optimal numbers. As we grow older, bacterial levels fall. The balance can be changed by common 20th century problems such as stress, pollution and food additives.

Eating two or three live bio-yogurts a week may benefit normally healthy people too.

Where bio-yogurt comes into its own is in the treatment of vaginal thrush. *Lactobacillus acidophilus* can colonize the vagina – so if you have a vaginal bacterial imbalance (e.g. anaerobic vaginosis; thrush) smearing on live yogurt containing *Lactobacillus acidophilus* will help reinstate a healthy bacterial balance.

Other claims that yogurt reduces the risk of cancer or reduces cholesterol levels are not yet fully substantiated.

Inflammation and ulceration of the stomach (gastritis; peptic ulcers) are now known to result from infection with a bug called *Helicobacter pylori*. This bacterium is present in 90 per cent of people with ulceration, compared with 40 per cent of healthy controls.

Helicobacter releases toxins and acids which attack the protective mucus lining of the stomach. The bug burrows underneath the mucus mantle, allowing acids to follow. It is possible that bacteria in bio-yogurt may suppress Helicobacter activity and therefore protect against gastritis and ulceration.

As peptic ulceration and Helicobacter are strongly linked with stomach cancers, this provides a mechanism to explain anecdotal evidence that yogurt protects against serious gastric disease.

Wonder food or not, yogurt is undeniably a tasty, filling, nutritious food which, like milk, is an excellent source of protein, vitamins, calcium and trace minerals.

Analysis

100g low-fat, natural yogurt contains:

Calcium: 190mg – a third of our daily needs. Calcium is essential for muscle contraction, strong bones and teeth – especially during pregnancy and childhood. Women's calcium intake throughout their lives is important to help prevent or minimize osteoporosis in later life.

Phosphorus: 160mg – a third of our daily needs. Phosphorus is an essential component of bones and teeth and combines with calcium to form calcium phosphate. Molecules containing phosphorus help store and release energy during metabolism.

Vitamin B12: 0.2mcg – up to a fifth of our daily needs. Vitamin B12 is essential for the formation of red blood cells and for the healthy functioning of our nervous system.

Riboflavin: 0.25mg – up to a third of our daily needs. We need riboflavin for the production of energy during metabolism.

Magnesium: 19mg – up to a tenth of our daily needs. Magnesium is an essential mineral that helps muscles and nerves function. It is needed for replication of our genetic material and for healthy bones and teeth.

Zinc: 0.6mg – up to a tenth of our daily needs. Zinc is needed for sense of taste, growth, sexual maturation and the healthy healing of wounds.

ANALYSIS OF DIFFERENT YOGURTS PER 150g

YOGURT	CALORIES	PROTEIN	FAT	%FAT	CARBO-HYDRATE
Greek,					
Cow's strained	173 kcals	9.6g	13.7g	9.1%	3.0g
Sheep's set	160 kcals	6.6g	11.3g	7.5%	8.4g
Low fat					
Plain	84 kcals	7.7g	1.2g	0.8%	11.3g
Flavoured	135 kcals	5.7g	1.35g	0.9%	26.9g
Fruit	135 kcals	6.2g	1.1g	0.7%	26.9g
Whole milk					
Plain	119 kcals	8.6g	4.5g	3.0%	11.7g
Fruit	158 kcals	7.7g	4.2g	2.8%	23.6g
Low calorie					
diet	62 kcals	6.5g	0.3g	0.2%	9.0g
Soya yogurt	108 kcals	7.5g	6.3g	4.2%	5.9g

The fats

As you can see from the table, yogurts vary tremendously in fat content. Greek strained yogurt contains the most fat – but is deliciously thick and creamy.

Whilst trying to lose weight it is best to stick to low-fat brands. Once you are into the Body Maintenance Plan, you can reintroduce Greek-style yogurt into your cooking as an excellent substitute for cream. It will curdle easily so do not boil.

Try stabilizing yogurt used in cooking by mixing in 5ml of cornflour to each 150g of yogurt first.

Two-thirds of the fat in yogurt tends to be saturated fat, with the other third is predominantly monounsaturated fat.

Added sugar

Added sugar, toffee or chocolate in flavoured yogurts puts the calorie count up. Some brands contain as much as 15–25g sugar, the equivalent of 3–5 lumps per 150g pot.

It's best to eat plain, natural yogurt (low-fat or Greek style) with your own added fruit for sweetness. Alternatively, swirl in a teaspoon of acacia honey which will add a mere 20 kcals.

Additives

Low-calorie or diet yogurts contain artificial sweeteners which, if you want to follow a wholefood diet, are best avoided.

Most fruit and flavoured yogurts also contain stabilizers, emulsifiers, thickeners, preservatives, acidity regulators and colourants, too.

Making Your Own Yogurt

You can buy dry, powdered cultures of yogurt bacteria in health food shops. These are easily made up according to instructions.

Another method involves utilizing the bacteria available in bought, live yogurt.

Buy a carton of natural live yogurt to begin with. Then, each time you make a batch, put aside one tablespoon to act as a starter culture for each subsequent fermentation.

Fresh milk (cow, sheep or goat) is the most popular base. Semi-skimmed or skimmed milk is useful for weight-watchers, but it can be watery. It's also possible to make yogurt from water and skimmed milk powder.

Fresh Milk Yogurt

600ml semi-skimmed milk
30ml (2 tbsp) live natural yogurt

Pre-heat a wide-necked thermos flask (or an ovenproof dish plus lid) with boiling water. Heat the fresh milk to blood heat – 37°C.

Empty the flask of boiling water and add the warmed milk. Stir in the live yogurt and seal.

Leave overnight and the yogurt will be ready to use next morning.

If you are using an ovenproof dish rather than a thermos, the culture should be left somewhere warm overnight, such as an airing cupboard.

Dried Milk Yogurt

600ml water
75g powdered skimmed milk
30ml (2 tbsp) natural yogurt

Pre-heat a wide-necked thermos flask with additional boiling water. Boil the recipe water and let it cool to blood heat – 37°C. Whisk in the powdered skimmed milk and the yogurt.

Empty the flask, then pour in the yogurt culture mixture. Seal.

Leave overnight and the yogurt will be ready to eat next morning.

Red Wine and Coronary Heart Disease

Much fascinating research has examined the effects of wine on our health. Wine, especially red, is a major component of the Mediterranean diet.

Evidence suggests that a moderate daily intake of 2–3 glasses per day has a beneficial effect on our heart and our health. Natural substances found in the skin of grapes lowers the stickiness of blood and makes clot formation less likely.

When wine is combined with the cardio-protective effects of fish oils, garlic and exercise, our risk of coronary heart disease is lowered even further.

At least 19 studies around the world have shown that a moderate intake of alcohol reduces the risk of coronary heart disease by 40 per cent.

The evidence is so strong that the US Food and Drug Administration have recently allowed vintners to label red wines as good for the health. One expert has even stated that, as far as coronary heart disease goes:

'A half bottle of good red wine with lunch may be a better preventative medicine than all the cholesterol guidelines combined. Alcohol is a drug that should be used regularly, but at moderate doses of 20–30g per day.'

The alcohol content of wine may not be the sole explanation for these cardio-protective effects.

Red wine contains many compounds whose properties play an important role and a new study suggests that non-alcoholic red wine might offer the same kind of protection against coronary heart disease as alcoholic wines.

Coronary heart disease (CHD) has been around since the time of the ancient Egyptians but only now, 3,000 years later, has it reached epidemic proportions. It is the biggest killer in the Western world, accounting for at least 50 per cent of all deaths.

CHD results from hardening and furring up of coronary artery walls. This reduces blood flow and leads to less oxygen reaching the tissues. In the case of the heart muscle, which beats over 100,000 times per day, lack of oxygen rapidly leads to problems such as angina. If lack of oxygen is extreme, muscle cells will die and a heart attack occurs.

CHD is linked with several factors, the most common being a diet high in saturated fat, high blood cholesterol levels, high blood pressure, lack of exercise and smoking.

Compared with Britain and the USA, the French eat as much saturated fat, have similar high cholesterol levels, smoke as much (if not more), take little exercise and drink vastly more wine. Yet their incidence of CHD is lower than in any other industrialized country except Japan.

The French paradox is the term coined to describe this apparent compatibility of lifestyle vices with an inexplicably low incidence of CHD.

It is most evident in Gascony – home of the fatty saucisses de Toulouse and the ultimate cardiologist's nightmare – pâté de foie gras.

In Toulouse, the annual male CHD mortality rate is 78 per 100,000 (women 11 per 100,000) and wine intake averages half a bottle of wine per day. Some males drink as much as a litre of red wine per day, but always to wash down meals. It is hardly ever drunk on its own.

In Glasgow, a city not renowned for its love of red wine, the annual male CHD mortality rate is more than four times greater at 380 per 100,000. For women, there is a staggering twelve-fold increase in incidence (132 per 100,000). Unfortunately, Scottish wine intake is unknown. What is known is that most males drink lager, beer or spirits and don't take their alcohol with meals.

There is no adequate explanation for the French paradox, though red wine consumption is increasingly thought to play a role.

168

In one large study of around 129,000 people, the cause of death in participants was assessed in relation to alcohol preference – wine, spirits or beer. After controlling for the number of drinks per day, wine preference was associated with a significantly lower risk of cardiovascular death (a 30 per cent reduction for men and a 40 per cent reduction for women) compared to spirit preference. This suggests that components of wine other than the alcohol may be involved.

Another study demonstrated that, in the 17 countries where dietary consumption is known, only wine has a significant, protective effect against risk of early death.

Research has also shown that non-alcoholic compounds found in red wine (phenols) are able to act as antioxidants, which mop up free radicals and prevent them from doing damage to the cholesterol in our blood. Some are more potent than vitamin E and can also prevent the formation of blood clots. Both these effects help to protect against atherosclerosis.

Procyanidins are found in red wine at concentrations of up to 1gm/l. These polyphenols are powerful antioxidants and free-radical scavengers.

Phytoalexins are natural anti-fungal agents in the skins of grapes. Red wine involves macerating grape skins longer than when making white wines or champagne, and therefore has a much higher concentration.

Another explanation for the apparent, protective effect of red wine against CHD is that it makes the blood less sticky. This is supported by findings that platelets (blood cell fragments involved in the clotting process) are less sticky in French blood than in English blood. At least one compound isolated from red wine (resveratrol) is known to produce this beneficial effect, although it wears off when wine is withdrawn and a dangerous, rebound stickiness may occur.

Because the French mostly consume their red wine with meals, it is absorbed more slowly. This may prolong any protective, anti-sticky effect on the blood at a time when dietary saturated fats – known to increase blood stickiness – are being absorbed.

In moderation, alcohol also counteracts the effects of stress by promoting relaxation – but only at levels of alcohol consumption compatible with health.

Unfortunately, the beneficial effects of alcohol must be weighed up against the bad. The key is in moderation. Men who regularly drink 6 units of alcohol per day (6 glasses of wine) or binge on drink at weekends have almost twice the risk of sudden death compared to moderate or non–drinkers.

Heavy drinkers have an increased risk of death from several causes, including road traffic accidents, suicide, homicide, certain malignancies, stroke, heart rhythm disturbances, weakened heart muscle (cardiomyopathy) and cirrhosis of the liver.

Interestingly, although the incidence of liver disease in France is twice that of the USA, it only accounts for 3 per cent of French deaths.

Evening Primrose Oil

Oil of evening primrose has popped in and out of fashion. Launched as the ultimate cure for eczema, cyclical breast pain and possibly premenstrual syndrome (PMS), it has since proved controversial in these areas – and very promising in others.

Recently, the efficacy of evening primrose oil in treating eczema was called into doubt – but this does not mean it should be dismissed as a preventive treatment.

From experience, I have seen many patients who

develop dry, itchy, scaling skin problems as soon as they follow a strict diet and start to lose weight.

This effect is at its worst when they follow a low-fat regime e.g. 20 per cent calories as fat, which is the optimum for losing excess weight rapidly and safely.

The clinical condition is similar to mild eczema and can be prevented by taking evening primrose oil supplements. The lesions disappear very impressively – almost overnight.

Apart from making the skin feel rough and itchy, the scaliness as a result of following a low-fat diet is not in itself serious. It does however indicate that the dieter may be at risk of an essential fatty acid deficiency. This may lead to cyclical breast pain, irregular periods and premenstrual symptoms.

The lipid (fat) fraction of our diet supplies us with:
- building blocks for cell membranes
- fatty acids necessary for the functioning of the central nervous system
- precursors for important, hormone-like chemicals called prostaglandins
- substrates for hormone production
- molecules from which to make bile salts
- fat-soluble vitamins A, D, E (F)

A diet deficient in fats, or providing fats of the wrong sort, can produce symptoms such as:
- dry, itchy skin
- eczema
- psoriasis
- acne
- brittle hair and nails
- hair loss
- slower than normal growth rate in children
- slow wound healing
- breast pain – especially cyclical, before a period

171

- painful and heavy periods
- premenstrual syndrome

Some fats are obligatory for the smooth metabolic functioning of the body. Not surprisingly, these have been labelled by scientists as essential fatty acids.

Essential fatty acids (all are polyunsaturated)

1. Arachidonic acid. Omega-6 series
2. Linoleic acid. Omega-6 series
3. Linolenic acid. Omega-3 series

These are known collectively as vitamin F.

Fatty acid research is still evolving and recommended daily requirements of linolenic acid are difficult to obtain. Its derivative, gammalinolenic acid is found in abundance in oil of evening primrose and in human milk – this may be why breast-fed babies don't get eczema.

Arachidonic acid is widespread (meat, dairy products, shrimps, prawns) and a relative deficiency is unlikely except on fat-exclusion diets.

We need 5–10g linoleic acid per day. This is found in plant oils (e.g. groundnut, corn, soya bean, sunflower) and is also present in fairly high quantities in olive oil and chicken fat.

Low-fat dieters will not run into problems if they include fish such as herring, salmon, and mackerel in their diet (as well as the leaner fish such as cod, plaice, sole etc.) and consider adding oil of evening primrose if prone to skin, breast or period problems.

Fats and the Skin

We've known for 60 years that certain fatty acids are necessary for skin function, but only in the last decade has it been appreciated that they play a role in several common disorders.

Skin has a very high turnover and lacks certain enzymes which would otherwise synthesize fatty acid requirements on the spot. There are no local stores on which to draw and the skin is dependent on getting supplies from the blood.

The cholesterol series of essential fatty acids (Omega-6) seem to be more important in the skin than the EPA (Omega-3) series. In deficiency, hair becomes thin and falls out. The skin becomes scaly, rough and loses water easily. Also, the sebaceous glands become distorted, the ducts block off and sebum increases in viscosity, setting the scene for an outbreak of spots. Normal healing of wounds fails to occur, possibly as a result of poor collagen formation.

Ageing, stress, smoking, alcohol and a diet rich in sugar and saturated fats impair the metabolism of fatty acids in the skin, causing imbalances.

Other common imbalances are hereditary and made worse by a poor, Western-style diet.

These imbalances and deficiencies can be overcome with oil of evening primrose. This magic oil contains gammalinolenic acid (GLA) – a close relation to one of the essential fatty acids.

In one experiment, 179 patients with skin problems were given oil of evening primrose for 12 weeks. In 116 cases, dramatic improvement was seen. In particular, the effect on skin-itching was striking.

GLA comes as an oil in capsules. These can be snipped open and used in salad dressings, sprinkled on food or taken as a capsule supplement. GLA also has an effect if massaged into affected areas of skin.

Fats and Hormones

The same factors causing fatty acid deficiency in the skin can result in hormonal imbalances. In women, this shows itself as painful, heavy periods, premenstrual syndrome and cyclical breast pain.

If low- or very low-fat diets are followed, these problems may appear in susceptible people or worsen if already present. Again, dietary fatty acid imbalances are at fault.

Some dietary essential fatty acids are converted into hormone bases called prostaglandins – so named because they were originally discovered in the male prostate gland.

The Omega-6 or cholesterol series of fatty acids make prostaglandins of one type and the Omega-3 or EPA series make prostaglandins of another. There's no mechanism to interchange between the two, so it's important to eat the right balance of fatty acid building blocks in your diet to make prostaglandins in the correct proportions.

Prostaglandins have a number of roles. These include:
- contraction of the uterus
- the inflammatory response
- initiation or prevention of blood clotting
- regulation of the reproductive cycle – by conversion into hormones such as progesterone, oestrogen and testosterone

Inflammation and painful periods are often treated with anti-prostaglandin drugs called non-steroidal, anti-inflamatories (NSAIDs e.g. ibuprofen).

Imbalances resulting in breast pain and painful periods are also prevented by GLA in the diet – this overcomes the metabolic block or dietary deficiency causing the symptoms. The classic example is the victim of anorexia nervosa whose periods may stop altogether.

Evening Primrose Oil and Coronary Heart Disease

Trials are currently ongoing to see if evening primrose oil can fulfil its potential to reduce CHD.

By encouraging production of prostaglandins that thin the blood, and by neutralizing the effects of other prostaglandins that make blood more sticky, a protective effect seems likely.

Certainly, GLA can relieve symptoms in people with blocked arteries in the legs. It may also prevent the re-blocking of arteries in patients who have had arterial bypass operations.

GLA and Cancer

It was recently discovered that GLA has powerful anti-cancer properties. One drug derived from GLA is injected into the veins and attacks cancer cells directly. Another derivative, taken by mouth, seems to reduce the adverse effects of radiotherapy.

Organisms that secrete GLA in a more concentrated form than that found in oil of evening primrose have now been discovered – in of all places, a mouldy carrot in a basement cellar. These organisms are grown in a large fermenter and pure GLA extracted from the solution. The extracts have been shown to boost the body's natural immunity so it destroys malignant cells. GLA also seems to reduce the spread of cancer cells by an as yet poorly understood mechanism.

GLA and Other Diseases

When evening primrose oil or GLA plus EPA were given

to patients with painful rheumatoid arthritis, 60 per cent were able to give up their anti-inflammatory (NSAID) tablets altogether. Between 25–35 per cent were able to halve the dose of NSAIDs they needed.

Evening primrose oil and fish oil also seem to help sufferers of AIDS and ME. In one trial, 80 per cent of patients reported an improvement after three months, compared with less than 20 per cent of those taking inactive substances. The GLA and fish oil mix seems to alleviate symptoms such as fatigue, diarrhoea and weight loss, too.

In yet another trial, GLA has been shown to halt the progressive damage to nerve cells that occurs in advanced diabetes. This can produce symptoms of numbness, weakness and impaired vision. GLA overcomes an essential fatty acid deficiency to improve – and prevent – these serious symptoms.

Most importantly, treatment with evening primrose oil (and pure GLA) is well tolerated and without clinically significant side effects.

Other problems which oil of evening primrose may help are:

- insomnia
- nightmares
- schizophrenia.

CHAPTER 9

Body Awareness Programme Diets

The Body Awareness Programmes

The Body Awareness Programme contains three healthy eating packages which are tailored to suit everyone:

Body Awareness Food Exchange Diet

To allow anyone who is overweight to mix-and-match their foods within pre-determined portion levels.

The number of portions you can eat depend on:
- how overweight you are
- whether you are male or female
- how active you are

Body Awareness Mediterranean Slim Diet

This is a pre-determined eating regime which gives you an average of 1,200 kcals per day. By increasing your exercise levels, and by eating regularly throughout the day you will use up an average of 200 kcals more per day than usual and excess weight will fall off rapidly.

The Mediterranean Slim Diet combines all the latest nutritional advice. It is low in fat, especially saturated fat, and high in carbohydrate, fibre and antioxidants. This diet provides:

- 20% of energy as protein
- 20% as fat
- 55% as carbohydrate
- around 5% as red wine
- over 30g of fibre per day

If you drink red grape juice instead of red wine your carbohydrate intake will increase to 60%.

Body Awareness Maintenance Diet

If you are already at the right weight for your height but want to eat more healthily, this is the diet for you. The maintenance diet advises on the number of calories or food exchange portions to eat every day and includes a selection of delicious, Mediterranean diet recipes for you to try.

Just work out how much you can eat within your calorie allowance and tuck in!

Aims of the Body Awareness Programmes

All the Body Awareness diets have similar aims:
1. To eliminate as much processed and pre-packed foods as possible. The diets are based on natural whole foods packed with minerals, vitamins and fibre.
2. To increase your intake of unrefined carbohydrates.

3. To increase the amount of fresh fruit, salads and vegetables you eat to 400–800g daily.

4. To decrease the amount of fat, especially saturated fat, in your diet. Fats should make up no more than 30% of daily calories. That's around 75g for men and 53g for women.

5. To decrease the amount of red meat and eggs you eat. On the Body Awareness Mediterranean Slim Diet, meat is only eaten once per week – with red and white meat alternating.

6. To increase the amount of fish you eat.

7. To increase the amount of pulses, seeds and nuts in your diet.

8. To reduce the amount of simple sugars and sweets you eat.

9. To drink one glass of good red wine or red grape juice per day.

10. To include food supplements which are essential for maximum health, especially during weight loss:

- Gammalinolenic acid (oil of evening primrose; starflower oil).
- Vitamins C E and betacarotene. A supplement such as Vital 3 is recommended.
- Marine fish oils for those not wishing to eat fish at least three times per week.

Body Awareness Food Exchange Diet

Some readers may find it difficult to follow a rigid diet. A set eating plan can be restrictive, especially if you're working.

This isn't a problem with the Body Awareness Programme however, all you have to do is follow the Body Awareness Food Exchange Diet and lose weight with complete freedom to choose what you eat.

How Body Awareness Food Exchanges Work

Every day you are allowed a set number of carbohydrate, fruit and vegetable, milk, fish and meat portions to eat. These depend on your level of activity, whether you're male or female, and how much weight you have to lose.

If you are not very active or are below the average height for your age, stick to the bottom end of the portion range.

If you are quite active or are tall for your age, you can eat more portions within your range, especially carbohydrate ones.

Choose a wide variety of foods within each portion group – obviously, if you eat all your carbohydrate portions as pasta you would end up consuming a lot more calories than if you stuck to bread or crispbreads – so mix and match.

Overall, the Food Exchange Diet provides at least 50 per cent of your energy intake as carbohydrate – ideal for health and losing weight.

What the Portions Consist of:

Choose a wide variety of foods to eat. Weigh out your food accurately – guessing can add hundreds of extra calories and destroy all your hard work.

Complex Carbohydrates
1 portion equals:

- 3 tbsp breakfast cereal (unsweetened)
- 1 slice wholemeal bread/toast
- ½ wholemeal bread roll
- 1 mini wholemeal pitta bread
- ½ medium chapatti
- 3 slim crispbreads

- 50g cooked brown rice
- 50g cooked wholemeal pasta
- 100g potato, boiled or baked

Vegetables and Fruit
1 portion equals:

- 100g leafy green vegetables (e.g. spinach, broccoli)
- large mixed leaf salad
- 100g root vegetable, e.g. carrot, parsnip
- 50g olives
- 225g rhubarb
- 1 apple, 1 orange, 1 kiwi, 1 nectarine, 1 peach, 1 pear
- ½ grapefruit, ½ ogen melon, ½ large banana
- 2 dates, 2 figs (fresh or dried), 2 satsumas
- 4 passion fruit, 4 apricots, 4 plums, 4 prunes
- 100g berries (e.g. strawberries, raspberries, etc.)
- 100g grapes, cherries, pineapple
- 30g dried mixed fruit
- 100ml freshly squeezed fruit juice

Milk, Cheese and Yogurt
1 portion equals:

- 200ml semi-skimmed milk
- 300ml skimmed milk
- 40g hard cheese (size of a matchbox)
- 100g low-fat cottage cheese
- 100g low-fat or reduced-fat cheese
- 100g low-fat natural fromage frais or bio-yogurt

Fish, Beans, Nuts and Seeds
1 portion equals:

- 50g oily fish
- 100g non-oily white fish
- 100g lobster, crab
- 100g peeled prawns, scampi, shrimps

- 400g mussels weighed with shells
- 100g mussels without shells
- 100g cooked beans/lentils
- 15g nuts
- 15g seeds

Meat and Eggs
1 portion equals:

- 2 eggs, size 4 (maximum of 4 eggs per week)
- 75g lean red meat, all visible fat removed
- 100g poultry without skin

Cooking Methods
- Grill
- Bake
- Steam
- Boil
- Poach
- Casserole
- Dry (stir) fry by brushing pan with olive oil
- If roasting meat, drain off all juices and fats

Supplements: 500mg gammalinolenic acid
134mg vitamin E
150mg vitamin C   } e.g. Vital 3
15mg betacarotene
12mg iron (optional)
300mg calcium (optional)

As many fresh herbs as you wish.
As much lemon juice as you wish.
As many herbal/fruit teas as you wish.
As much mineral water as you wish.
Drink at least 3 litres of fluid per day.
15g olive oil–based spread if necessary per day.
Light brushing with olive oil whilst grilling or baking.

Estimated Daily Amount of Energy (kcals) You Need:

	TO MAINTAIN WEIGHT		TO LOSE WEIGHT SAFELY	
AGE	MALES	FEMALES	MALES	FEMALES
0–3 months	545	515		
4–6 months	690	645		
7–9 months	825	765		
10–12 months	920	865		
1–3 years	1230	1165		
4–6 years	1715	1545		
7–10 years	1970	1740		
11–14	2220	1845	2000	1600
15–18	2755	2110	2400	1800
19–59	**2550**	**1920**	**1700**	**1200**
60–74	2355	1900	1500	1200
75 plus	2100	1810	1400	1100

PLUS INCREASED EXERCISE

Age: 11–14 Years

The portion quantities suggested below are intended as a guide only. During this period of rapid growth, it is unwise to restrict energy intake too severely.

Ideally, children should aim to maintain the same weight (and not actually lose weight) as they continue to grow in height. This will produce a natural streamlining effect as growth continues.

Encourage increased exercise as well as a slight reduction in food intake. It's best for a child to slim under medical supervision.

Estimated normal daily energy requirement age 11–14 years:
Male (♂)   2220 kcals
Female (♀)   1845 kcals

Suggested daily energy intake to slim down safely:
Male (♂)   2000 kcals plus increased exercise
Female (♀)   1600 kcals plus increased exercise

Age 11–14 years

Portions of Each Food Group Suggested Per Day

	Carbo-hydrate		Veg Fruit		Milk Cheese		Fish Beans		Meat Eggs	
	♂	♀	♂	♀	♂	♀	♂	♀	♂	♀
How much weight do you need to lose?										
None	10–16	8–12	5–10	5–9	3–6	3–6	2	2	0–1	0–1
< 6kg (< 1st)	8–14	6–10	5–9	5–8	3–4	3–5	1–2	1–2	0–1	0–1
>6 kg (> 1st)	9–14	7–10	5–9	5–8	3–4	3–5	1–2	1–2	0–1	0–1

Age: 15–18 Years

During this period of sexual maturation it is still unwise to restrict energy intake too severely. Anorexia, relatively common during adolescence, results in long-term, serious effects on health – including undesirable effects on the ovaries and bones.

Aim to keep your weight steady as your height increases. There doesn't need to be an actual loss of weight unless you are more than 6kg (1 stone) over your ideal weight. Work out what your Body Mass Index (*see Chapter 2*) is now, and what it should be for your estimated final height. This will give you an idea of how much you should finally weigh – and how much weight, if any, you need to lose.

Increase your level of physical activity – exercise levels

often drop dramatically on entering the sixth form or leaving school.

Estimated normal daily energy requirement:
Male (♂)   2755 kcals
Female (♀)   2110 kcals

Suggested daily energy intake to slim down safely:
Male (♂)   2400 kcals plus increased exercise
Female (♀)   1800 kcals plus increased exercise

Age 15–18 years

Portions of Each Food Group Suggested Per Day

	Carbo-hydrate		Veg Fruit		Milk Cheese		Fish Beans		Meat Eggs	
	♂	♀	♂	♀	♂	♀	♂	♀	♂	♀
How much weight do you need to lose?										
None	15–20	10–15	5–10	5–10	3–6	3–5	2–4	2–3	0–1	0–1
< 6kg (< 1st)	12–18	8–13	5–9	5–8	3–5	3–4	1–3	1–3	0–1	0–1
> 6kg (> 1st)	13–19	9–14	5–9	5–8	3–5	3–4	1–3	1–3	0–1	0–1

Age: 19–59 Years

It is now safe to lower your energy intake more dramatically as you have finished your rapid growth spurt. A drop in calories of 700–900 kcals per day will result in a quick and satisfying weight loss.

Most overweight adults do not get enough exercise. You need to raise your heart beat to your maximum safe pulse rate for at least 20 consecutive minutes, three times per week (*see Chapter 6*). By increasing your exercise level, you will achieve a lower weight and improved health at top speed.

Estimated normal daily energy requirement:
Male (♂)　　　2550 kcals
Female (♀)　　1920 kcals

Suggested daily energy intake to lose 6kg (1stone) in weight safely:
Male (♂)　　　1700 kcals plus increased exercise
Female (♀)　　1200 kcals plus increased exercise

Age 19–59 years

Portions of Each Food Group Suggested Per Day

	Carbo-hydrate		Veg Fruit		Milk Cheese		Fish Beans		Meat Eggs	
	♂	♀	♂	♀	♂	♀	♂	♀	♂	♀
How much weight do you need to lose?										
None	15–20	10–14	6–12	5–10	2–3	2–3	2–4	2–3	0–1	0–1
< 6kg (< 1st)	8–12	5–8	5–10	5–8	1–2	1–2	1–2	1–2	0–1	0–1
> 6kg (> 1st)	10–14	6–10	6–10	6–8	1–2	1–2	1–2	1–2	0–1	0–1

Age: 60–74 Years

Your metabolism is now slowing significantly at a rate of up to three per cent a year. If you don't cut down on the amount you eat, your weight will naturally start to go up as your basal metabolic rate lowers.

By eating around 700–900 kcals per day less than you need you should see a steady drop in weight.

Some people in this age group need to stick to a carefully calculated 1,000 kcals per day if their metabolism is particularly sluggish. It's worth having your thyroid gland function checked if you find it difficult to lose weight.

It's important for long-term health to continue a steady – but not too vigorous – exercise regime.

Estimated normal daily energy requirement:
Male (♂)   2355 kcals
Female (♀)   1900 kcals

Suggested daily energy intake to lose 6kg (1stone) in weight safely:
Male (♂)   1500 kcals plus increased exercise
Female (♀)   1200 kcals plus increased exercise

Age 60–74 years

Portions of Each Food Group Allowed Per Day

	Carbo-hydrate		Veg Fruit		Milk Cheese		Fish Beans		Meat Eggs	
	♂	♀	♂	♀	♂	♀	♂	♀	♂	♀
How much weight do you need to lose?										
None	12–17	8–13	6–12	5–10	2–3	2–3	2–3	2–3	0–1	0–1
< 6kg (< 1st)	6–11	5–8	5–8	5–7	1–2	1–2	1–2	1–2	0–1	0–1
> 6kg (> 1st)	7–13	6–9	6–8	6–7	1–2	1–2	1–2	1–2	0–1	0–1

Age: 75 Years and Over

Your basal metabolic rate is now up to 12 per cent slower than when you were in your twenties. Try to cut down on the amount you eat whilst continuing with gentle exercise – especially non-weight bearing exercise (e.g. cycling, swimming). Otherwise, your weight will slowly increase as your metabolism slows further.

Estimated normal daily energy requirement:
Male (♂)   2100 kcals
Female (♀)   1810 kcals

Suggested daily energy intake to lose 6kg (1stone) in weight safely:

Male (♂)   1400 kcals plus increased exercise
Female (♀)   1100 kcals plus increased exercise

Age 75 years and over

Portions of Each Food Group Allowed Per Day

	Carbo-hydrate		Veg Fruit		Milk Cheese		Fish Beans		Meat Eggs	
	♂	♀	♂	♀	♂	♀	♂	♀	♂	♀
How much weight do you need to lose?										
None	10–15	10–13	5–10	5–8	2–3	2–3	2–3	2–3	0–1	0–1
< 6kg (< 1st)	6–10	5–7	5–8	4–6	2	2	2	2	0–1	0–1
> 6kg (> 1st)	8–11	6–8	6–8	5–6	2	2	2	2	0–1	0–1

Dieting Tips

Try to spread your meals throughout the day to maintain your optimum metabolic rate. Ideal times for eating are: 8 a.m., 10 a.m., midday, 2 p.m., 4 p.m. and 6 p.m.

Try not to eat anything but fruit after 8 p.m. Your metabolism is slowing down and any calories you eat late in the day are more likely to plump up your fat storage cells.

By eating little and often, your metabolism is kept working at its maximum rate and more calories are burned overall. This also maintains your blood sugar levels so you feel full for longer – it's blood sugar fluctuations that cause sensations of hunger.

The daytime meals can easily be taken to work in food boxes. Keep a small, black pepper grinder at the office as this will liven up all your savoury snacks.

If you are cooking rice, beans, potatoes or pasta for the evening meal, make double the quantity required so that it can also be used for a salad lunch the following day. By doing this, the next day's lunch is easily and quickly prepared.

Try getting up an hour earlier than normal and preparing your daytime meals fresh each day. By sleeping one less hour per day, you will burn up even more calories.

If you find it difficult going without this extra sleep, still try to get up that hour earlier but go to bed an hour earlier too — after your relaxation period. This has the added bonus of making you less tempted to snack later in the evening.

In general, try to eat meat as a main meal only once a week, vegetarian meals three times a week and fish as a main meal three times a week.

Fish is important as its beneficial effects to your health are unrivalled.

You are allowed one glass of red wine with your evening meal. This can be replaced with a similar quantity of red grape juice if you prefer.

After your evening meal (preferably eaten at around 6 p.m.) you are allowed unlimited herbal teas. You may also nibble your way slowly through 100g of fresh grapes, preferably red ones.

Your metabolic rate is naturally lower towards the evening and you will tend to be less active. This is your time for relaxation, hobbies and pampering.

Both the Body Awareness Food Exchange Diet and the detailed Body Awareness Mediterranean Slim Diet are natural and easy to follow. You will have no trouble sticking to either of them.

Important: these diets can only work quickly and properly if you boost your metabolic rate. This means increasing your muscle to fat ratio through increased physical activity. Exercise for at least 20 minutes continuously, at least three times per week.

Set against this, you need frequent relaxation periods too so your body can recuperate. They will help you feel better about yourself and help to reinforce your long-term, healthy-eating and weight-loss goals. Relaxation periods are incorporated into the Body Awareness Programme for you.

After only one month of eating healthily and exercising regularly, you will lose around 6kg (1stone) in weight and feel fitter, sleeker and healthier. You will burst with new-found energy and feel on top of the world.

The Body Awareness Programme is the diet for the twenty-first century — and one supported by all the research and data available to science today. It is compatible with World Health Organization guidelines for healthy eating and their universal population nutrient goals.

Breads

Over the last few years, an exciting variety of Continental breads have become available in supermarkets. Whenever bread is mentioned during the menu plans, you can have around 50g of either of the following, but adjust your calorie intake record accordingly:

Whole grain bread (219 kcals per 100g, 80 kcals per slice)
Ciabatta (259 kcals per 100g)
Pitta (261 kcals per 100g)
Focaccia (327 kcals per 100g)
Pugliese (315 kcals per 100g)
Sesame bread sticks (492 kcals per 100g, 34 kcals per individual stick)

If you need to use a spread on your bread, use an olive oil-based one. In general however, the sandwiches included in the diet have fillings which are moistened with low fat fromage frais or natural bio yogurt, so a spread is often unnecessary.

Every evening, check what you require for the next day's menu plan as some advanced preparation may be necessary, e.g. cooking twice as much pasta for an evening meal so you can make a cold pasta salad for the following day's lunch.

Body Awareness Mediterranean Slim Diet

Over the 30-day diet plan, the Body Awareness Mediterranean Slim Diet gives you an average intake of:

- 1200 kcals per day
- Over 30g of fibre per day
- 55% carbohydrate
- 20% protein
- 20% fat
- 5% alcohol

If you drink red grape juice instead of red wine with your evening meal, your carbohydrate intake goes up to 60%.

This diet plan is suitable for any woman with 6kg (1 stone) or less to lose. If you:

- have a physically demanding job
- have over 6kg (1 stone) in weight to lose
- are male

you may, if you wish, eat an extra 300kcals per day on top of the slim plan menus. These additional calories should be eaten mainly as carbohydrate for maximum health and slimming benefit. For example:

- 30g Apricot Nut Seed Muesli (110 kcals)

plus

- 1 slice of wholegrain toast with a scraping of olive oil-based spread (100 kcals)

191

plus
- 1 medium banana (100 kcals)

or a double portion of rice/pasta per day.

Select what you can fit into your allowance from the calorie counter provided in the appendices of this book. Also *see* Dieting Tips, page 188.

Low-fat Diets

A dietary intake of 20 per cent fat is as low as I recommend for health reasons. We need a certain amount of fat to maintain our body functions. The Body Awareness Diet is high in monounsaturated oil (e.g. olive oil) and eicosapentanoic acid (fish oil).

A daily supplement of oil of evening primrose will guard against the skin scaling and hormonal imbalances (e.g. irregular periods, cyclical breast pain, premenstrual syndrome) which some low-fat dieters have suffered when following other low-fat diets.

The Body Awareness Mediterranean Slim Diet assumes you start on a Saturday. You may, however, begin on any day of the week, as long as you start with the programme for the relevant day.

On Saturdays and Sundays, extra activities and slightly more adventurous meals and relaxation techniques are incorporated. If you work at weekends or if your time is at a premium, you can always swop a mid-week regime for a weekend regime without any worries about upsetting your Body Awareness Programme.

Daily Allowances on the Mediterranean Slim Diet

Unlimited mineral water — sparkling, plain, or try adding a twist of fresh lemon or lime juice.

Unlimited herbal or fruit teas, drunk without milk or sweetener.

Either: 300ml semi-skimmed milk (138 calories)

Or: 300ml skimmed milk (98 calories)

Tea or coffee using your milk allowance. Limit yourself to a total of 3 cups per day. Try not to use sugar or sweeteners. This is your chance to retrain your taste buds. If you drink unsweetened natural fruit/herbal teas regularly, you will not miss traditional tea and coffee at all.

In total, drink at least 3 litres of fluid per day.

Supplements: 500mg gammalinolenic acid
134mg vitamin E
150mg vitamin C
15mg betacarotene

The antioxidant vitamins E, C and betacarotene are most easily obtained in one pack with the Vital 3 food supplement. Alternative supplements are available if you prefer to buy your antioxidant vitamins individually.

Some dieters may want to supplement their diet with iron as well. This is recommended for people who have:

- a past medical history of anaemia
- heavy periods
- previously followed an unhealthy diet high in saturated fats and low in fresh fruit and vegetables

Dieting females should consider taking calcium supplements to reduce the risk of osteoporosis.

Body Awareness Mediterranean Slim Diet 30-day Plan

Recipes shown in **bold** type can be found in the recipe section starting on page 245.

DAY 1: Saturday
SUPPLEMENTS
500mg Gammalinolenic acid
12mg iron (optional)
Vitamin E 134mg
Vitamin C 150mg ⎱ e.g. Vital 3
Betacarotene 15mg ⎰

BREAKFAST e.g. 8 a.m.
30g **Apricot Nut Seed Muesli**
150ml low-fat, natural bio yogurt
1 sachet fruit/herbal tea (e.g. grapefruit and orange)

MID-MORNING e.g. 10 a.m.
1 orange
1 sachet fruit/herbal tea (e.g. orange grove)

LUNCH (Eat half at midday, half at 2 p.m.)
Prawn sandwich
   2 slices wholegrain bread
   60g cooked tiger prawns
   4 tbsp light fromage frais
   1 tbsp fresh squeezed lemon juice
   1 tsp fresh garlic and herbs, chopped
   Dash of cayenne pepper
Mixed leaf salad with 1 tbsp mixed seeds and lemon juice
1 beef tomato
1 sachet fruit/herbal tea (e.g. Mediterranean citrus)

MID-AFTERNOON e.g. 4 p.m.
2 apricots, fresh or dried

2 dates, fresh or dried
1 sachet fruit/herbal tea (e.g. fennel and lemon balm)

DINNER e.g. 6–8 p.m.
Grilled fish (e.g. salmon steak) with Lemon and Herbs
100g cooked pasta (e.g. spinach tagliatelle)
Steamed broccoli (as much as you want)
100g strawberries
1 glass (100ml) good red wine or red grape juice

EVENING
100g grapes
1 sachet herbal tea (e.g. tranquillity)

If possible, eat the main meal of the day at midday.

EXERCISE
e.g. gym weights or a brisk walk

DAY 2: Sunday
SUPPLEMENTS
500mg Gammalinolenic acid
12mg iron (optional)
Vitamin E 134mg
Vitamin C 150mg } e.g. Vital 3
Betacarotene 15mg

BREAKFAST
1 slice wholegrain toast
1 dried apricot, 1 dried prune, 1 dried fig, 1 date, soaked
overnight in Lapsang Souchong tea

MID-MORNING
1 large red apple
1 sachet fruit/herbal tea (e.g. apple and blackberry)

LUNCH (Eat half at midday, half at 2 p.m.)
Cheese and Nut Pasta Salad
    100g cooked pasta, cold
    1 tbsp freshly chopped basil or coriander leaves
    100g low fat cottage cheese
    1 tbsp chopped walnuts
    2 tbsp light fromage frais
    Freshly ground black pepper
Mixed leaf salad with 1 tbsp mixed seeds and lemon juice
1 beef tomato
1 sachet fruit/herbal tea (e.g. grapefruit and orange)

MID-AFTERNOON
1 orange
1 sachet fruit/herbal tea (e.g. lime and lemon)

DINNER
Chicken with Lemon and Olives
100g cooked brown rice
Spinach, lightly steamed (as much as you want)
Mixed leaf salad with 1 tbsp mixed seeds and lemon juice
1 nectarine
1 glass (100ml) good red wine or red grape juice

EVENING
100g grapes
1 sachet fruit/herbal tea (e.g. vespers)

If possible, eat the main meal of the day at midday.

RELAXATION
e.g. flotation therapy

DAY 3: Monday
SUPPLEMENTS
500mg Gammalinolenic acid
12mg iron (optional)

Vitamin E 134mg
Vitamin C 150mg } e.g. Vital 3
Betacarotene 15mg

BREAKFAST
1 low–fat natural bio yogurt mixed with 30g **Apricot Nut Seed Muesli**
1 sachet fruit/herbal tea (e.g. bright and early)

MID–MORNING
1 kiwi fruit
1 sachet fruit/herbal tea (e.g. mango and apple)

LUNCH (Eat half at midday, half at 2 p.m.)
Mediterranean Rice Salad
   100g cooked brown rice
   2 tbsp basil leaves, chopped
   1 tbsp pine nuts (or walnuts)
   1 tbsp freshly squeezed lemon juice
   1 tbsp Parmesan cheese, freshly grated
   1 clove garlic, crushed
   Freshly ground black pepper
Mixed leaf salad with 1 tbsp mixed seeds and lemon juice
1 beef tomato
1 sachet fruit/herbal tea (e.g. camomile and lemon grass)

MID–AFTERNOON
1 pear
1 sachet fruit/herbal tea (e.g. wild cherry)

DINNER
Roasted Red Pepper Devils
100g cooked pasta (e.g. tonnarelli) with herbs and garlic
Green beans, lightly steamed (as much as you want)
100g fresh cherries
1 glass (100ml) good red wine or red grape juice

EVENING
100g grapes
1 sachet fruit/herbal tea (e.g. night time)

If possible, eat the main meal of the day at midday.

EXERCISE
e.g. cycling, gym cardiovascular workout or aerobics

DAY 4: Tuesday
SUPPLEMENTS
500mg Gammalinolenic acid
12mg iron (optional)
Vitamin E 134mg
Vitamin C 150mg   } e.g. Vital 3
Betacarotene 15mg

BREAKFAST
One whole grapefruit, cut in half, drizzled with 1 tsp acacia honey and grilled
1 slice wholemeal toast with 1 tbsp yeast extract (top with cucumber slices if desired)
1 sachet fruit/herbal tea (e.g. grapefruit and orange)

MID-MORNING
1 large green apple
1 sachet fruit/herbal tea (e.g. apple and cinnamon)

LUNCH (Eat half at midday, half at 2 p.m.)
Tuna and Cucumber sandwich
   2 slices wholemeal bread
   100g tuna canned in brine, drained
   1 tsp fresh mixed herbs and garlic, chopped
   Baby lettuce leaves
   1 spring onion, chopped
   4 tbsp light fromage frais
   Freshly ground black pepper
Mixed leaf salad with 1 tbsp mixed seeds and lemon juice
4 dates (fresh or dried)
1 sachet fruit/herbal tea (e.g. fennel)

MID-AFTERNOON
1 peach
1 sachet fruit/herbal tea (e.g. rosehip)

DINNER
Grilled Trout with Walnuts and Dill
1 grilled beef tomato
Steamed courgettes (as much as you want)
100g boiled new potatoes with fresh mint
Mixed leaf salad with 1 tbsp mixed seeds and lemon juice
100g ripe plums
1 glass (100ml) good red wine or red grape juice

EVENING
100g grapes
1 sachet fruit/herbal tea (e.g. camomile and spearmint)

If possible, eat the main meal of the day at midday.

RELAXATION
e.g. aromatherapy bath

DAY 5: Wednesday
SUPPLEMENTS
500mg Gammalinolenic acid
12mg iron (optional)
Vitamin E 134mg
Vitamin C 150mg   } e.g. Vital 3
Betacarotene 15mg

BREAKFAST
One slice wholemeal toast topped with 1 grilled beef tomato, sliced
1 tsp chopped, mixed fresh herbs and garlic
Freshly ground black pepper
1 sachet fruit/herbal tea (e.g. morning time)

MID-MORNING
1 orange
1 sachet fruit/herbal tea (e.g. lemon verbena)

LUNCH (Eat half at midday, half at 2 p.m.)
Pepper and egg sandwich
   2 slices wholemeal bread
   ¼ red pepper, chopped
   1 boiled egg, chopped
   4 tbsp light fromage frais or natural bio yogurt
   Mixed fresh herbs and garlic, chopped
   Freshly ground black pepper
1 large red apple
1 sachet fruit/herbal tea (e.g. mixed fruit)

MID-AFTERNOON
1 kiwi fruit
1 sachet fruit/herbal tea (e.g. passion fruit and vanilla)

DINNER
Aubergines Parmesan
Mixed leaf salad with 1 tbsp mixed seeds and lemon juice
¼ stick warm, crusty French bread
100g raspberries
1 glass (100ml) good red wine or red grape juice

EVENING
100g grapes
1 sachet fruit/herbal tea (e.g. golden slumbers)

If possible, eat the main meal of the day at midday.

EXERCISE
e.g. gym weights or a brisk walk

DAY 6: Thursday
SUPPLEMENTS
500mg Gammalinolenic acid
12mg iron (optional)
Vitamin E 134mg
Vitamin C 150mg   } e.g. Vital 3
Betacarotene 15mg

BREAKFAST
30g **Apricot Nut Seed Muesli**
150ml low-fat natural bio yogurt
1 sachet fruit/herbal tea (e.g. nettle)

MID-MORNING
1 orange
1 sachet fruit/herbal tea (e.g. mixed fruit)

LUNCH (Eat half at midday, half at 2 p.m.)
Greek salad sandwich
    2 slices wholegrain bread
    30g feta cheese, crumbled
    1 tbsp coriander leaves, freshly chopped
    2 anchovy fillets, chopped
    4 black olives, stoned and chopped
    1 beef tomato, sliced
    Baby lettuce leaves
1 peach
1 sachet fruit/herbal tea (e.g. Mediterranean citrus)

MID-AFTERNOON
1 large green apple
1 sachet fruit/herbal tea (e.g. apple and cinnamon)

DINNER
Grilled fish (e.g. monkfish) with Lemon and Herbs
100g cooked brown rice with chopped fresh herbs
Spinach, lightly steamed (as much as you want)
Mixed leaf salad with 1 tbsp mixed seeds and lemon juice
100g strawberries
1 glass (100ml) good red wine or red grape juice

EVENING
100g grapes
1 sachet fruit/herbal tea (e.g. rosehip)

If possible, eat the main meal of the day at midday.

RELAXATION
e.g. basic relaxation exercise

DAY 7: Friday
SUPPLEMENTS
500mg Gammalinolenic acid
12mg iron (optional)
Vitamin E 134mg
Vitamin C 150mg ⎫ e.g. Vital 3
Betacarotene 15mg ⎭

BREAKFAST
1 slice wholegrain toast with yeast extract, topped with
cucumber slices if desired
½ small ogen/Galia melon
1 sachet herbal tea (e.g. tropical fruit)

MID-MORNING
1 large red apple
1 sachet herbal tea (e.g. apple and blackberry)

LUNCH (Eat half at midday, half at 2 p.m.)
Fruity rice salad
   100g cooked, brown rice
   100g low-fat cottage cheese with pineapple
   1 tbsp chopped mixed herbs (oregano, coriander,
   parsley)
Mixed leaf salad with 1 tbsp mixed seeds and lemon juice
1 beef tomato
1 sachet fruit/herbal tea (e.g. tropical fruit)

MID-AFTERNOON
1 orange
1 sachet fruit/herbal tea (e.g. camomile)

DINNER
Pasta alla Puttanesca
Mixed leaf salad with 1 tbsp mixed seeds and lemon juice
½ small ogen/Galia melon
1 glass (100ml) good red wine or red grape juice

EVENING
100g grapes
1 sachet fruit/herbal tea (e.g. tranquillity)·

If possible, eat the main meal of the day at midday.

EXERCISE
e.g. cycling, gym cardiovascular workout or aerobics

DAY 8: Saturday
SUPPLEMENTS
500mg Gammalinolenic acid
12mg iron (optional)
Vitamin E 134mg
Vitamin C 150mg   } e.g. Vital 3
Betacarotene 15mg

BREAKFAST
1 slice wholegrain toast
100g wild mushrooms, sliced and fried in 1 tsp extra virgin
olive oil
1 tbsp chopped fresh herbs and garlic
Freshly ground black pepper
1 sachet herbal tea (e.g. bright and early)

MID-MORNING
1 small orange
1 sachet herbal tea (e.g. lime and lemon)

LUNCH (Eat half at midday, half at 2 p.m.)
Tuna and Pasta Salad
   100g cooked pasta
   100g tuna canned in brine, drained
   100g low fat cottage cheese with chives

1 beef tomato, chopped
1 tbsp parsley, freshly chopped
Freshly ground black pepper
Mixed leaf salad with 1 tbsp mixed seeds and lemon juice
1 peach
1 sachet fruit/herbal tea (e.g. Mediterranean citrus)

MID-AFTERNOON
1 large apple
1 sachet fruit/herbal tea (e.g. mango and apple)

DINNER
Grilled Lemon Sole with Coriander and Green Pepper
Mangetout, lightly steamed (as much as you want)
Baby carrots, lightly boiled (as much as you want)
100g boiled new potatoes with fresh mint
100g strawberries
1 glass (100ml) good red wine or red grape juice

EVENING
100g grapes
1 sachet fruit/herbal tea (e.g. wild strawberry)

If possible, eat the main meal of the day at midday.

RELAXATION
e.g. flotation therapy

DAY 9: Sunday
SUPPLEMENTS
500mg Gammalinolenic acid
12mg iron (optional)
Vitamin E 134mg
Vitamin C 150mg } e.g. Vital 3
Betacarotene 15mg

BREAKFAST
30g **Apricot Nut Seed Muesli** with milk allowance
1 sachet fruit/herbal tea (e.g. passionfruit and vanilla)

MID-MORNING
1 kiwi fruit
1 sachet fruit/herbal tea (e.g. blackcurrant)

LUNCH (Eat half at midday, half at 2 p.m.)
Tomato, Orange and Ginger Soup
50g focaccia, ciabatta or wholegrain bread *or*
¼ stick warm crusty French bread
100g cherries
1 sachet fruit/herbal tea (e.g. wild cherry)

MID-AFTERNOON
1 orange
1 sachet fruit/herbal tea (e.g. lime and lemon)

DINNER
100g **Roast Rosemary and Garlic Lamb**
Cannellini beans (from lamb recipe)
Steamed broccoli (as much as you want)
100g baked potato
100g cherries or raspberries
1 glass (100ml) good red wine or red grape juice

EVENING
100g grapes
1 sachet fruit/herbal tea (e.g. golden slumbers)

If possible, eat the main meal of the day at midday.

EXERCISE
e.g. cycling, gym cardiovascular workout or aerobics

DAY 10: Monday
SUPPLEMENTS
500mg Gammalinolenic acid
12mg iron (optional)
Vitamin E 134mg
Vitamin C 150mg   } e.g. Vital 3
Betacarotene 15mg

BREAKFAST
1 pink grapefruit
1 slice wholemeal toast with 1 tbsp mashed cannellini beans from last night *or* a scraping of yeast extract. Top with slices of cucumber if wished
1 sachet fruit/herbal tea (e.g. nettle)

MID-MORNING
1 apple
1 sachet fruit/herbal tea (e.g. apple and blackberry)

LUNCH (Eat half at midday, half at 2 p.m.)
Salmon pitta
    1 mini wholemeal pitta bread (e.g. St Michael)
    60g smoked salmon or gravadlax
    1 tsp dill, freshly chopped
    1 tbsp low-fat yogurt
    Large mixed salad with 1 tbsp mixed seeds and lemon juice
1 beef tomato
1 sachet fruit/herbal tea (e.g. camomile and spearmint)

MID-AFTERNOON
1 kiwi fruit
1 sachet fruit/herbal tea (e.g. fennel)

DINNER
Ratatouille
100g cooked brown rice
Lightly steamed green beans (as much as you want)
Large mixed salad with 1 tbsp mixed nuts/seeds and lemon juice
1 peach
1 glass (100ml) good red wine or red grape juice

EVENING
100g grapes
1 sachet fruit/herbal tea (e.g. night time)

If possible, eat the main meal of the day at midday.

RELAXATION
e.g. aromatherapy massage

DAY 11: Tuesday
SUPPLEMENTS
500mg Gammalinolenic acid
12mg iron (optional)
Vitamin E 134mg
Vitamin C 150mg } e.g. Vital 3
Betacarotene 15mg

BREAKFAST
Scrambled egg with red pepper and tomato
1 slice wholemeal toast
1 sachet fruit/herbal tea (e.g. morning time)

MID-MORNING
1 medium orange
1 sachet fruit/herbal tea (e.g. Mediterranean citrus)

LUNCH (Eat half at midday, half at 2 p.m.)
Pineapple rice salad
   100g cooked brown rice
   ¼ green pepper, chopped
   100g fresh pineapple, chopped
   1 tbsp mixed herbs and garlic, freshly chopped
   4 tbsp light fromage frais
   Freshly ground black pepper
1 sachet fruit/herbal tea (e.g. mixed fruit)

MID-AFTERNOON
1 small banana *or* 100g fresh pineapple
1 sachet fruit/herbal tea (e.g. nettle)

DINNER
Mackerel with Mustard and Herbs
100g lightly steamed Florence fennel
100g potatoes, boiled or baked

Large mixed leaf salad with 1 tbsp mixed seeds and lemon juice
100g strawberries *or* 100g fresh pineapple
1 glass (100ml) good red wine or red grape juice

EVENING
100g grapes
1 sachet fruit/herbal tea (e.g. vespers)

If possible, eat the main meal at midday.
EXERCISE
e.g. gym weights or a brisk walk

DAY 12: Wednesday
SUPPLEMENTS
500mg Gammalinolenic acid
12mg iron (optional)
Vitamin E 134mg
Vitamin C 150mg   } e.g. Vital 3
Betacarotene 15mg

BREAKFAST
30g **Apricot Nut Seed Muesli**
150ml low-fat natural bio yogurt
1 sachet fruit/herbal tea (e.g. tropical fruit)

MID-MORNING
1 orange
1 sachet fruit/herbal tea (e.g. blackcurrant)

LUNCH (Eat half at midday, half at 2 p.m.)
Italian cheese and tomato sandwich
   2 slices wholegrain bread
   30g grated Mozzarella cheese
   1 beef tomato
   2 tbsp light fromage frais
   1 tbsp mixed herbs and garlic, chopped
   Freshly ground black pepper

Mixed leaf salad with 1 tbsp mixed seeds and lemon juice
1 sachet fruit/herbal tea (e.g. lemon grove)

MID-AFTERNOON
1 pear
1 sachet fruit/herbal tea (e.g. orange grove)

DINNER
Pasta with Tomato, Cinnamon and Bay
Steamed courgettes (as much as you want)
Mixed leaf salad with 1 tbsp mixed seeds and lemon juice
1 nectarine
1 glass (100ml) good red wine or red grape juice

EVENING
100g grapes
1 sachet fruit/herbal tea (e.g. golden slumbers)

If possible, eat the main meal at midday.

RELAXATION
e.g. basic relaxation exercise

DAY 13: Thursday
SUPPLEMENTS
500mg Gammalinolenic acid
12mg iron (optional)
Vitamin E 134mg
Vitamin C 150mg   } e.g. Vital 3
Betacarotene 15mg

BREAKFAST
1 apricot, 1 fig, 1 prune, 1 date (fresh or dried)
1 tbsp walnuts
150ml low-fat natural bio yogurt
1 sachet fruit/herbal tea (e.g. morning time)

MID-MORNING
1 orange
1 sachet fruit/herbal tea (e.g. grapefruit and orange)

LUNCH (Eat half at midday, half at 2 p.m.)
Mediterranean tomato herb roll
   1 small, crusty baguette roll
   1 beef tomato, sliced
   1 tsp wholegrain mustard
   1 tbsp mixed oregano, basil and parsley, freshly chopped
   4 tbsp light fromage frais
   Freshly ground black pepper
Mixed leaf salad with 1 tbsp mixed seed and lemon juice
1 sachet fruit/herbal tea (e.g. camomile and spearmint)

MID-AFTERNOON
1 nectarine
1 sachet fruit/herbal tea (e.g. rosehip)

DINNER
Mediterranean-style Monkfish
Lightly steamed broccoli (as much as you want)
100g boiled new potatoes with fresh mint
Mixed leaf salad with 1 tbsp mixed seeds and lemon juice
1 kiwi fruit, sliced
1 glass (100ml) good red wine or red grape juice

EVENING
100g grapes
1 sachet fruit/herbal tea (e.g. tranquillity)

If possible, eat the main meal at midday.

EXERCISE
Cycling, gym cardiovascular workout or aerobics

DAY 14: Friday
SUPPLEMENTS
500mg Gammalinolenic acid
12mg iron (optional)
Vitamin E 134mg
Vitamin C 150mg   }   e.g. Vital 3
Betacarotene 15mg

BREAKFAST
1 slice wholemeal toast
1 grilled beef tomato
Mixed fresh garlic and herbs, chopped
Freshly ground black pepper
1 sachet fruit/herbal tea (e.g. mixed fruit)

MID-MORNING
1 orange
1 sachet fruit/herbal tea (e.g. orange grove)

LUNCH (Eat half at midday, half at 2 p.m.)
Pitta, cheese and date sandwich
   1 mini wholemeal pitta bread
   100g natural low-fat cottage cheese
   30g dates *or* apricots, chopped
   1 tbsp mixed fresh herbs, chopped
Mixed leaf salad with 1 tbsp mixed seeds and lemon juice
1 sachet fruit/herbal tea (e.g. camomile)

MID-AFTERNOON
1 large green apple
1 sachet fruit/herbal tea (e.g. Mediterranean citrus)

DINNER
Avocado, Herb and Vegetable Bake
1 beef tomato, baked
100g cooked brown rice
Spinach, lightly steamed (as much as you want)
100g strawberries
1 glass (100ml) good red wine or red grape juice

EVENING
100g grapes
1 sachet fruit/herbal tea (e.g. night time)

If possible, eat the main meal at midday.

RELAXATION
e.g. face pack or facial

DAY 15: Saturday
SUPPLEMENTS
500mg Gammalinolenic acid
12mg iron (optional)
Vitamin E 134mg
Vitamin C 150mg $\Big\}$ e.g. Vital 3
Betacarotene 15mg

BREAKFAST
30g **Apricot Nut Seed Muesli**
150ml low-fat natural bio yogurt
1 sachet fruit/herbal tea (e.g. orange grove)

MID-MORNING
1 large red apple
1 sachet fruit/herbal tea (e.g. apple and cinnamon)

LUNCH (Eat half at midday, half at 2 p.m.)
Open pear, cheese and walnut sandwiches
   2 slices wholegrain bread
   1 ripe pear, cut in half, cored and sliced
   Topped with 100g cottage cheese and 1 tbsp walnuts, chopped
1 sachet fruit/herbal tea (e.g. wild raspberry)

MID-AFTERNOON
1 orange
1 sachet fruit/herbal tea (e.g. grapefruit and orange)

DINNER
Sardines with Wine and Parsley
100g boiled new potatoes with fresh mint
Mixed leaf salad with 1 tbsp mixed seeds and lemon juice
100g strawberries
1 glass (100ml) good red wine or red grape juice

EVENING
100g grapes

1 sachet fruit/herbal tea (e.g. vespers)

If possible, try to eat the main meal at midday.

EXERCISE
e.g. gym weights or brisk walk

DAY 16: Sunday
SUPPLEMENTS
500mg Gammalinolenic acid
12mg iron (optional)
Vitamin E 134mg
Vitamin C 150mg   } e.g. Vital 3
Betacarotene 15mg

BREAKFAST
1 slice wholemeal toast
½ small ogen/Galia melon
1 sachet fruit/herbal tea (e.g. morning time)

MID-MORNING
1 orange
1 sachet fruit/herbal tea (e.g. Mediterranean citrus)

LUNCH (Eat half at midday, half at 2 p.m.)
Luxury prawn salad
    100g Tiger prawns (or lobster, crab, etc.)
    4 tbsp light fromage frais
    1 tbsp mixed herbs and garlic, freshly chopped
    Sprigs of watercress
    1 tbsp mixed sprouting beans
    1 tbsp hazelnuts, chopped
Mixed leaf salad with 1 tbsp mixed seeds and lemon juice
50g focaccia, ciabatta, wholegrain bread *or* ¼ stick warm,
crusty French bread
1 beef tomato
1 sachet fruit/herbal tea (e.g. rosehip)

213

MID-AFTERNOON
1 nectarine
1 sachet fruit/herbal tea (e.g. wild blackcurrant)

DINNER
150g lean **Orange Chicken with Herbs**
100g cooked brown rice
Steamed spinach (as much as you want)
Mixed leaf salad with 1 tbsp mixed seeds and lemon juice
½ small ogen/Galia melon
1 glass (100ml) good red wine or red grape juice

EVENING
100g grapes
1 sachet fruit/herbal tea (e.g. night time)

If possible, try to eat the main meal at midday.

RELAXATION
e.g. flotation therapy

DAY 17: Monday
SUPPLEMENTS
500mg Gammalinolenic acid
12mg iron (optional)
Vitamin E 134mg
Vitamin C 150mg   } e.g. Vital 3
Betacarotene 15mg

BREAKFAST
30g **Apricot Nut Seed Muesli** with milk allowance
1 sachet fruit/herbal tea (e.g. wild raspberry)

MID-MORNING
1 orange
1 sachet fruit/herbal tea (e.g. orange grove)

LUNCH (Eat half at midday, half at 2 p.m.)
Greek salad sandwich
   2 slices wholegrain bread

30g feta cheese, crumbled
4 black olives, stoned and chopped
2 tbsp light fromage frais
1 spring onion, chopped
1 beef tomato, sliced
1 tsp oregano, freshly chopped
Sprigs of watercress
1 sachet fruit/herbal tea (e.g. lime and lemon)

MID-AFTERNOON
1 apple
1 sachet fruit/herbal tea (e.g. wild raspberry)

DINNER
Mediterranean Fennel Bake
100g cooked pasta (e.g. spaghetti with sun-dried tomatoes)
Green beans, lightly steamed (as much as you want)
Mixed leaf salad with 1 tbsp mixed seeds and lemon juice
100g strawberries
1 glass (100ml) good red wine or red grape juice

EVENING
100g grapes
1 sachet fruit/herbal tea (e.g. golden slumbers)

If possible, try to eat the main meal at midday.

EXERCISE
e.g. cycling, gym cardiovascular workout or aerobics

DAY 18: Tuesday
SUPPLEMENTS
500mg Gammalinolenic acid
12mg iron (optional)
Vitamin E 134mg
Vitamin C 150mg   } e.g. Vital 3
Betacarotene 15mg

BREAKFAST
1 slice wholegrain toast topped with 100g low-fat cottage cheese
1 tsp toasted sesame seeds
1 beef tomato, sliced
1 sachet fruit/herbal tea (e.g. camomile)

MID-MORNING
1 orange
1 sachet fruit/herbal tea (e.g. orange grove)

LUNCH (Eat half at midday, half at 2 p.m.)
Pasta pesto salad
    100g cooked pasta
    2 tbsp basil leaves, freshly chopped
    1 tbsp pine nuts (or walnuts), chopped
    1 tbsp freshly squeezed lemon juice
    4 tbsp light fromage frais
    1 clove garlic, crushed
    Freshly ground black pepper
Mixed leaf salad with 1 tbsp mixed seeds and lemon juice
1 sachet fruit/herbal tea (e.g. lemon and lime)

MID-AFTERNOON
1 apple
1 sachet fruit/herbal tea (e.g. apple and blackberry)

DINNER
Lemon Sole in Red Grape Sauce
Broccoli, lightly steamed (as much as you want)
100g boiled new potatoes with fresh mint
Mixed leaf salad with 1 tbsp mixed seeds and lemon juice
100g ripe plums
1 glass (100ml) good red wine or red grape juice

EVENING
100g grapes
1 sachet fruit/herbal tea (e.g. night time)

If possible, try to eat the main meal at midday.

RELAXATION
e.g. aromatherapy bath

DAY 19: Wednesday
SUPPLEMENTS
500mg Gammalinolenic acid
12mg iron (optional)
Vitamin E 134mg
Vitamin C 150mg ⎫
Betacarotene 15mg ⎭ e.g. Vital 3

BREAKFAST
4 large prunes soaked overnight in Lapsang Souchong tea
1 slice wholegrain toast
1 sachet fruit/herbal tea (e.g. morning time)

MID-MORNING
1 orange
1 sachet fruit/herbal tea (e.g. banana and cinnamon)

LUNCH (Eat half at midday, half at 2 p.m.)
Apricot, cheese and coriander sandwich
   2 slices wholegrain bread
   100g low-fat cottage cheese
   1 tsp pine nuts (or walnuts)
   2 apricots (fresh or dried), chopped
   1 tbsp coriander leaves, freshly chopped
   Sprigs watercress
1 beef tomato
Mixed leaf salad with 1 tbsp mixed seeds and lemon juice
1 sachet fruit/herbal tea (e.g. Mediterranean citrus)

MID-AFTERNOON
1 large apple
1 sachet fruit/herbal tea (e.g. apple and blackberry)

DINNER
Grilled Jerusalem Artichokes with Feta Cheese
1 grilled red pepper

100g cooked brown rice
100g green beans, lightly steamed
100g strawberries
1 glass (100ml) good red wine or red grape juice

EVENING
100g grapes
1 sachet fruit/herbal tea (e.g. night time)

If possible, try to eat the main meal at midday.

EXERCISE
e.g. gym weights or a brisk walk

DAY 20: Thursday
SUPPLEMENTS
500mg Gammalinolenic acid
12mg iron (optional)
Vitamin E 134mg
Vitamin C 150mg $\Big\}$ e.g. Vital 3
Betacarotene 15mg

BREAKFAST
30g **Apricot Nut Seed Muesli** with milk allowance
1 sachet fruit/herbal tea (e.g. bright and early)

MID-MORNING
1 apple
1 sachet fruit/herbal tea (e.g. apple)

LUNCH (Eat half at midday, half at 2 p.m.)
Salmon and dill sandwich
   2 slices wholegrain bread
   60g smoked salmon *or* gravadlax
   4 tbsp light fromage frais
   1 tbsp dill leaves, freshly chopped
   Thinly sliced cucumber (as much as you want)
1 beef tomato
Mixed leaf salad with 1 tbsp mixed seeds and lemon juice
1 sachet fruit/herbal tea (e.g. mixed fruit)

MID-AFTERNOON
1 orange
1 sachet fruit/herbal tea (e.g. fennel and lemon balm)

DINNER
Baked Whole Fish with Lemon and Herbs
100g baked potato
Spinach, broccoli or courgettes, lightly steamed (as much
as you want)
100g fresh apricots or plums
1 glass (100ml) good red wine or red grape juice

EVENING
100g grapes
1 sachet fruit/herbal tea (e.g. night time)

If possible, try to eat the main meal at midday.

RELAXATION
e.g. basic relaxation exercise

DAY 21: Friday
SUPPLEMENTS
500mg Gammalinolenic acid
12mg iron (optional)
Vitamin E 134mg
Vitamin C 150mg ⎫ e.g. Vital 3
Betacarotene 15mg ⎭

BREAKFAST
1 kiwi fruit, sliced
150ml low-fat natural bio yogurt
1 slice wholegrain toast
1 sachet fruit/herbal tea (e.g. fennel)

MID-MORNING
1 nectarine
1 sachet fruit/herbal tea (e.g. blackcurrant)

LUNCH (Eat half at midday, half at 2 p.m.)
Waldorf salad pitta
   1 mini wholemeal pitta bread
   2 sticks celery, chopped
   1 apple, chopped
   1 tbsp walnuts, chopped
   1 spring onion, chopped
   1 tbsp garlic and herbs, freshly chopped
   4 tbsp light fromage frais
1 beef tomato
Mixed leaf salad with 1 tbsp mixed seeds and lemon juice
1 sachet fruit/herbal tea (e.g. apple and cinnamon)

MID-AFTERNOON
1 orange
1 sachet fruit/herbal tea (e.g. grapefruit and lemon)

DINNER
Pasta Al Funghi
100g green beans or spinach, lightly steamed
Mixed leaf salad with 1 tbsp mixed seeds and lemon juice
100g strawberries
1 glass (100ml) good red wine or red grape juice

EVENING
100g grapes
1 sachet fruit/herbal tea (e.g. vespers)

If possible, try to eat the main meal at midday.

EXERCISE
e.g. cycling, gym cardiovascular workout or aerobics

DAY 22: Saturday
SUPPLEMENTS
500mg Gammalinolenic acid
12mg iron (optional)

Vitamin E 134mg
Vitamin C 150mg   } e.g. Vital 3
Betacarotene 15mg

BREAKFAST
30g **Apricot Nut Seed Muesli**
150ml low-fat natural bio yogurt
1 sachet fruit/herbal tea (e.g. mango and apple)

MID-MORNING
1 orange
1 sachet fruit/herbal tea (e.g. orange grove)

LUNCH (Eat half at midday, half at 2 p.m.)
Lentil and Apricot Soup
50g focaccia, ciabatta or wholegrain bread
Mixed leaf salad with 1 tbsp mixed seeds and lemon juice
1 sachet fruit/herbal tea (e.g. rosehip)

MID-AFTERNOON
1 kiwi fruit
1 sachet fruit/herbal tea (e.g. strawberry and vanilla)

DINNER
Cod in Yogurt, Tomato and Basil Sauce
Steamed courgettes *or* broccoli (as much as you want)
100g boiled new potatoes with fresh mint
Mixed leaf salad with 1 tbsp mixed seeds and lemon juice
100g strawberries or raspberries
1 glass (100ml) good red wine or red grape juice

EVENING
100g grapes
1 sachet fruit/herbal tea (e.g. night time)

If possible, try to eat the main meal at midday.

RELAXATION
e.g. flotation therapy

DAY 23: Sunday
SUPPLEMENTS
500mg Gammalinolenic acid
12mg iron (optional)
Vitamin E 134mg
Vitamin C 150mg   }   e.g. Vital 3
Betacarotene 15mg

BREAKFAST
1 grapefruit, grilled
1 slice wholemeal toast with yeast extract
Top with cucumber slices if desired
1 sachet fruit/herbal tea (e.g. passion fruit and vanilla)

MID-MORNING
1 kiwi fruit
1 sachet fruit/herbal tea (e.g. tropical fruit)

LUNCH (Eat half at midday, half at 2 p.m.)
French Onion Soup
2 slices wholegrain toast
Mixed leaf salad with 1 tbsp mixed seeds and lemon juice
1 sachet fruit/herbal tea (e.g. Mediterranean citrus)

MID-AFTERNOON
1 large red apple
1 sachet fruit/herbal tea (e.g. wild cherry)

DINNER
Lamb with Herbs, Lemon and Black Olives
100g cooked brown rice
Mixed leaf salad with 1 tbsp mixed seeds and lemon juice
100g raspberries/strawberries or cherries
1 glass (100ml) good red wine or red grape juice

EVENING
100g grapes
1 sachet fruit/herbal tea (e.g. golden slumbers)

If possible, try to eat the main meal at midday.

EXERCISE
e.g. cycling, gym cardiovascular workout or aerobics

DAY 24: Monday
SUPPLEMENTS
500mg Gammalinolenic acid
12mg iron (optional)
Vitamin E 134mg
Vitamin C 150mg   } e.g. Vital 3
Betacarotene 15mg

BREAKFAST
1 slice wholegrain toast
1 apricot, 1 date, 1 fig, 1 prune, soaked overnight in Lapsang Souchong tea
1 sachet fruit/herbal tea (e.g. grapefruit and orange)

MID-MORNING
1 large green apple
1 sachet fruit/herbal tea (e.g. wild blackcurrant)

LUNCH (Eat half at midday, half at 2 p.m.)
Open Italian cheese and tomato sandwiches
   2 slices wholegrain bread
   1 beef tomato, sliced
   60g Mozzarella cheese
   1 tbsp mixed basil, oregano and parsley, freshly chopped
Mixed leaf salad with 1 tbsp mixed seeds and lemon juice
Freshly ground black pepper
1 orange
1 sachet fruit/herbal tea (e.g. orange grove)

MID-AFTERNOON
1 peach
1 sachet fruit/herbal tea (e.g. tropical fruit)

DINNER
Pasta with Tomato, Tuna and Parsley Sauce
Mixed leaf salad with 1 tbsp mixed seeds and lemon juice

100g plums
1 glass (100ml) good red wine or red grape juice

EVENING
100g grapes
1 sachet fruit/herbal tea (e.g. vespers)

If possible, try to eat the main meal at midday.

RELAXATION
e.g. aromatherapy massage

DAY 25: Tuesday
SUPPLEMENTS
500mg Gammalinolenic acid
12mg iron (optional)
Vitamin E 134mg
Vitamin C 150mg   } e.g. Vital 3
Betacarotene 15mg

BREAKFAST
30g **Apricot Nut Seed Muesli**
150ml low–fat natural bio yogurt
1 sachet fruit/herbal tea (e.g. tropical fruit)

MID–MORNING
1 peach
1 sachet fruit/herbal tea (e.g. mango and apple)

LUNCH (Eat half at midday, half at 2 p.m.)
Pasta with asparagus
   100g cooked pasta
   6 spears cooked asparagus, chopped
   2 spring onions, chopped
   1 tbsp mixed garlic and herbs, freshly chopped
   4 tbsp light fromage frais
   1 tbsp freshly squeezed lemon juice
   Freshly ground black pepper
Mixed leaf salad with 1 tbsp mixed seeds and lemon juice

1 apple
1 sachet fruit/herbal tea (e.g. apple and blackberry)

MID-AFTERNOON
1 pear
1 sachet fruit/herbal tea (e.g. fennel)

DINNER
Mackerel with Ginger and Fennel
100g boiled new potatoes with fresh mint
100g asparagus spears, lightly steamed
1 kiwi fruit
1 glass (100ml) good red wine or red grape juice

EVENING
100g grapes
1 sachet fruit/herbal tea (e.g. golden slumbers)

If possible, try to eat the main meal at midday.

EXERCISE
e.g. gym weights or a brisk walk

DAY 26: Wednesday
SUPPLEMENTS
500mg Gammalinolenic acid
12mg iron (optional)
Vitamin E 134mg
Vitamin C 150mg } e.g. Vital 3
Betacarotene 15mg

BREAKFAST
Pizza toast
   1 slice wholegrain toast
   1 large grilled tomato, mashed
   1 tbsp mixed garlic and herbs, freshly chopped
   1 clove garlic, crushed
   Freshly ground black pepper
1 sachet fruit/herbal tea (e.g. morning time)

MID-MORNING
1 nectarine
1 sachet fruit/herbal tea (e.g. tropical fruit)

LUNCH (Eat half at midday, half at 2 p.m.)
Egg, pepper and potato salad
    100g boiled potatoes, cubed
    1 spring onion, chopped
    1 boiled egg, chopped
    ¼ red pepper, chopped
    4 tbsp light fromage frais
    1 tbsp mixed garlic and herbs, freshly chopped
    Freshly ground black pepper
Mixed leaf salad with 1 tbsp mixed seeds and lemon juice
1 beef tomato
1 sachet fruit/herbal tea (e.g. strawberry and vanilla)

MID-AFTERNOON
1 orange
1 sachet fruit/herbal tea (e.g. lemon grove)

DINNER
Aubergines Parmesan
¼ stick warm, crusty French bread
Mixed leaf salad with 1 tbsp mixed seeds and lemon juice
100g fresh apricots
1 glass (100ml) good red wine or red grape juice

EVENING
100g grapes
1 sachet fruit/herbal tea (e.g. night time)

If possible, try to eat the main meal at midday.

RELAXATION
e.g. basic relaxation exercise

DAY 27: Thursday
SUPPLEMENTS
500mg Gammalinolenic acid

12mg iron (optional)
Vitamin E 134mg
Vitamin C 150mg $\Big\}$ e.g. Vital 3
Betacarotene 15mg

BREAKFAST
1 slice wholegrain toast
2 dried apricots, chopped
1 dried fig, chopped
2 dates, fresh or dried
4 tbsp light fromage frais
1 sachet fruit/herbal tea (e.g. tropical fruit)

MID-MORNING
1 apple
1 sachet fruit/herbal tea (e.g. blackberry and apple)

LUNCH (Eat half at midday, half at 2 p.m.)
Coriander, cheese and walnut sandwich
   2 slices wholegrain bread
   100g natural low-fat cottage cheese
   2 tbsp light fromage frais
   1 tbsp walnuts, chopped
   1 tbsp coriander leaves, freshly chopped
   Sprigs of watercress
   Freshly ground black pepper
1 sachet fruit/herbal tea (e.g. lime and lemon)

MID-AFTERNOON
1 orange
1 sachet fruit/herbal tea (e.g. grapefruit and orange)

DINNER
Fish (e.g. haddock or salmon) in Filo Parcels
Spinach, lightly steamed (as much as you want)
100g baked potato
Mixed leaf salad with 1 tbsp mixed seeds and lemon juice
100g strawberries or raspberries
1 glass (100ml) good red wine or red grape juice

EVENING
100g grapes
1 sachet fruit/herbal tea (e.g. camomile and spearmint)

If possible, try to eat the main meal at midday.

EXERCISE
e.g. cycling, gym cardiovascular workout or aerobics

DAY 28: Friday
SUPPLEMENTS
500mg Gammalinolenic acid
12mg iron (optional)
Vitamin E 134mg
Vitamin C 150mg } e.g. Vital 3
Betacarotene 15mg

BREAKFAST
30g **Apricot Nut Seed Muesli** with milk allowance
1 kiwi fruit, sliced
1 sachet fruit/herbal tea (e.g. mixed fruit)

MID-MORNING
1 orange
1 sachet fruit/herbal tea (e.g. grapefruit and orange)

LUNCH (Eat half at midday, half at 2 p.m.)
Salmon sandwich
    2 slices wholegrain bread
    60g smoked salmon or gravadlax
    4 tbsp light fromage frais
    1 tbsp dill leaves, freshly chopped
    Freshly ground black pepper
    Mixed leaf salad with 1 tbsp mixed seeds and lemon
    juice
1 nectarine
1 sachet fruit/herbal tea (e.g. lemon verbena)

MID-AFTERNOON
1 large red apple

1 sachet fruit/herbal tea (e.g. mango and apple)

DINNER
Pasta with Lemon Cream
Spinach lightly steamed (as much as you want)
Mixed leaf salad with 1 tbsp mixed seeds and lemon juice
100g strawberries
1 glass (100ml) good red wine or red grape juice

EVENING
100g grapes
1 sachet fruit/herbal tea (e.g. camomile and spearmint)

If possible, try to eat the main meal at midday.

RELAXATION
e.g. face pack or facial

DAY 29: Saturday
SUPPLEMENTS
500mg Gammalinolenic acid
12mg iron (optional)
Vitamin E 134mg
Vitamin C 150mg   } e.g. Vital 3
Betacarotene 15mg

BREAKFAST
1 slice wholegrain toast with yeast extract
½ small ogen/Galia melon
1 sachet fruit/herbal tea (e.g. mango and apple)

MID-MORNING
1 orange
1 sachet fruit/herbal tea (e.g. Mediterranean citrus)

LUNCH (Eat half at midday, half at 2 p.m.)
Mediterranean Bean Soup
50g focaccia, ciabatta or wholegrain bread
Mixed leaf salad with 1 tbsp mixed seeds and lemon juice
1 sachet fruit/herbal tea (e.g. lemon grove)

MID-AFTERNOON
1 large green apple
1 sachet fruit/herbal tea (e.g. apple and cinnamon)

DINNER
Baked Orange and Rosemary Trout
100g cooked brown rice
Broccoli, lightly steamed (as much as you want)
Mixed leaf salad with 1 tbsp mixed seeds and lemon juice
½ small ogen/Galia melon
1 glass (100ml) good red wine or red grape juice

EVENING
100g grapes
1 sachet fruit/herbal tea (e.g. vespers)

If possible, try to eat the main meal at midday.

EXERCISE
e.g. gym weights or a brisk walk

DAY 30: Sunday
SUPPLEMENTS
500mg Gammalinolenic acid
12mg iron (optional)
Vitamin E 134mg
Vitamin C 150mg   } e.g. Vital 3
Betacarotene 15mg

BREAKFAST
30g **Apricot Nut Seed Muesli**
1 sachet fruit/herbal tea (e.g. fennel)

MID-MORNING
1 peach
1 sachet fruit/herbal tea (e.g. tropical fruit)

LUNCH
Kedgeree
   100g cooked brown rice

1 hard-boiled egg, chopped
60g flaked, smoked haddock (additive-free)
1 tbsp parsley, freshly chopped
1 tbsp coriander, freshly chopped
1 spring onion, chopped
1 tsp coriander seed, ground
¼ tsp cumin seed, ground
4 tbsp light fromage frais
Mix together. Season with freshly ground black pepper,
grated nutmeg and fresh lemon juice to taste.
Mixed leaf salad with 1 tbsp mixed seeds and lemon juice
1 sachet fruit/herbal tea (e.g. camomile and spearmint)

MID-AFTERNOON
1 large red apple
1 sachet fruit/herbal tea (e.g. apple and cinnamon)

DINNER
Coq au Vin Rouge
100g boiled new potatoes with fresh mint
Broccoli, lightly steamed (as much as you want)
Mixed leaf salad with 1 tbsp mixed seeds and lemon juice
100g strawberries
1 glass (100ml) good red wine or red grape juice

EVENING
100g grapes
1 sachet fruit/herbal tea (e.g. golden slumbers)

If possible, try to eat the main meal at midday.

RELAXATION
e.g. flotation therapy

Body Awareness Maintenance Plan

The Body Awareness Maintenance Plan is designed for readers who:
- have a healthy Body Mass Index (*see Chapter 10*) but want to eat more healthily
- have recently lost weight and want to maintain their new-found shape

If you don't have a weight problem but want to eat more healthily the chart below shows the estimated number of calories you need for weight maintenance according to your age and sex. If you are at your correct weight (BMI), have not recently dieted and want to eat more healthily, note how many calories to aim for and skip the following pages. Move straight to Tips on Healthy Eating (page 241).

Estimated Amount of Energy (kcals) You Need:

	TO MAINTAIN WEIGHT		TO LOSE WEIGHT SAFELY	
AGE	MALES	FEMALES	MALES	FEMALES
11–14	2220	1845	2000	1600
15–18	2755	2110	2400	1800
19–59	2550	1920	1700	1200
60–74	2355	1900	1500	1200
75 plus	2100	1810	1400	1100

PLUS INCREASED EXERCISE

These figures are averages. Fifty per cent of people need fewer calories than these to maintain their weight, while fifty per cent need more.

If you've recently lost weight, after all your hard work and sheer willpower has paid off, you don't want to see that lost weight slowly (or rapidly) creeping back. Maintaining your new figure is the most challenging part of losing weight. Once you start re-introducing foods and calories, your metabolism – which has learned to work

232

more efficiently than usual – will automatically try to convert these extra calories into body fat stores.

Most experts agree that you need:

- a **low-fat diet** such as the Body Awareness Mediterranean Slim Diet to take weight off
- and **exercise** to keep it off.

So whatever you do, don't give up your exercise plan. Continue exercising for twenty minutes continuously at least three times per week **for the rest of your life**.

Weight training helps to build muscle and compensates for the natural loss of lean tissue as you get older. Because muscle tissue burns energy more rapidly than fat cells, increased muscle mass leads to an increased basal metabolic rate. The extra calories you eat after reaching your goal weight are therefore more likely to burn and less likely to stick if you follow an exercise programme.

Many successful dieters opt for aerobic exercise. A regular aerobics class will keep you slim, healthy and sleek. Cycling, swimming and jogging are good aerobic exercises, too.

Make a note of the estimated maintenance calorie intake for a person of your age and sex from the chart on page 232.

If you've recently followed a calorie-restricted diet such as the Body Awareness Mediterranean Slim Diet or the Food Exchange Diet, this calorie estimate is a lot higher than your metabolism is used to. If you immediately start eating at this level, you will put on weight.

During your time of famine, your metabolism slipped into super-efficient mode. Every calorie eaten was used and no energy wasted as excess heat. On eating again, every spare calorie is diverted to replenish your raided body fat stores in the typical scenario of yo-yo dieting.

But don't worry – the Body Awareness Programme won't let this happen to you.

You need to increase your calorie intake slowly so your metabolism is lulled into a sense of security. As food slowly becomes more plentiful, wasteful metabolic pathways will switch back on in your brown fat cells. More food energy will be dissipated as heat, and less of your extra calories will stick as fat.

Introducing Extra Calories into Your Diet Without Regaining Weight

You are going to increase your calorie intake slowly until you reach a weight/calorie equilibrium. Remember to keep up your exercise programme to encourage an increased metabolic rate.

The difference between the number of daily calories you were on to lose weight and the calories the average person of your sex and age needs to maintain a healthy weight is called your calorie deficit.

You will slowly increase your calorie intake through five phases lasting from 10–30 days each. At each phase, your calorie intake will increase by approximately 20 per cent of your calorie deficit.

Some previously overweight people need less calories than the average person. Some readers will therefore stabilize their weight at an intermediate phase without increasing their calorie intake to the full maintenance level.

The portion tables beginning on page 184 for each age range include estimated portions from each food group needed to maintain a healthy weight. Start by introducing a few extra portions every ten days. Weigh yourself regularly and you will soon work out how many portions within each food group you need to maintain your new body weight.

Important

As you start eating more:

- Ensure that at least 50–60 per cent of your increased calorie intake is in the form of complex carbohydrate (e.g. wholegrain bread, brown rice, wholemeal pasta) and fruit. (See the Portion Exchange list of carbohydrate foods; or count calories – see Appendix 8, p 443.)
- Make sure you don't increase your fat intake above 30 per cent of calories. Saturated fat should make up no more than 10 per cent of your energy intake. This means keeping your intake of red meat, eggs and dairy products low.
- Keep up the exercise.
- Use the calorie-counted Mediterranean-style meals included in this book to help make up your calorie allowance.
- Use the Food Analysis Chart to estimate your calorie intake of other foods you eat.
- Always weigh food accurately. Guessing can lead to eating more calories than you think you are.

Phase 1

To start reintroducing more calories to your diet, go up to your estimated Phase 1 calorie intake according to your age and sex (see table). Phase 1 gives your dieting calorie allowance plus 20 per cent of your calorie deficit.
Weigh yourself after ten days.
If your weight goes down or remains stable:
- go up to your Phase 2 intake and eat an extra 20 per cent of your calorie deficit.
If your weight goes up:
- stay at Phase 1 and eat the same number of calories for another ten days. Then weigh again.

   If your weight has gone up again, check that you are counting your calories accurately by keeping a food diary

Estimated Calorie Intake from Slimming Levels Through Four Intermediate Phases to Maintenance Calorie Intake (kcals per day)

AGE

	11–14 ♂	11–14 ♀	15–18 ♂	15–18 ♀	19–59 ♂	19–59 ♀	60–74 ♂	60–74 ♀	Over 75 ♂	Over 75 ♀
Slimming	2000	1600	2400	1800	1700	1200	1500	1200	1400	1100
Phase 1	2045	1650	2470	1860	1870	1340	1670	1340	1540	1240
Phase 2	2090	1700	2540	1925	2040	1490	1840	1480	1680	1380
Phase 3	2130	1750	2610	1990	2210	1630	2010	1620	1820	1520
Phase 4	2175	1800	2680	2050	2380	1780	2180	1760	1960	1670
Maintenance	2220	1845	2755	2110	2550	1920	2355	1900	2100	1810

for a week. Drop back on your calorie intake to your dieting allowance and increase the amount of exercise you take. When you achieve your goal weight, re-start Phase 1.

Phase 2

Total calories = Diet allowance + 40 per cent of calorie deficit. Weigh yourself after 14 days.

If your weight goes down or remains stable:
• go up to Phase 3 and eat an extra 20 per cent of your calorie deficit.

If your weight goes up:
• stay at Phase 2 and eat the same number of calories for another ten days then weigh again.

If your weight increases further, check that you are counting your calories accurately by keeping a food diary for a week. Drop back to your Phase 1 calorie intake and increase the amount of exercise you do. When you achieve your goal weight again, re-start Phase 2.

Phase 3

Total calories = diet allowance + 60 per cent of calorie deficit. Stay at this phase for at least three weeks. Weigh yourself at least once per week.

If your weight goes down or remains stable:
• go up to Phase 4 and eat an extra 20 per cent of your calorie deficit.

If your weight goes up:
• drop back to Phase 2 for a few more weeks so your metabolism acclimatizes further. Everyone's metabolic rate and maintenance calorie needs vary. You may find that the Phase 2 calorie intake is the right maintenance for you.

When you reach your goal weight again, experiment

with accurately recorded calorie intakes lying between your Phase 2 and Phase 3 allowances until you discover a maintenance calorie intake which is right for you.

Phase 4

Total calorie intake = Diet allowance plus 80 per cent of calorie deficit. Stay at this phase for at least one month. Weigh yourself at least once per week.

If your weight goes down:

This is unlikely. You may have increased your exercise calorie needs above average. Try eating a little more carbohydrate and experiment until you find a calorie intake that allows you to maintain your goal weight.

If your weight remains stable:

• increase your calorie allowance to your estimated maintenance calorie needs (see chart).

If your weight goes up:

• drop back to your Phase 3 intake for a few more weeks so your metabolism can acclimatize further. Everyone differs and you may find that your Phase 3 calorie intake is the right maintenance intake for you.

When you reach your goal weight again, experiment with accurately recorded calorie intakes lying between your Phase 3 and Phase 4 allowances until you discover a maintenance calorie intake which is right for you.

Maintenance Phase

Total calorie intake = Diet allowance plus 100 per cent of calorie deficit = Estimated maintenance allowance.

If your weight goes down:

This is unlikely. You may have increased your exercise calorie needs above average. Try eating a little more carbohydrate and experiment until you find a calorie intake which allows you to maintain your goal weight.

If your weight goes up:

- drop back to your Phase 4 intake for a few more weeks so your metabolism can acclimatize further. Everyone's calorie needs vary and you may find that your Phase 4 calorie intake is the right maintenance intake for you.

When you reach your goal weight again, experiment with accurately recorded calorie intakes lying between your Phase 4 and Maintenance allowances until you discover a maintenance calorie intake which is right for you.

If your weight remains stable:

- stay at this maintenance level of calorie intake and weigh yourself regularly. At the first sign of putting on weight, cut back on calories or increase your exercise levels – or both.

Weight can creep back on if you drop your guard. Don't relax your vigilance. Aim to weigh yourself at least once per week for the rest of your life. And adjust your calorie and exercise levels accordingly.

Tips to Help Keep Your Weight Down

These tips will help you eat less.

- If possible, try to eat the main meal of the day at lunchtime.
- Relax before your meals and take your time to eat. Adopt the French habit of spending several hours over your food.
- Slowly drink a glass of mineral water before you start your meal.
- Chew each mouthful of food longer than usual.
- Pause regularly whilst eating and put down your knife and fork between mouthfuls.
- Re-discover the art of mealtime conversation.
- Serve smaller helpings than you think you need.
- Use a smaller plate than usual.

239

- Always sit down at a laid table to eat. Don't eat 'on the hoof' or whilst standing up.
- Concentrate on enjoying your food. Don't read or watch TV at the same time – you will swallow mechanically without appreciating your food and end up eating through feelings of fullness.
- Try not to eat whilst driving. This can become a habit on long journeys.
- Drink fruit/herbal teas. These are delicious, relaxing or stimulating depending on which you choose and, as they are drunk without milk, are calorie-free.
- Mix chilled white or red wine with sparkling mineral water to make refreshing spritzers.
- When you crave another glass of wine, have mineral water with a dash of lime or lemon juice instead. Elderflower cordial diluted 1:15 with water is an excellent white wine substitute.
- Try to avoid excessive fresh fruit juices outside of your diet allowances. These quickly add on calories.
- Use low-calorie versions of everything possible when cooking or eating. Skimmed milk has almost 50% less calories per pint than whole milk. On a half pint per day allowance, you can save 450 calories a week.
- Cut down on cooking fats. Don't roast or deep-fry. Instead, grill, bake or dry-fry using a non-stick pan.
- Low-fat yogurt is an ideal substitute for cream in most recipes, although it will curdle if you let it boil.
- When you feel the urge to eat between meals, do some vigorous exercise and work up a sweat – or try cleaning your teeth with strong, tingling toothpaste.
- Keep a food diary and write down everything you eat if the scales start creeping up.

Tips on Healthy Eating

The Body Awareness Food Exchange Diet gives guidelines on how many portions of each food to eat during the
maintenance phase.

- Consider adding antioxidant supplements to your diet (e.g. betacarotene, vitamins E and C).
- Avoid processed and pre-packed foods as much as possible. Follow a wholefood diet with fresh ingredients.
- Buy low-fat versions of everything possible, e.g. milk.
- Use olive oil-based spreads instead of butter.
- Use olive oil for cooking or salad dressings.
- Eat more complex carbohydrates. Ensure at least 50 per cent of your daily energy intake is carbohydrate.
- Eat more vegetables and fruit (5–10 portions per day).
- Ensure your intake of fibre is high. Fibre fills you up, speeds the action of the bowels, absorbs fats in the gut so less are absorbed (which helps to lower blood cholesterol levels) and helps to protect against bowel cancers.
- Have at least one (if not more) vegetarian days per week.
- Eat fewer eggs – a maximum of two per week.
- Eat red meat and poultry only once a week.
- Choose lean cuts of meat and trim off all visible fat.
- Eat more fish, e.g. three times per week.
- Eat more pulses.
- Eat more seeds and nuts – at least 30g per day.
- Reduce the amount of refined sugars and sweets you eat. These should make up no more than 10 per cent of your diet and preferably less. Most of us eat at least 14 per cent of daily energy from refined sugars (e.g. biscuits, cakes, chocolate, sweets, fizzy drinks, etc.).
- Cut down on the amount of salt you add to your food. You can get all the salt you need just from eating enough bread and cereals. The WHO recommended maximum salt intake is 6g per day. Most of us eat at least 7g per day. Most recipes in this book contain rock salt in the list of ingredients, but

only add salt sparingly whilst cooking. Try not to add it to food on the table.

- Try not to eat after 8 p.m.
- Choose fruit, sorbets or low-fat cheese and biscuits instead of creamy, sweet desserts.
- Drink wine, especially red wine, rather than beer or spirits.
- Keep an eye on your alcohol intake and ensure that it is within safe limits (21 units per week for males, 14 units per week for non-pregnant females).

Tips on Eating Out

Most restaurants have now heard of the healthy eating revolution even if they're doing nothing about it. Many chefs now specialize in Mediterranean-style whole foods.

When eating out, don't be afraid to ask for what you want. I've only ever eaten once in a restaurant where a simple request was greeted frostily. It soon became clear that boil-in-the-bag was the only food the management were serving and I didn't want to eat there again anyway.

The Good Food Guide is the ultimate bible for locating the best, most amenable and most enjoyable restaurants in your locality. You also have the ultimate weapon at hand: if a restaurant doesn't come up to expectations, write and tell the *Guide*. The chances are that other readers will have reported that particular restaurant wasn't up to scratch either.

When analysing the menu, decide whether you can afford a blow-out or whether caution dictates you should:

- Pass on the pre-prandial bread roll and butter.
- Avoid deep-fried foods and go for grilled, baked or steamed dishes instead.
- Go for an adventurous vegetarian option.
- Eat fish instead of red meat.
- Eat white meat with skin removed rather than red meat.

- Ask for all visible fat to be trimmed before cooking.
- Ask to have buttery or creamy sauces left off.
- Request a simple lemon, herb and olive oil dressing for fish, poultry, salads, etc.
- Don't choose anything that's wrapped in pastry, fried, battered or stuffed – unless it's with simple fresh herbs.
- Opt for Chinese, Malaysian or Japanese dishes that are usually low in hidden fat.
- Choose chicken and vegetable dishes with bean or oyster sauce and avoid sweet and sour creations.
- Choose steamed fish – Oriental cooking usually excels here. Try steamed scallops with ginger and spring onions, for example.
- Go for plain boiled rice rather than special fried rice or pilau.
- Avoid pasta with creamy sauces (e.g. carbonara). Opt for tomato, fish or clam sauces instead – and request that added oil is scant.
- Choose pizzas with plain tomato, garlic and vegetable toppings rather than meat or cheese.
- When going Indian, avoid heavy curries that are dripping with ghee (clarified butter).
- Choose plain tandoori or tikka dishes (without massala sauce).
- Sizzling dishes (korais) can be low in added fat if requested.
- Chapattis, naans and parathas are an excellent, healthy alternative to pilau rice.
- Choose fresh fruit or sorbet for dessert.

Tips for Burning Extra Calories

- Walk briskly rather than dawdling.
- Use the stairs rather than the lift.
- Buy a bicycle (and safety helmet) or an exercise bike and use it regularly.

- Buy a dog (but only if you love animals) and give it plenty of exercise.
- When out with the dog, try an alternate jog 1 minute – walk 1 minute – jog 1 minute – walk 1 minute routine.
- Swim regularly.
- Take up a team sport such as rowing, netball, football, etc.

CHAPTER 10

Body Awareness Mediterranean-style Recipes

The recipes included in this book are based on the Mediterranean Diet and are designed to be delicious, healthy and easy to prepare. They contain ingredients such as extra virgin olive oil, fresh herbs, fish, lean meat, fresh fruit and vegetables, yogurt, fromage frais, wine, and un-refined complex carbohydrates.

All recipes are calorie-counted so you can estimate the number of calories you eat in a day. The Food Analysis Chart (see page 443) lists the energy values of common healthy foods you are likely to eat whilst following the Body Awareness Programme.

I recommend that you keep a food diary for at least one week, but preferably longer. Write down everything you eat, even the odd peanut and nibble of cheese – it all adds up. You may be surprised at how much – or how little – you need to maintain your body weight.

When using these recipes, go easy on added salt. Add yogurt to sauces or casseroles off the heat. Don't add yogurt to liquids at boiling point or it may curdle. This doesn't affect the flavour but some people find it looks unappetizing. If this is the case, try using creamy Greek-style yogurt instead. This has a higher fat content and is more stable. To stabilize yogurt so it's less likely to curdle, stir in 1 teaspoon (5ml) of cornflour per 150ml of yogurt before using it in a recipe.

When yogurt is used as a topping for fish baked *en papillote*, the protein will coagulate. If you prefer, try using fromage frais instead, or pour over the yogurt mixed with herbs and seasoning after the fish is removed from the oven.

Index of Recipes

Kcals per serving unless otherwise specified.

Miscellaneous

Apricot Nut Seed Muesli 110 kcals per 30g portion
Mixed Seeds and Nuts to Sprinkle on Salads 25 kcals/tbsp
Scrambled Eggs with Red Pepper and Tomato 120 kcals
Kedgeree 325 kcals

Sauces, Dips and Dressings

Garlic Mayonnaise (Aïoli) 120 kcals per tbsp
Chilli Mayonnaise (Rouille)
      Version 1 60 kcals per tbsp
      Version 2 95 kcals per tbsp
Pesto 120 kcals per tbsp
Greek Almond and Garlic Relish 75 kcals per tbsp
Greek Barbecue Marinade 120 kcals per tbsp
Walnut Sauce 60 kcals per tbsp
Italian Olive Relish 40 kcals per tbsp
Italian Tarragon Relish 55 kcals per tbsp

Raita 170 kcals (70 kcals if very low-fat yogurt is used)
Olive, Anchovy and Caper Relish 50 kcals per tbsp
Potted Anchovies 390 kcals
Anchovy Paste 60 kcals per tbsp
Hummus 60 kcals per tbsp

Salads and Starters

Mixed Leaf Salad With Feta Cheese and Hazelnuts
185 kcals
Greek Salad 315 kcals
Green Lentil, Ginger and Coriander Salad 265 kcls
Mediterranean Potato Salad 255 kcals
Potato Salad with Lemon and Chives 110 kcals
Salad Niçoise 350 kcals
Tuna and Pasta Salad 220 kcals
Mediterranean Bean Salad 310 kcals
Aromatic Bean Salad 120 kcals
Bean and Fennel Salad 150 kcals
Apple, Walnut and Grape Salad 190 kcals
Mediterranean Rice Salad 200 kcals
Pesto Rice Salad 225 kcals
Pineapple Rice Salad 160 kcals
Avocado, Cheese and Tomato Salad 400 kcals
Hippocratic Salad of Crab, Olives and Toasted Pine Nuts 290 kcals
Aubergine and Olive Salad 180 kcals
Tuna, Pasta and Basil Salad 170 kcals
Waldorf Pasta with Apple, Cheese, Celery and Walnuts 220 kcals
Marinated Herring Salad 300 kcals
Ceviche 160 kcals
Melon, Tomato and Herb Salad 60 kcals
Walnut and Coriander Pâté 300 kcals
Stuffed Vine Leaves (Dolmades) 55 kcals per dolmade

Grilled Jerusalem Artichokes with Feta Cheese 300 kcals

Mediterranean Scallops 160 kcals

Flashed Oysters with Lemon, Garlic and Herbs 50 kcals

Flashed Oysters with Yogurt and Breadcrumbs 25 kcals

Salmon Tartare 120 kcals

Soups

Mediterranean Bean Soup 250 kcals

Mediterranean Fish Soup 380 kcals

Seafood and Sweetcorn Chowder with Dill 240 kcals

Spanish Salad Soup 175 kcals

Tomato, Orange and Ginger Soup 110 kcals

Jerusalem Artichoke and Hazelnut Soup 360 kcals

Mushroom, Garlic and Fennel Soup 160 kcals

French Onion Soup 80 kcals

Lentil and Apricot Soup 290 kcals

Tomato and Garlic Soup 160 kcals

Vegetable, Basil and Garlic Soup 325 kcals

Prawn, Basil and Lemon Grass Soup 75 kcals

Prawn, Avocado and Cucumber Soup 190 kcals

Seafood Recipes

Mediterranean Herb Oil 120 kcals per tbsp

Baked Whole Fish with Lemon and Herbs 385 kcals

Baked Fish with Wine and Garlic 400 kcals

Grilled Fish Steaks with Lemon and Herbs 150 kcals

Bouillabaisse 375 kcals

Mixed Seafood in Tomato, Fennel and Chilli Sauce 380 kcals

Fish in Filo Parcels 330 kcals
Soused Gravadlax Mackerel 340 kcals
Mackerel with Mustard and Herbs 370 kcals
Sicilian Mackerel 435 kcals
Mackerel with Ginger and Fennel 370 kcals
Sardines from Crete 500 kcals
Sardines with Wine and Parsley 400 kcals
Trout Almondine 240 kcals
Grilled Trout with Walnuts and Dill 290 kcals
Baked Orange and Rosemary Trout 225 kcals
Salmon in Dill Sauce 240 kcals
Mediterranean-style Cod 160 kcals
Cod in Yogurt, Tomato and Basil Sauce 170 kcals
Cod in Green Sauce 240 kcals
Grilled Lemon Sole with Coriander and Green Pepper 160 kcals
Sole in Red Grape Sauce 220 kcals
Sea Bass with Fennel 250 kcals
Sea Bass with Spring Onion and Ginger 260 kcals
Pickled Peppered Herrings 230 kcals
Swordfish Steaks with Pink Grapefruit 290 kcals
Mediterranean-style Monkfish 250 kcals
Monkfish and Herb Kebabs 200 kcals
Paella 400 kcals
Drunken Sea Bream with Fennel 250 kcals
Mediterranean-style Red Mullet 350 kcals
Grey Mullet with Herbs and Cheese 300 kcals
Gurnard with Walnut Sauce 500 kcals
John Dory in Orange and Cointreau Sauce 210 kcals
John Dory in Marsala 260 kcals
Poached Turbot with Wine and Lime 160 kcals

Mussels

Moules Marinières 320 kcals

Mussels with Cider, Saffron and Leeks 250 kcals
Greek Mussels 190 kcals
Mussels in Spiced Cream 290 kcals
Mussels in Lemon Cream 315 kcals
Mussels with Coriander, Walnuts and Cheese 65 kcals per mussel
Mussels with Garlic and Parsley 50 kcals per mussel
Genoese Mussels 30 kcals per mussel
Mussels with Basil and Tomato 20 kcals per mussel
Crispy Mussels 35 kcals per mussel

Lobster

Baby Lobster Salad 220 kcals
Lobster Salad with Basil and Strawberries 240 kcals
Tarragon Lobster with Madeira 400 kcals

Chicken

Chicken with Tomato and Basil Sauce 300 kcals
Tarragon Chicken 215 kcals
Chicken Marengo 255 kcals
Coq au Vin Rouge 260 kcals
Chicken with Lemon and Olives 240 kcals
Orange Chicken with Herbs 400 kcals

Lamb

Lamb Shish Kebabs 330 kcals
Lamb and Aubergine Kebabs 330 kcals
Spicy Lamb Kebabs with Lemon Balm 300 kcals
Roast Rosemary and Garlic Lamb with Cannellini Beans 460 kcals

Lamb Lasagna 575 kcals
Mediterranean Moussaka 300 kcals
Lamb with Herbs, Lemon and Black Olives 450 kcals
Lamb Alla Romana 450 kcals
Lamb Curry 525 kcals

Vegetarian Main Courses

Green Herbed Omelette 225 kcals
Ratatouille 120 kcals
Roasted Red Pepper Devils 150 kcals
Aubergines Parmesan 400 kcals
Stuffed Cinnamon Aubergines 160 kcals
Aubergine and Spinach Bake 485 kcals
Italian Pepper Salad (Peperonata) 250 kcals
Peppery Scrambled Eggs (Piperade) 250 kcals
Cheese and Lentil Herb Loaf 330 kcals
Asparagus, Walnut and Mushroom Roast 390 kcals
Mediterranean Fennel Bake 180 kcals
Baked Potatoes with Herbs, Spinach and Cheese
330 kcals
Avocado, Herb and Vegetable Bake 350 kcals
Mediterranean Chickpeas 400 kcals

Pasta

Pasta with Pesto 600 kcals
Pasta with Walnuts and Coriander 575 kcals
Pasta with Fennel and Mixed Mediterranean Herbs
435 kcals
Pasta with Tomato and Mozzarella Sauce 600 kcals
Pasta with Tomato, Cinnamon and Bay 380 kcals
Pasta with Garlic Oil and Chilli 425 kcals
Pasta Al Funghi 450 kcals

Pasta with Mixed Vegetables 475 kcals
Pasta with Lemon Cream 400 kcals
Pasta with Anchovies 600 kcals
Pasta with Smoked Salmon and Fennel 450 kcals
Pasta with Mussels, Tomato and Garlic 450 kcals
Pasta Alla Puttanesca 520 kcals
Pasta with Tomato, Tuna and Parsley Sauce 460 kcals

Pizza

Traditional White Luxury Egg Dough 530 kcals
Basic Pizza Dough 400 kcals
Wholemeal Pizza Dough 320 kcals
Original Tomato and Herb La Marinara 55 kcals topping
Original Cheese and Tomato La Margherita 125 kcals topping
Original Anchovy La Napoletana 180 kcals topping
Original Mushroom Pizza Al Funghi 140 kcals topping
Original Four Seasons Pizza 170 kcals topping

Bread

Coriander and Garlic Pitta Bread 220 kcals
Olive Bread 3170 kcals per large loaf
Walnut Bread 2850 kcals per large loaf
    With Apricots 3010 kcals per large loaf
Olive and Coriander Focaccia
    1689 kcals per large flat loaf
    845 kcals per small flat loaf

Miscellaneous

Apricot Nut Seed Muesli

Makes 700g of muesli mix, enough for 23 × 30g servings of approx 100 kcals each. Top with some of your daily milk allowance or with low-fat fromage frais or yogurt.

    50g rolled oats
    50g toasted wheatflakes
    50g rye flakes
    50g barley flakes
    50g bran buds/flakes
    25g bran
    100g dried apricots, chopped
    50g dried dates, chopped
    50g dried figs, chopped
    25g brazil nuts, chopped
    25g hazelnuts, chopped
    50g walnuts, chopped
    50g pine nuts
    25g sunflower seeds
    25g pumpkin seeds
    25g sesame seeds

1. Mix all ingredients together and store in an air-tight container.
2. Shake well before weighing out each serving as the bran tends to settle to the bottom.

Mixed Seeds and Nuts to Sprinkle on Salads

    50g sunflower seeds, toasted and/or raw
    50g pumpkin seeds, toasted and/or raw
    100g mixed nuts

50g pine kernels
50g sesame seeds, toasted
50g poppy seeds

Makes enough for approx 70 tablespoons of mixed nuts/seeds to sprinkle on salads at approx 25 kcals per tablespoon.

Scrambled Eggs with Red Pepper and Tomato

Makes 4 small (1 egg) portions at 120 kcals each.
　　2 tsp extra virgin olive oil
　　2 clove garlic, crushed
　　1 red pepper, cut into strips
　　1 beef tomato, chopped
　　4 x size 1 eggs, beaten
　　Freshly ground black pepper

　　Garnish: fresh parsley

1. Lightly brush the base of a saucepan with olive oil.
2. Fry the garlic, red pepper and tomato until soft.
3. Add the beaten eggs and continue to cook, stirring all the time with a wooden spatula to scramble the egg.
4. Season well with black pepper and garnish with parsley.

Kedgeree

Serves 4 at approx 325 kcals each.
　　400g cooked brown rice
　　4 hard-boiled eggs, chopped
　　300g flaked smoked haddock (colouring free)
　　4 tbsp fresh parsley, chopped
　　4 tbsp fresh coriander, chopped

254

4 spring onions, finely chopped
4 tsp garam massala (or freshly ground curry powder)
150g light fromage frais
Freshly ground black pepper

Garnish: watercress, grated nutmeg and fresh lemon juice

1. Mix all ingredients well and serve piled onto a platter.
2. Garnish with watercress and grated nutmeg and sprinkle with lemon juice.
NB: The recipe on Day 30 of the Mediterranean Slim Diet is slightly lower in calories as it contains less smoked haddock.

Sauces, Dips and Mayonnaise

Garlic Mayonnaise (Aïoli)

This Provençal garlic mayonnaise is stirred into soups or stews at the table to add an extra bite to meals. Go easy on aïoli of you're watching calories as the sting in the tail is the calorie count– approx 120 kcals per tablespoon for either version.

Version 1
   8 cloves garlic
   2 egg yolks
   450ml extra virgin olive oil
   Juice of 1 lemon
   Rock salt and freshly ground black pepper

1. Crush the garlic in a pestle and mortar.
2. With a hand whisk, stir in the egg yolks.
3. Drizzle in the olive oil, whisking continuously until you have a thick, yellow, aromatic mayonnaise. Stir in the lemon juice and season with salt and pepper to taste.

Alternatively, place all ingredients except the olive oil into a liquidizer. Turn on and drizzle the oil in slowly.

Version 2
  2 thick slices of white bread, crusts removed
  60ml (4tbsp) semi-skimmed milk
  8 cloves garlic, crushed
  300ml extra virgin olive oil
  Rock salt and freshly ground black pepper

1. Soak the bread in milk for five minutes.
2. Squeeze out excess liquid and place the bread in a mortar or liquidizer with the garlic.
3. Crush with a pestle or blend together. Slowly drizzle in the olive oil until you have a thick sauce. Season to taste.

This bread–based sauce may separate, in which case either add 1 tbsp boiling water and beat vigorously, or beat in 2 egg yolks.

Chilli Mayonnaise (Rouille)

This Provençal chilli sauce is used to spice up soups and stews. It is often stirred into fish soups with Aïoli and croûtons.

Version 1
Approx 60 kcals per tablespoon.
  3 cloves garlic, crushed
  1 slice bread, crusts removed
  30ml (2 tbsp) semi-skimmed milk
  2 hot, red fresh chilli peppers, seeded and finely chopped
  45ml (3 tbsp) extra virgin olive oil
  Rock salt and freshly ground black pepper

1. Crush the garlic to a paste in a pestle and mortar.

2. Add the bread and chopped chillies and pound until smooth.

3. Whisk in the olive oil until the mixture is smooth, red and shiny with the texture of French mustard. Season to taste.

Version 2

Approx 95 kcals per tablespoon.

2 hot red fresh chilli peppers, seeded and finely chopped
or 2 dried red chillies, soaked to soften and seeded
2 cloves garlic, crushed
½ small sweet red pepper, seeded and chopped
2 egg yolks
250ml extra virgin olive oil
Rock salt and freshly ground black pepper

1. Pound or blend together the chillies, garlic and red pepper.

2. Stir in the egg yolks and seasoning.

3. Slowly whisk in the olive oil until a sauce with the consistency of mayonnaise is obtained.

Pesto Sauce

Truly the food of the Gods. This is so lovely and addictive you will find yourself eating it straight from the bowl. Pesto can be stirred into soups or stews or used as a delicious dressing on pasta or potatoes. Approx 120 kcals per tablespoon.

Pesto can be sweetened slightly by adding the mashed flesh of one grilled beef tomato, to make red pesto sauce.

50g fresh basil leaves, washed and dried without bruising
3 cloves garlic, crushed
50g pine kernels or walnuts, chopped
30g Parmesan cheese, freshly grated
30g Pecorino cheese (or more Parmesan), freshly grated

180ml extra virgin olive oil
Rock salt and freshly ground black pepper

For a smooth sauce:
1. Place the basil, salt, pepper and garlic in a blender and reduce to a smooth, green purée.
2. Add the pine kernels and cheese and blend slightly.
3. Drizzle in the olive oil until you have a smooth, creamy textured sauce.

For a coarser textured sauce:
1. Grind the basil leaves against the side of a marble pestle with a wooden mortar.
2. Add the garlic and crush together with a little olive oil.
3. Add the pine kernels and crush together with more olive oil.
4. Pound in the cheese and the remaining olive oil. Season to taste.

Greek Almond and Garlic Relish (Skordalia)

This Greek garlic sauce is traditionally used to enliven plain, grilled fish or boiled prawns. It can also be spooned over vegetables and potatoes. Approx 75 kcals per table-spoon.

1 slice white bread, crusts removed
30ml (2 tbsp) white wine vinegar
4 large cloves garlic, crushed
150ml extra virgin olive oil
100g ground almonds
Rock salt and freshly ground black pepper

1. Soak the bread in the vinegar.
2. Crush the garlic to a purée in a pestle and mortar or blender.
3. Stir in the oil, a little at a time.

4. Blend in the soaked bread and ground almonds. Season to taste.

Greek Barbecue Marinade (Salmoriglio)

This oil and lemon sauce from southern Italy is brushed over fish or meat during barbecuing or grilling. It gives a fresh, lemony tang and prevents the flesh drying out. It can also be used as a quick marinade for fish. Approx 120 kcals per tablespoon.

250ml extra virgin olive oil
Freshly squeezed juice of 2 lemons
2 cloves garlic, crushed
1 tbsp fresh lemon thyme, lemon balm or oregano, chopped
1 tbsp fresh parsley, chopped
Rock salt and freshly ground black pepper

1. Whisk the oil until it begins to thicken.
2. Add in the lemon juice, garlic and fresh herbs and continue whisking.
3. Season to taste, pour into a saucepan and warm over a low heat whilst using to baste as required.

Walnut Sauce

This sauce can be used to stuff pasta shapes, to dress pasta or as a dip for vegetable crudités. Approx 60 kcals per tablespoon.

1 slice white bread, crusts removed
45ml (3 tbsp) semi-skimmed milk
225g walnuts
2 cloves garlic, crushed
2 tbsp extra virgin olive oil
2 tbsp walnut oil
4 tbsp thick fromage frais

Rock salt and freshly ground black pepper

1. Soak the bread in the milk, then squeeze out excess liquid.
2. Crush the walnuts in a pestle or blender until finely ground.
3. Blend in the bread, crushed garlic, oils and fromage frais. Mix well to achieve a homogenous sauce. If you are using the sauce to dress rather than stuff pasta and it seems too dry, add a little extra walnut or olive oil. Season to taste.

Italian Olive Relish (Aulivi Cunsati)

A Sicilian olive sauce used to accompany grilled fish or meat. This is best made one or two days in advance so the flavours can infuse. Approx 40 kcals per tablespoon.

    400g green olives, stoned and crushed
    3 tbsp fresh dill weed, finely chopped
    1 tbsp chives, finely chopped
    Newly sprouted tops of 6 mint sprigs, finely chopped
    4 cloves garlic, crushed
    ½ inch ginger root, finely chopped
    2 celery sticks, finely chopped
    ½ red chilli pepper, seeded and finely chopped
    150ml (10 tbsp) extra virgin olive oil
    5 tbsp balsamic vinegar
    1 tbsp acacia honey
    Rock salt and freshly ground black pepper

1. Place all the ingredients in an earthenware bowl and mix thoroughly. If preferred, blend to a smooth paste in a liquidizer.
2. Cover and leave to stand, if possible, for 24 hours.
3. Stir again just before serving.

Italian Tarragon Relish (Salsa di Dragoncello)

This recipe from Sienna is delicious spooned over boiled potatoes or as an accompaniment to grilled meat or fish. It is especially good with barbecued chicken. Approx 55 kcals per tablespoon.

    2 slices white bread, crusts removed
    45ml (3 tbsp) balsamic or tarragon vinegar
    A handful of fresh tarragon leaves, finely chopped
    2 cloves garlic, crushed
    120ml (8 tbsp) extra virgin olive oil
    Freshly ground black pepper

1. Soak the bread in the vinegar, then place in a blender.
2. Add the chopped tarragon and garlic and blend.
3. Drizzle in the olive oil until you have a smooth, even sauce. Season with plenty of black pepper.

Raita

This eastern Mediterranean dip can be served as a salad, a sauce with grilled fish or curries and as a dip with vegetable crudités. It may also be diluted with chilled water and served as a summer soup. Divided into four servings, the calorie count is approx 170 kcals each (70 kcals if very low-fat yogurt is used instead). Serves 4.

    1 medium cucumber, peeled and grated
    3 cloves garlic, crushed
    2 tbsp fresh mint, chopped
    1 tbsp chives, chopped
    1 tbsp freshly squeezed lemon juice
    500ml strained Greek yogurt
    1 tsp acacia honey (optional)
    Rock salt and freshly ground black pepper
    Freshly ground nutmeg

1. Mix all ingredients together in an earthenware bowl.
2. Season with salt and black pepper to taste. Serve topped with freshly ground nutmeg.

Olive, Anchovy and Caper Relish (Tapenade)

This strongly flavoured sauce has a beautiful, purple colour and is a good alternative to caviar. Spread tapenade on toast, stir into fish soups or serve as an accompaniment to boiled eggs. Makes about 300ml. Approx 50 kcals per tablespoon.

   100g ripe black olives, stoned
   10 canned anchovy fillets, drained
   3 tbsp capers
   120ml (8 tbsp) extra virgin olive oil
   30ml (2 tbsp) French brandy
   15ml (1 tbsp) freshly squeezed lemon juice
   Freshly ground black pepper

1. Place the olives, anchovies and capers in a blender with 2 tbsp olive oil. Start to blend.
2. Slowly drizzle in the remaining olive oil until the mixture starts to thicken.
3. Add the brandy and lemon juice. Season to taste.

Potted Anchovies (Bagna Cauda)

This hot anchovy dip from Piedmont, northern Italy, is literally called a 'hot bath'. It is served with bread sticks (grissini) and large quantities of fresh crudités, including chicory, celery, fennel, red and yellow peppers, carrot, radishes and broccoli. *Bagna cauda* is also added to scrambled eggs to create a spicy lunch. Approx 390 kcals per serving if all the oil is eaten. Serves 4.

12 cloves of garlic, peeled and finely sliced
45ml (3 tbsp) semi-skimmed milk
12 large, salted anchovies, soaked and filleted *or*
2 x 50g cans of anchovy fillets in olive oil
40g olive oil spread
75ml (5 tbsp) extra virgin olive oil (to include the canned anchovy oil)
75ml (5 tbsp) walnut oil (or more olive oil if preferred)

1. Simmer the garlic with the milk until soft – be careful not to burn.
2. Add the chopped flesh of the anchovy fillets, plus a little olive oil.
3. Keeping the heat low, stir and mash the anchovies until they start to disintegrate.
4. Add the olive oil spread and slowly pour in the remaining olive oil to form a brown sauce under a layer of oil.
5. Bring the sauce to the boil and place in a small fondue pot over a burner or nightlight.
6. To eat, dip bread sticks and vegetables into the hot oil, stirring up the sauce sediment.

Anchovy Paste (Anchoïade)

This delicious sauce is an excellent alternative for lovers of gentleman's relish or yeast extract spreads. Spread over hot toast and serve as an aperitif. Anchoïade is traditionally served with celery and boiled eggs. Approx 60 kcals per tablespoon.

12 large, salted anchovies, soaked and filleted, *or*
2 x 50g tins anchovy fillets, drained
2 cloves garlic, crushed
½ tsp red wine vinegar
Freshly ground black pepper
60ml (4 tbsp) extra virgin olive oil (or oil from anchovy cans)

1. Pound together or mash the anchovy fillets, garlic and vinegar.

2. Add drizzles of olive oil until a coarse paste of the desired consistency is obtained. Season to taste.

Hummus

This chickpea and sesame dip is often served with vegetable crudités or as part of a Greek meze course. The dried chickpeas should be soaked in water overnight or until their weight has more or less doubled. Approx 60 kcals per tablespoon.

150g dried chickpeas, soaked overnight
3 tbsp extra virgin olive oil
Freshly squeezed juice and zest of 2 lemons
3 cloves garlic, crushed
120g tahini (sesame) paste
Rock salt and freshly ground black pepper

Garnish: chopped parsley or paprika pepper

1. After soaking the chickpeas, change their water and simmer for 1½ hours or until soft. Drain, saving the liquor residue.

2. Put 5 tbsp cooking liquor in a blender with the olive oil, lemon juice, zest and garlic. Start to blend.

3. Add the chickpeas and tahini paste slowly. If the blender clogs, add more liquor until a grainy, creamy purée is obtained.

4. Season to taste. More olive oil or tahini paste can be added to vary the flavour as desired.

Salads and Starters

These recipes may be served as healthy starters, as a main

course with lots of hot, crusty bread, or as part of a selection in a buffet-style lunch.

Try adding edible flower heads to salad leaves for a welcome splash of colour. Petals you can safely use after thorough washing include: nasturtium, bergamot, borage, calendula, chives, clove pinks, violets, pansies, primroses, rose, marigold, sunflower, meadow crane's-bill, lawn daisy. Don't use flower heads that have been sprayed with fertiliser or pesticides.

Mixed Leaf Salad with Feta Cheese and Hazelnuts

Absolutely delicious. Makes enough for 4 at approx 185 kcals each.

225g mixed salad leaves
A handful of flat leaf parsley
A handful of coriander
50g crumbled Feta cheese
120g newly sprouted pulses, e.g. bean shoots, alfalfa
50g roasted hazelnuts, crushed

Minimal Dressing
1 tbsp hazelnut, extra virgin olive oil or walnut oil
1 tbsp lemon juice or herb vinegar
1 tbsp whole grain mustard
1 clove garlic, crushed
1 tsp acacia honey
Rock salt and freshly ground black pepper

1. Combine all the salad ingredients in a serving bowl and mix well, being careful not to bruise the leaves.
2. Mix the salad dressing ingredients thoroughly. Season to taste.
3. Pour the dressing over the salad, toss and serve immediately.

Greek Salad

A traditional Greek salad makes a satisfying meal. It can be made quickly and goes well with pitta bread or boiled new potatoes and fish. Serves 4 at approx 315 kcals each (this could be reduced by using less olive oil in the dressing).

225g mixed green salad leaves
8 whole radishes, trimmed
12 black olives, rinsed and stoned
12 green olives, rinsed and stoned
1 red onion, thinly sliced and separated into rings
1 red sweet pepper, seeded and cut into strips
1 green pepper, seeded and cut into strips
¼ cucumber, thinly sliced
8–12 sweet baby tomatoes
1 can anchovy fillets, drained and rinsed
225g Feta cheese

Dressing
1 tbsp red wine vinegar
3 tbsp extra virgin olive oil
1 clove garlic, crushed
1 tsp whole grain mustard
1 tsp acacia honey
1 tbsp mixed fresh herbs, chopped (parsley, basil, oregano, thyme)
Rock salt and freshly ground black pepper

1. Arrange all the salad ingredients, except the anchovies, in a large, wooden bowl.
2. To make the vinaigrette place all dressing ingredients in a screw-topped jar and shake vigorously. Pour over the salad ingredients and toss well.
3. Decorate the salad with a lattice of anchovy fillets.

Green Lentil, Ginger and Coriander Salad

This salad is best made while the cooked, green lentils are still hot so the flavours infuse. It can be served warm with fish or chicken dishes, or allowed to chill when the flavours have marinated. The amount of ginger, lemon juice and coriander leaves can be varied according to personal preference. Serves 4 at approx 265 kcals per portion.

225g green lentils
1 large carrot, grated
45ml (3 tbsp) extra virgin olive oil
1 medium onion, finely chopped
2 cloves garlic, crushed
30ml (2 tbsp) freshly squeezed lemon (or lime) juice
1 tbsp coriander seed, crushed
1–2 tbsp fresh coriander, finely chopped
2.5cm (1 inch) piece fresh root ginger, peeled and finely chopped

1. Simmer the lentils in 600ml water for around 30 minutes, until they are cooked but still firm. Add the grated carrot and cook for a further five minutes. Drain.
2. Heat half the olive oil and fry the onion, garlic and crushed coriander seeds until beginning to colour.
3. Add the fried onion mixture and the remaining ingredients to the drained lentils. Mix well and season to taste. If serving hot, keep warm for flavours to infuse.

Mediterranean Potato Salad

The potatoes are best dressed with vinaigrette while still hot so the flavours can penetrate the flesh. The warm potato salad can be served plain at this stage if wished. Alternatively, leave to cool, then add the red pepper, olives and eggs for a delicious potato salad with a difference. Serves 4 at approx 255 kcals each.

    450g potatoes
    ½ sweet red pepper, seeded and coarsely chopped
    2 hard-boiled eggs, shelled and coarsely chopped
    8 black olives, rinsed, stoned and finely chopped
    Rock salt and freshly ground black pepper

Dressing
    4 tbsp extra virgin olive oil
    2 tbsp freshly squeezed lemon juice
    1 tsp whole-grain mustard
    1 clove garlic, crushed
    1 tbsp chopped, fresh coriander (or basil, parsley, etc.)
    3 spring onions, finely chopped

    Garnish: Coriander leaves; black olives; mustard and cress

1. If using new potatoes leave their skins on, otherwise peel. Cut the potatoes into chunks and boil for 15 to 20 minutes until cooked but firm. Drain.
2. Combine the dressing ingredients and mix well. Pour onto the hot potatoes and toss.
3. Season to taste and, if desired, serve hot at this point.
4. Alternatively, allow to cool. Then add the chopped boiled eggs, red pepper and olives. Garnish with feathery coriander leaves and olives.

Potato Salad with Lemon and Chives

Serves 4 at approx 110 kcals each.
    450g unpeeled new potatoes
    1 large sprig of fresh mint
    2 tbsp fresh chives, chopped
    4 spring onions, chopped

Dressing
1 clove garlic, crushed
1 tbsp freshly squeezed lemon juice and grated zest
150ml light fromage frais
Rock salt and freshly ground black pepper

1. Boil the new potatoes with the mint until just tender. Drain and discard the mint.
2. Mix together the dressing ingredients and pour over the potatoes whilst they are still hot.
3. Sprinkle on the chives and spring onions. Serve hot or cold.

Salad Niçoise

This classic dish from Nice makes a satisfying and filling lunch, or a tantalizing hors d'oeuvres. Serves 4 at approx 350 kcals each.

450g French green beans, topped and tailed
2 little gem lettuce hearts
8 small, boiled new potatoes (cold), halved
200g tuna fish in olive oil, drained
2 hard-boiled eggs, shelled and chopped
8 sweet baby tomatoes
8 black olives, stoned and halved
1 small onion, thinly sliced and separated into rings
1 small can anchovy fillets, drained and rinsed
Several flat parsley leaves
Several coriander leaves
A few chives

Dressing
4 tbsp extra virgin olive oil
1–2 tbsp balsamic vinegar
1 clove garlic, crushed
1 tsp whole grain mustard
1 tsp acacia honey

1 tbsp fresh parsley, finely chopped
1 tbsp fresh basil, finely chopped
Rock salt and freshly ground black pepper

1. Cut the green beans in half longways, and steam for 5 to 10 minutes until tender but still crisp. Drain, and plunge into ice cold water.

2, Place all the salad dressing ingredients in a screw-topped jar. Season and shake well.

3. Line a salad bowl with lettuce leaves. Arrange the potatoes and green beans on top.

4. Pile the tuna fish into the middle of the bowl. Decorate round the edges with chopped egg, tomatoes, black olives and onion. Make a lattice of anchovy fillets over the top.

5. Shake the salad dressing and drizzle all over. Garnish with chives, coriander and parsley.

Tuna and Pasta Salad

Serves 4 as a starter at approx 110 kcals each or 2 as a lunch at approx 220 kcals each.

225g mixed salad leaves
1 x 200g fresh tuna steak, grilled with herbs and lemon juice and allowed to cool, then flaked or
200g tinned tuna chunks in brine, drained
225g cooked, wholemeal pasta shapes
100g low-fat, natural cottage cheese
1 beef tomato, chopped
2 spring onions, chopped
2 tbsp fresh parsley, chopped
1 tbsp freshly squeezed lemon juice
4 tbsp light fromage frais
Freshly ground black pepper

1. Mix all ingredients except the salad leaves together and season well.

2. Arrange the salad leaves in a bowl and top with the tuna and pasta mixture.

Aromatic Bean Salad

Serves 4 at approx 120 kcals each.
    400g cooked mixed beans
    1 beef tomato, chopped
    2 cloves garlic, crushed
    2 tbsp fresh coriander, chopped
    A few coriander seeds, crushed
    2 tbsp fresh parsley, chopped
    2 tbsp freshly squeezed lemon juice
    2 tbsp freshly squeezed orange juice
    4 tbsp light fromage frais
    Rock salt and freshly ground black pepper

Mix together all ingredients and season well.

Bean and Fennel Salad

Serves 4 at approx 150 kcals each.
    400g cooked flageolet beans
    200g Florence fennel, chopped into matchsticks
    100g carrot, grated
    1 tsp fresh ginger root, grated
    2 tbsp fresh dill, chopped
    2 tbsp fresh parsley, chopped
    2 tbsp freshly squeezed lemon juice
    2 cloves garlic, crushed
    1 tbsp extra virgin olive oil
    Freshly ground black pepper

Mix together all ingredients and allow to marinate for several hours before eating.

271

Apple, Walnut and Grape Salad

Serves 4 at approx 190 kcals each.
  225g mixed leaf salad
  2 large red apples, cored and diced
  4 sticks celery, chopped
  50g walnuts, chopped
  100g seedless red grapes, halved

Dressing
150ml natural, low-fat bio yogurt
2 spring onions, finely chopped
1 clove garlic, crushed
Freshly squeezed juice of one lemon
2 tbsp fresh parsley, chopped
Freshly ground black pepper

1. Mix all the salad ingredients together.
2. Mix together the salad dressing ingredients and stir well. Pour over the salad and serve immediately.

Mediterranean Bean Salad

This bean salad was supposedly a favourite of Napoleon while he was in exile on the island of St. Helena. Serves 4 at approx 310 kcals per portion.
  225g dried haricot or cannellini beans, soaked overnight
  1 bay leaf
  1 sprig rosemary
  1 sprig thyme
  1 carrot, grated
  4 spring onions, finely chopped
  1 tbsp fresh parsley, chopped
  1 tbsp fresh basil, chopped
  1 tbsp fresh tarragon, chopped
  1 tbsp fresh oregano, chopped

Dressing

4 tbsp extra virgin olive oil
1 tbsp balsamic or tarragon vinegar
1 tsp whole grain mustard
1 tsp acacia honey
Rock salt and freshly ground black pepper

1. Bring 600ml water to the boil. Add the beans, bayleaf, rosemary and thyme. Cover and simmer for 1½ to 2 hours until cooked. Top up with water if necessary to prevent boiling dry. Drain and discard the boiled herbs.
2. Mix the salad dressing ingredients in a screw-top jar and shake well. Season to taste.
3. Combine the beans, grated carrot, chopped spring onions and remaining herbs. Pour over the dressing. Mix well.
4. Cover with cling film, allow to cool, then refrigerate before serving.

Mediterranean Rice Salad

Serves 4 at approx 200 kcals each.

400g cooked brown rice
1 red pepper, chopped
4 spring onions, finely chopped
100g cooked fresh new broad beans (not frozen)
30 black olives, stoned and chopped

Dressing

150ml low-fat, natural bio yogurt
1 tbsp fresh lemon juice
2 tbsp fresh parsley, chopped
1 tbsp fresh mint, chopped
1 tbsp fresh coriander leaf, chopped
1 tbsp fresh oregano, chopped
Freshly ground black pepper

1. Mix together the rice and other salad ingredients.
2. Mix together the salad dressing ingredients, stir well and season. Pour dressing over rice salad and mix together.

Pesto Rice Salad

Serves 4 at approx 225 kcals each.
   2 cloves garlic, crushed
   30g pine nuts (or walnuts), chopped
   4 tbsp fresh basil leaves, chopped
   4 tbsp freshly squeezed lemon juice
   4 tbsp light fromage frais
   400g cooked brown rice
   30g Parmesan cheese, freshly grated

1. Pound together the garlic, nuts and basil with the lemon juice and fromage frais.
2. Mix well with the rice and Parmesan cheese.

Pineapple Rice Salad

Serves 4 at approx 160 kcals each.
   400g cooked brown rice
   1 green pepper, chopped
   100g fresh pineapple, skinned and chopped
   4 tbsp freshly chopped mixed herbs
   4 tbsp light fromage frais
   Freshly ground black pepper

Mix together all the ingredients. Season well with black pepper.

Avocado, Cheese and Tomato Salad

This delightfully simple dish is made in minutes. Serves 4 at approx 400 kcals each.

    2 avocados, peeled, stoned and cut in half
    2 beef tomatoes, sliced
    120g Gouda cheese with cumin seeds (or Mozzarella), sliced

Dressing
    2 tbsp walnut oil
    1 tbsp freshly squeezed lemon juice
    1 tbsp fresh basil, finely chopped
    Rock salt and freshly ground black pepper

1. Incompletely slice the avocado halves lengthways, leaving the last 1cm (½ inch) at the narrowest end intact. Place upside down on individual serving plates. Apply pressure to the cut end so the avocado slices separate and form a fan-shape.
2. Tuck alternating slices of tomato and cheese between the avocado fan slices.
3. Combine the dressing ingredients in a screw-top jar, season well and shake. Drizzle over the avocado halves.

Hippocratic Salad of Crab, Olives and Toasted Pine Nuts

I enjoyed this unusual salad on the island of Kos whilst admiring Hippocrates' tree and re-affirming my oath. Serves 4 at approx 290 kcals each.

    50g pine nuts
    225g mixed lettuce leaves
    225g cold, small new potatoes, cooked in their skins and halved
    30g black olives, stoned and finely chopped

225g fresh crab meat

Dressing
2 tbsp extra virgin olive oil
1 tbsp white wine vinegar
1 tsp wholegrain mustard
1 spring onion, finely chopped
1 tsp acacia honey
Rock salt and freshly ground black pepper

Garnish: freshly chopped parsley

1. Gently toast the pine nuts until slightly coloured. Sprinkle with salt and leave to cool.
2. Mix all the dressing ingredients in a screw-topped jar, season and shake well.
3. Toss the mixed lettuce leaves in a bowl with a third of the dressing.
4. Arrange the halved, new potatoes on top and coat with half the remaining dressing.
5. Mix the remaining dressing and olives into the crab meat and pile on top of the potatoes. Garnish with toasted pine nuts and chopped parsley. Serve immediately.

Aubergine and Olive Salad

An unusual salad served by one of the best bistros in Nice. Serves 4 at approx 180 kcals each.

450g aubergines, cubed
4 tbsp extra virgin olive oil
1 medium onion, chopped
1 chilli pepper, seeded and chopped
50g pickled onions, chopped
50g pickled gherkins, chopped
30g capers
2 tsp acacia honey
4 tbsp red wine vinegar

1 tbsp pine kernels
50g green olives, stoned
1 tsp fresh basil leaves, chopped
1 tsp fresh dill weed, chopped
Rock salt and freshly ground black pepper

1. Sweat the aubergines in olive oil until soft and starting to brown. Remove with a slotted spoon and dry on absorbent paper.
2. Fry the onions, chilli pepper, pickled onions, gherkins and capers for 5 minutes. Add the honey and vinegar and cook for a further 5 minutes.
3. Add the aubergines, pine kernels, olives and chopped herbs. Season. Serve warm or cold.

Tuna, Pasta and Basil Salad

A simple, filling and tasty salad for lunch. Serves 4 at approx 170 kcals each.

200g tuna, drained and flaked
100g low-fat cottage cheese
1 beef tomato, chopped
1 tbsp fresh basil, chopped
1 tbsp fresh parsley, chopped
350g cold, cooked pasta
Freshly ground black pepper

1. Combine the tuna, cottage cheese, tomato and herbs and season well.
2. Add the pasta and toss to mix all ingredients.

Waldorf Pasta with Apple, Cheese, Celery and Walnuts

A filling and delicious salad for lunch. Serves 4 at approx 220 kcals each.

    1 large red apple, cored and chopped
    1 tbsp freshly squeezed lemon juice
    350g cold, cooked pasta
    100g low-fat cottage cheese
    50g Parmesan cheese, freshly grated
    2 sticks celery, chopped
    30g chopped walnuts
    Several coriander leaves, roughly shredded
    1 tbsp fresh parsley, chopped
    Freshly ground black pepper

1. Toss the chopped apple with lemon juice to prevent discoloration.
2. Add all the remaining ingredients, toss and season well.

Marinated Herring Salad

An unusual, hot marinated dish. Provides 8 servings at approx 300 kcals per serving. This will keep for several days in the fridge.

    8 x 100g herring fillets

Marinade
    300ml dry white wine
    4 tbsp white wine vinegar
    1 tsp acacia honey
    2 large spring onions, finely chopped
    1 bay leaf
    12 peppercorns, green, red and black mixed, crushed
    1 tbsp fresh dill weed, chopped

Dressing

300ml Greek strained yogurt
1–2 tbsp freshly squeezed lemon juice
2 tbsp wholegrain mustard
1 tbsp acacia honey
Rock salt and freshly ground black pepper

Garnish: freshly chopped dill weed

1. Place all the marinade ingredients in a saucepan. Cover and simmer gently for 20 minutes.
2. Place the herring fillets in a shallow dish and pour over the boiling marinade. Cover and leave until cold.
3. Remove the fish and skin the fillets. Chop into bite-sized chunks or leave whole as desired.
4. Mix the yogurt, lemon juice, mustard and honey together, seasoning to taste.
5. Pour the yogurt mixture over the herring fillets and serve chilled with salad and boiled potatoes.

Ceviche

Ceviche is a delicious concoction of marinated raw fish. The cod must be very fresh – caught that morning rather than shrink-wrapped and bought from a supermarket several days old. The fish is left to marinate in the fridge overnight, ready for an unusual lunch next day. Serves 4 at approx 160 kcals each.

445g very fresh cod

Marinade

1 tbsp onion, finely chopped
1 green chilli, seeded and chopped
150ml freshly squeezed mixed lemon and lime juice
Rock salt and freshly ground black pepper

Salad

2 tbsp extra virgin olive oil

1 green pepper, seeded and sliced
1 beef tomato, chopped
1 tbsp fresh parsley, chopped
1 tbsp fresh coriander, chopped
2 large spring onions, finely chopped

1. Skin and bone the cod. Cut into goujons 1cm (½ inch) wide and 4–6 cm (1½–2½ inch) long. Arrange in a shallow dish with the onion and chilli. Season well.
2. Pour over the lemon and lime juice and mix well. Refrigerate for at least 12 hours, preferably overnight. Turn occasionally.
3. When serving, remove the fish from the lemon/lime juice. Pour over the olive oil and turn the fish to coat fully.
4. Add the herbs and sliced salad ingredients. Serve with crisp iceberg lettuce and crusty bread.

Melon, Tomato and Herb Salad

Deliciously cooling on a hot summer's day. Serves 4 at approx 60 kcals each.

225g cantaloupe melon
1 beef tomato, chopped into chunks
100g peeled cucumber, grated
2–4 tbsp freshly chopped fragrant herbs (mint, lemon balm, basil)
300ml low-fat, natural bio yogurt
Freshly ground black pepper

1. Remove the melon flesh using a melon baller or by cutting into bite-sized chunks.
2. Combine the melon, tomato and cucumber and mix well.
3. Add the herbs to the yogurt and season to taste with black pepper.

4. Arrange the fruit in bowls and spoon on the yogurt and herb mix. Garnish with dainty sprigs of herb leaves.

Walnut and Coriander Pâté

This delicious pâté is best served chilled with wholegrain toast and watercress. Serves 4 at approx 300 kcals each.

100g walnuts
30g sesame seeds
175g thick fromage frais (or cream cheese)
2 cloves garlic, crushed
1 tbsp fresh coriander, chopped
1 tbsp walnut oil
2 tbsp semi-skimmed milk
Rock salt and freshly ground black pepper

1. Lightly toast the walnuts and sesame seeds for 5 minutes under the grill.
2. Grind the nuts and seeds in a pestle and mortar until coarse. Remove half the mix and continue grinding the other half until fine.
3. Mix together the fromage frais, garlic and coriander. Season well.
4. Moisten the nuts with the walnut oil then add to the fromage frais mixture. Thin with a little milk if necessary. Chill before serving.

Other combinations of nuts and herbs can be used, e.g. hazelnut and dill, hazelnut and oregano, almond and lemon balm, or walnut, hazelnut and sage. Alternatively, use whatever is at hand.

Stuffed Vine Leaves (Dolmades)

A classic Mediterranean dish – a little fiddly to make but worth the effort. The broken leaves used to line the base of the pan become sweet, sour and tangy. Although many cooks discard them, they are one of the most delicious parts of this dish. Approx 55 kcals per dolmade. Makes 20.

20 large, whole vine leaves

Filling

1 medium onion, finely chopped
1 clove garlic, crushed
1 tbsp extra virgin olive oil
150g long grain rice
1 tbsp tomato paste
1 tsp fresh mint or fresh rosemary, finely chopped
1 tsp fresh dill weed or thyme, finely chopped
¼ tsp powdered cinnamon
Pinch of grated nutmeg
½ tsp fresh ginger root, chopped
30g pine kernels or chopped walnuts
30g raisins
1 tsp honey
Juice of half a lemon
Rock salt and freshly ground black pepper

Cooking juice

Several broken vine leaf pieces
Juice of half a lemon
1 tbsp extra virgin olive oil
1 tsp honey
1 clove garlic, crushed
150ml water

1. If using fresh vine leaves, soften them in boiling, salted water for one minute. If using pickled leaves, wash them under a running tap, then soak them in water for at least five minutes. Cut off any stalks and carefully open out the leaves.
2. Fry the onion and garlic in the olive oil until starting to colour. Stir in the rice, tomato paste and 150ml water. Simmer until all the liquid is absorbed.

3. Add the remaining filling ingredients, season to taste and mix well.

4. Place a tablespoon of rice filling on the centre of each vine leaf. Roll up loosely, as the rice will continue to swell with further cooking.

5. Line a large frying pan with the broken vine leaves. In a cup, mix together the lemon juice, oil, garlic and honey.

6. Arrange the stuffed vine leaves in the frying pan, forming two layers if necessary. Spoon over the cooking juice.

7. Pour over 150ml water. Cover and weight the dolmades with a plate and simmer for a further 30 minutes. Add extra water if the pan becomes dry. Cook further until the rice is fully cooked, depending on the type used. Serve hot, as a starter or main course with salad and natural yogurt, or cold, as a starter or aperitif.

Grilled Jerusalem Artichokes with Feta Cheese

Since I discovered this recipe in a dimly lit restaurant, it has become a favourite starter. The artichokes should be eaten immediately as they will rapidly discolour on exposure to air. Serves 4 at approx 300 kcals each.

225g mixed lettuce leaves
4 large Jerusalem artichokes, as un-knobbly as possible
50g hazelnuts, crushed
200g Greek feta cheese
1 tbsp extra virgin olive oil, for basting

Dressing
1 tbsp extra virgin olive oil
1 tbsp hazelnut oil
1 tbsp garlic vinegar
1 tsp acacia honey
Rock salt and freshly ground black pepper

Garnish: freshly chopped parsley

1. Cook the artichokes in boiling water until tender. Meanwhile, place all ingredients for the dressing in a screw-top jar and shake well. Season to taste.

2. Cut the cooked artichokes in half and place upside down on a grill pan. Brush with olive oil and grill under a high heat until beginning to blacken.

3. Turn the artichoke halves the right way up and brush the cut surfaces with olive oil. Grill until beginning to blacken. They will start to puff up and may ooze slightly. Meanwhile, toast the hazelnuts under the grill.

4. Arrange the lettuce leaves on individual plates. Dot with feta cheese and pour over the dressing. Add the artichoke halves, sprinkle them with toasted hazelnuts and garnish with plenty of chopped parsley.

Mediterranean Scallops

A quick, aromatic dish. Do not overcook the scallops or they will toughen and become rubbery. Serves 4 as a starter (160 kcals) or 2 as a main course (320 kcals each).

    16 medium scallops
    4 tbsp extra virgin olive oil
    4 cloves garlic, crushed
    1 tsp coriander seeds, crushed
    1 sprig rosemary
    1 bay leaf
    1 tsp fresh parsley, chopped
    1 tsp fresh basil, chopped
    1 tsp fresh coriander leaves, chopped
    2 tbsp freshly squeezed lemon juice

1. Remove the scallops from their shells and tear away any black bits. Cut the scallops in half horizontally and rinse well.

2. Heat the oil in a heavy-based frying pan. Add the garlic

and crushed coriander seeds. Fry until the garlic is just turning golden.

3. Add the fresh herbs and scallops and stir continuously until the scallop flesh just sets, turning from translucent to opaque white. This doesn't take very long.

4. Sprinkle over the lemon juice and give the mix a final good stir. Serve immediately with hot, crusty bread and salad.

Flashed Oysters with Lemon, Garlic and Herbs

I have difficulty eating raw oysters and much prefer them flashed under the grill so the flesh is just set. Oysters are excellent done this way with a topping of Hollandaise sauce, but this version is far healthier. Approx 50 kcals per oyster.

24 oysters
100ml (6½ tbsp) extra virgin olive oil
100ml (6½ tbsp) dry white wine
2 cloves garlic, crushed
1 tbsp wholegrain mustard
3 tbsp freshly squeezed lemon juice
2 tbsp freshly chopped mixed herbs (e.g. chives, parsley, basil, coriander)
Freshly ground black pepper

Garnish: sprigs of watercress

1. Place the olive oil, white wine, garlic, mustard and herbs in a screw-top jar and shake well. If possible, leave several hours for the flavours to marinate.

2. Open the oysters, discarding one shell. Arrange on a grill pan. Season each well with black pepper.

3. Shake the marinade jar to emulsify the contents and spoon two teaspoons over each oyster.

4. Flash the oysters under a hot grill for 2 to 3 minutes until set.

Flashed Oysters with Yogurt and Breadcrumbs

An even healthier version of flashed oysters. This works out at approx 25 kcals per oyster if Greek strained yogurt is used, or 18 kcals with very low-fat yogurt.

24 oysters
300ml Greek strained or low-fat yogurt
2 tbsp wholegrain mustard
2 tbsp fresh parsley, chopped
1 tbsp coriander leaves, chopped
2 tbsp freshly squeezed lemon juice
A handful of fresh, wholemeal breadcrumbs
Freshly ground black pepper

Garnish: freshly chopped parsley

1. Mix together the yogurt, mustard, parsley, coriander and lemon juice.
2. Open the oysters, discarding one shell. Arrange on a grill pan. Season each well with black pepper.
3. Spoon one tablespoon of yogurt mixture over each oyster.
4. Sprinkle breadcrumbs over the oysters, using as much or as little as you like.
5, Flash under a hot grill for 2 to 3 minutes until set and the breadcrumbs toasted.

Salmon Tartare

This starter must be made with exceptionally fresh fish. Serves 4 at 120 kcals per serving.

225g fresh raw salmon, minced
2 tsp freshly squeezed lime juice
2 spring onions, finely chopped
120g low-fat fromage frais
1 tbsp wholegrain mustard
1 tbsp fresh chives, finely chopped
2 tbsp fresh dill weed, finely chopped
Rock salt and freshly ground black pepper

Garnish: dill sprigs

1. Mix together the minced salmon, lime juice and spring onion. Season well and mould into four flattened rounds.
2. Mix together the fromage frais, mustard, chives and dill to make the sauce.
3. Spoon the sauce onto a plate, carefully place the salmon round in the centre and garnish with sprigs of dill. Serve with toast and a green salad.

Soups

Croûtons

All soups are enhanced by the addition of croûtons. In their simplest form, these are squares of bread toasted under the grill. If you can afford the calories, the following recipe makes delicious, garlicky crisp breads that convert a hearty soup into a main meal. Up to 90 kcals per round of bread, depending how much oil is absorbed. Serves 4.

12 thin slices French bread
2 cloves garlic, cut in half
8 tbsp extra virgin olive oil

1. Rub the bread with the cut edges of garlic.
2. Heat the oil until starting to bubble. Add the garlic

pieces, now crushed, and the bread. Fry until golden and crisp, turning regularly.

3. Dry the fried bread on absorbent paper.

For extra luxury, top with grated cheese and flash under the grill.

Garlic and Sesame Croûtons

    1 egg white
    1 clove garlic, crushed
    1 tbsp sesame seeds
    1 tbsp soy sauce (optional)
    125g bread, cut into 1cm (½ inch) cubes
    8 tbsp extra virgin olive oil

1. Whisk together the egg white, garlic, sesame seeds and soy sauce.

2. Dip the bread cubes in the mixture to coat lightly.

3. Heat the olive oil until beginning to bubble. Fry the bread cubes until crispy and golden.

4. Drain the croûtons on absorbent paper.

Mediterranean Bean Soup (Zuppa di Fagioli)

A Tuscan bean soup popular in Florence, Italy. Delicious and filling with an authentic Mediterranean flavour. Serves 4 at approx 250 kcals each.

    225g dried cannellini beans
    2 cloves garlic, peeled and crushed
    1 large onion, peeled and coarsely chopped
    2 tbsp extra virgin olive oil
    1 large carrot, chopped
    1 large leek, chopped

1 celery stick, chopped
1 beef tomato, chopped
1 tbsp tomato paste
1.5 litres vegetable/chicken stock or water
1 sprig fresh rosemary
1 sprig fresh thyme
Juice of half a lemon
Rock salt and freshly ground black pepper

Garnish: freshly grated Parmesan cheese and herbs

1. Soak the beans overnight. Change the water, and bring
to the boil. Skim off any foam. Cook for 10 minutes.
Change the water and boil for another 10 minutes. Drain.
2. Fry the garlic and onion in olive oil until translucent.
Add the remaining vegetables and fry for five minutes.
3. Transfer vegetables, herbs, beans and water/stock to a
saucepan. Cover and simmer for an hour until the beans
are tender.
4. Discard the herb sprigs and remove one ladleful of
cooked vegetables. Liquidize the rest of the soup. Season
with rock salt and freshly ground black pepper.
5. Return the ladleful of vegetables to the liquidized soup
with the lemon juice and simmer gently for ten minutes.
Adjust seasoning, garnish and serve.

Mediterranean Fish Soup (La Soupe de Poissons)

This is the sort of authentic fish soup found in every
maritime French restaurant. Every one is different – and
unfortunately I've tasted a few bitter ones. There are two
simple rules for success: don't use oily fish such as mackerel
or herring, and remove the heads and bones from the soup
before liquidizing. Serves 4 handsomely at around

380 kcals each. Could easily be diluted with more fish stock to go further.

   1kg mixed fish, e.g. cod, whiting, gurnard, mullet, dogfish, unpeeled prawns
   Chopped vegetables for stock – 1 carrot, 1 onion, 1 celery stick, 1 bay leaf, 6 crushed peppercorns, 2 cloves
   2 large onions, peeled and chopped
   3 celery sticks, chopped
   1 large leek, sliced
   3 sticks Florence fennel, chopped
   6 cloves garlic, crushed
   4 tbsp extra virgin olive oil
   2 tbsp brandy
   2 beef tomatoes, chopped
   1 tbsp tomato purée
   Juice and zest of half an orange
   1 large carrot, grated
   ½ red pepper, seeded and chopped
   1 bay leaf
   6 stamens saffron
   4 tbsp dry vermouth
   2 tbsp chopped, fresh herbs, e.g. parsley, thyme, oregano, rosemary
   1 tsp finely chopped red chilli pepper *or*
   1 tsp cayenne pepper
   Rock salt and freshly ground black pepper

Garnish: aïoli, rouille, grated Parmesan, garlic croûtons or chopped fresh parsley, as desired.

1. Fillet the fish. Use the heads and bones to make a fish stock by boiling with 1.5 litres water and stock vegetables for 15 minutes. Strain. If time allows, let the stock cool before straining.
2. Sweat the onion, celery, leek, fennel and garlic in olive oil until they soften and start to colour. If preferred, add more oil but this will increase the calorie count.
3. Pour on the brandy and allow to evaporate away.

4. Add the tomatoes, tomato purée, orange juice and zest, grated carrot, red pepper, bay leaf, saffron and fish fillets. Cook until the fish flesh clouds, stirring and turning continuously.

5. Add the strained fish stock, vermouth and fresh herbs. Bring to the boil and simmer for 30 minutes.

6. Remove the bay leaf and liquidize the soup. Season and stir in the chilli pepper.

Serve with garlic croûtons and bowls of rouille, aïoli and freshly grated Parmesan cheese, varying amounts of which are stirred into individual servings to taste.

Seafood and Sweetcorn Chowder with Dill

This fish soup serves 4 at approx 240 kcals each.

    1 medium onion, finely chopped
    2 medium potatoes, peeled and diced
    420ml semi-skimmed milk
    2 bay leaves
    445g white fish fillets, skinned and diced
    100ml dry white wine
    225g cooked sweetcorn
    4 tbsp fresh dill, chopped
    50g peeled prawns or crab meat
    Rock salt and freshly ground black pepper

1. Place the onions, potatoes, milk and bay leaves in a saucepan. Simmer gently for 10 to 15 minutes until the potatoes are cooked.

2. Add the diced fish, wine, sweetcorn, dill and prawns/crab meat and cook gently for 10 minutes. Season.

3. Remove the bay leaves and serve with hot, crusty bread.

Spanish Salad Soup (Gazpacho)

I prefer to leave the tomato seeds in this summer soup for their extra roughage and vitamins. Serves 4 at approx 235 kcals each. The olive oil can be omitted to reduce each serving to approx 175 kcals.

900g beef tomatoes, coarsely chopped (seeded if preferred)
½ cucumber, thinly peeled and coarsely chopped
2 red peppers, cored, seeded and chopped
1 chilli pepper, seeded and chopped (optional)
3 garlic cloves, crushed
1 small onion, coarsely chopped
9 basil leaves
2 tablespoon balsamic vinegar
6 tbsp extra virgin olive oil
300ml vegetable stock
1 tsp acacia honey
1 tbsp freshly squeezed lemon juice
Tabasco or Worcestershire sauce, to taste
Rock salt and freshly ground black pepper

Garnish: Mascarpone cheese, finely diced red pepper and sprigs of basil

1. Mix ingredients up to, and including, the olive oil and leave to marinate overnight in the fridge.
2. Add the vegetable stock and liquidize until ultra-smooth.
3. Season to taste with the honey, lemon juice and Tabasco or Worcestershire sauce just before serving.
4. Serve chilled garnished with swirls of Mascarpone cheese, diced pepper and sprigs of basil.

Tomato, Orange and Ginger Soup

This soup is equally delicious served hot in front of a roaring log fire, or served cold on a summer picnic. Serves 4 at approx 110 kcals per serving.

To make the bouquet garni, tie the following together with cotton thread:
    Small sprig of rosemary
    1 bay leaf
    1 sprig of thyme
    2.5cm (1 inch) piece of fresh ginger root, heavily scored with a knife

    1 medium onion, chopped
    1 clove garlic, crushed
    2 tbsp extra virgin olive oil
    225g medium carrots, coarsely chopped
    450g beef tomatoes, chopped
    1 bouquet garni, as above
    600ml vegetable stock
    100ml freshly squeezed orange juice
    Rock salt and freshly ground black pepper

    Garnish: handful of fresh, chopped parsley

1. Fry the onion and garlic in the oil until slightly coloured.
2. Add all ingredients except the orange juice and simmer for 20 minutes.
3. Remove the bouquet garni then liquidize, or sieve if you prefer a velvety smooth soup.
4. Before serving (hot or cold), add the fresh orange juice, a little at a time, until the desired flavouring is obtained.

Jerusalem Artichoke and Hazelnut Soup

Choose the least knobbly Jerusalem artichokes as these are easier to peel. Serves 4 at approx 360 kcals per serving.

    450g Jerusalem artichokes
    Juice of 1 lemon
    1 medium onion, coarsely chopped
    2 tbsp extra virgin olive oil
    300ml vegetable stock
    300ml dry white wine
    100g roasted hazelnuts
    2 tbsp hazelnut oil
    Rock salt and freshly ground black pepper
    200ml Greek strained yogurt

    Garnish: crushed roasted hazelnuts

1. Peel and dice the artichokes. Submerge in a bowl of cold water to which the lemon juice has been added until you are ready to cook them to prevent them discolouring.
2. Fry the onions in the olive oil until softened.
3. Drain the artichokes and lightly fry in olive oil for five minutes without colouring.
4. Pour on the vegetable stock and wine. Bring to the boil and simmer for 20 minutes.
5. Meanwhile, crush the hazelnuts and blend with the hazelnut oil.
6. Liquidize the soup, stir in the Greek yogurt and season.
7. Stir the hazelnut paste into the soup, reheat and adjust seasoning.

Mushroom, Garlic and Fennel Soup

A million times better than tinned mushroom soup. Serves 4 at approx 160 kcals each.

For an alternative flavour, substitute a handful of finely chopped fresh dill weed for the ginger and fennel seeds.

1 large onion, peeled and chopped
3 cloves garlic, crushed
3 tbsp extra virgin olive oil
450g chestnut mushrooms, chopped
600ml semi-skimmed milk
2.5cm (1 inch) ginger root, chopped
24 fennel seeds, crushed
150ml Greek strained yogurt
Rock salt and freshly ground black pepper

Garnish: chopped fresh parsley

1. Sauté the onions and garlic in olive oil until just starting to colour. Add the mushrooms and sweat for 5 minutes.
2. Add the milk, ginger and fennel seeds and bring to the boil. Simmer for 20 minutes.
3. Liquidize the soup until smooth and stir in the yogurt. Season with salt and plenty of black pepper. Garnish with chopped parsley.

French Onion Soup

A classic French soup. Serves 4 at approx 80 kcals each. Classically, this soup is poured over rounds of toasted bread and cheese and sprinkled with chopped parsley.

2 large onions, peeled and finely sliced
2 cloves garlic, crushed
2 tbsp extra virgin olive oil
900ml vegetable stock
2 tbsp mixed fresh herbs, chopped
2 tsp yeast extract
Rock salt and freshly ground black pepper

Garnish: croûtons or toasted crusty bread, grated cheese, parsley

1. Sauté the onions and garlic in the oil until golden brown.
2. Add the remaining ingredients and bring to the boil.
3. Cover and simmer for 15 minutes.

Lentil and Apricot Soup

This sweet, spicy cream soup is similar to a mild mulligatawny. Serves 4 at approx 290 kcals each.

1 medium onion, chopped
2 cloves garlic, crushed
½ tsp cumin seeds, freshly ground
1 tsp coriander seeds, freshly ground
1 tbsp extra virgin olive oil
125g red lentils
125g dried apricots
1 large potato, cubed
1 medium carrot, grated
½ red sweet pepper, finely chopped
300ml dry white wine
250ml low-fat yogurt

Garnish: sprigs of parsley, chopped dried apricots

1. In a large saucepan, sauté the onion, garlic, cumin and coriander in olive oil until the onion starts to colour.
2. Add all remaining ingredients, except the yogurt, and 900ml water. Bring to the boil. Cover and simmer for 30 minutes.
3. Liquidize until smooth. Stir in the yogurt and season to taste.

Tomato and Garlic Soup

Guaranteed to keep the vampires at bay, cooked garlic loses a lot of its potency. Serves 4 at approx 160 kcals each.

2 medium onions, finely chopped
2 tbsp extra virgin olive oil
8–12 large cloves garlic, crushed
2 medium potatoes, peeled and cubed
1 kg tomatoes, peeled and chopped
1½ litres water or vegetable stock
1 bay leaf
Rock salt and freshly ground black pepper
4 slices stale French bread

Garnish: chopped parsley and freshly grated Parmesan cheese

1. Fry the onions in olive oil until turning golden.
2. Add the garlic and potatoes and fry for a further five minutes.
3. Add the chopped tomatoes and continue to cook for ten minutes.
4. Add the water/vegetable stock and bay leaf. Bring to the boil and simmer for half an hour. Season with salt and freshly ground black pepper.
5. Place a slice of stale bread in each warmed soup bowl and pour over the garlic soup. Garnish with chopped parsley and Parmesan.

Vegetable, Basil and Garlic Soup (Soupe au Pistou)

An excellent warming dish for winter. Serves 4 heartily at approx 325 kcals each.

100g mixed dried beans (e.g. haricot, cannellini, kidney, black-eyed)

1 large onion, peeled and roughly chopped
4 cloves garlic, crushed
2 tbsp extra virgin olive oil
350g beef tomatoes, chopped
1 large potato, peeled and cubed
225g courgettes, cubed
225g green beans, cut into 2cm lengths
225g fresh broad beans, shelled
16 fresh basil leaves, chopped
50g walnuts, chopped
Rock salt and freshly ground black pepper

Garnish: Freshly grated Parmesan cheese, garlic croûtons, basil

1. Soak the beans in water overnight.
2. Fry the onion and 2 cloves of garlic in olive oil.
3. Add the tomatoes and potatoes and cook for five minutes.
4. Add 1 litre water and drained, soaked beans. Bring to the boil and simmer for 15 minutes.
5. Add the remaining vegetables. Simmer for 20 minutes.
6. Meanwhile, mash the basil, 2 cloves of garlic and a dribble of olive oil in a pestle and mortar. Add the walnuts and crush together to make a simple pesto.
7. Stir the pesto sauce into the soup and season. Garnish with croûtons, Parmesan cheese and basil leaves.

Prawn, Basil and Lemon Grass Soup (Dom Yam Kung)

This delicious, spicy soup comes from Thailand where it is served in its own steamboat. Burning coals underneath and a central flue keep the soup hot. Serves 4 at approx 75 cals each.

700g cooked, shell-on prawns

2.5cm (1 inch) root ginger, peeled and scored
4 stalks lemon grass, sliced into 2 cm (¾ inch) lengths
8 citrus leaves (e.g. lemon, lime, clementine). Ask your greengrocer for leaves from delivery boxes or grow young plants from pips.
6 tbsp lime or lemon juice
2 green chillies, finely chopped
6 spring onions, finely chopped
16 fresh basil, mint or tarragon leaves, shredded
A handful of fresh coriander leaves, chopped
Rock salt and freshly ground black pepper

1. Peel the prawns. Make a fish stock by boiling the heads and shells in 1.5 litres water for 15 minutes. Strain.
2. Bring the fish stock, root ginger, lemon grass and citrus leaves to the boil. Simmer for five minutes.
3. Add the lime juice, green chillies and spring onion. Simmer for 5 minutes.
4. Add the peeled prawns and herbs. Simmer for a few minutes, then season to taste. Serve immediately.

Prawn, Avocado and Cucumber Soup

An unusual, chilled summer soup with a delicate flavour. Serves 4 at approx 190 kcals each.
300ml vegetable stock
225g shell-on prawns
1 clove garlic, crushed
1 large, ripe avocado, peeled
1 small cucumber, peeled
Freshly squeezed juice from half a lemon
450ml low-fat natural bio yogurt
2 tbsp freshly chopped dill
Rock salt and freshly ground black pepper

Garnish: slices of cucumber, 1 shell-on prawn per person and sprigs of dill

1. Bring the vegetable stock to the boil.
2. Peel the prawns, saving the shells.
3. Add the shells and garlic to the vegetable stock and simmer for 15 minutes. Strain and allow to cool.
4. Liquidize the avocado and cucumber flesh together with the lemon juice to prevent discoloration.
5. Slowly add the strained stock, yogurt and dill to the processor and continue liquidizing until smooth.
6. Pour the soup into a bowl and season. Add the prawns and lightly stir to mix. Serve well chilled with crusty bread and green salad.

Seafood

Mediterranean Herb Oil

This oil is excellent for basting fish during grilling. It takes two weeks to mature and stores well. Use within one year.

    600ml extra virgin olive oil
    12 black peppercorns
    12 green peppercorns
    12 fennel seeds
    12 coriander seeds
    1 sprig rosemary
    1 sprig thyme
    1 sprig tarragon
    1 sprig oregano
    2 bay leaves
    4 cloves garlic, peeled and scored
    2 red chilli peppers
    1 tsp rock salt

1. Place all ingredients in a clear wine bottle and cork. Shake well.
2. Leave for two weeks, if possible in a sun-lit place. Shake and turn every day.

Basic Court Bouillon

Seafood dishes are enhanced by the use of a fragrant, home-made fish stock or traditional court bouillon for poaching or making a sauce. This court bouillon will last several days in a fridge. It is an excellent base liquor for making many of the soup dishes in this book. In an emergency, a fish or vegetable stock cube may be substituted instead.

  600ml dry white wine
  Freshly squeezed juice of half a lemon
  1 large onion, chopped into quarters
  1 carrot, grated
  1 leek, cut into four lengthways and washed
  A few celery leaves
  1 fresh bay leaf
  1 sprig fresh rosemary
  1 sprig fresh thyme
  4 black peppercorns
  4 green peppercorns
  2 cloves garlic, crushed

1. Add all ingredients to a large saucepan with 600ml water, cover and bring to the boil.
2. Simmer all ingredients for half an hour.
3. Allow to cool, then strain.

Basic Fish Stock

Add up to 1kg trimmings (heads, skins, bones and fins) from non-oily fish to the above court bouillon ingredients. Add enough extra water/wine to cover.

Baked Whole Fish with Lemon and Herbs

This aromatic dish can be served hot with new potatoes and broccoli or cold with mayonnaise and salad. Serves 4 at approx 385 kcals each.

    1.5kg whole round fish (e.g. sea bass, grey mullet, trout)
    1 tbsp extra virgin olive oil (or herb-flavoured olive oil)
    Freshly squeezed juice of one lemon
    2 tbsp fresh parsley, chopped
    2 tbsp chopped mixed fresh herbs (e.g. fennel, dill, thyme, rosemary)
    1 stalk lemon grass
    Rock salt and freshly ground black pepper

    Garnish: green olives

1. Ask your fishmonger to gut, bone and decapitate the fish, whilst leaving the flesh whole. Trim off fins and sharp spikes. Wash the fish well, inside and out and strip off any scales.
2. Pre-heat the oven to 190°C/375°F/gas mark 5.
3. Brush the fish inside and out with olive oil or herb-flavoured oil. Season well.
4. Fill the body cavity with fresh herbs and sprinkle with lemon juice. Lay the lemon grass lengthways down the centre of the fish. Season again.
5. Wrap the fish well in foil and bake for 30 to 45 minutes.

Baked Fish with Wine and Garlic

This dish is remarkably easy to prepare. It can be served with boiled potatoes, rice, pasta or crusty bread plus plenty of broccoli, courgettes or salad. Serves 4 at approx 400 kcals each.

    1.5kg whole round fish (e.g. Arctic char)

1 tbsp extra virgin olive oil
1 tbsp chopped mixed fresh herbs (e.g. fennel, dill, thyme,
rosemary)
100ml dry white wine
Rock salt and freshly ground black pepper

Garnish: freshly chopped parsley

1. Ask your fishmonger to gut, bone and decapitate the
fish, whilst leaving the flesh whole. Trim off fins and sharp
spikes. Wash the fish well, inside and out and strip off any
scales.
2. Pre-heat the oven to 190°C/375°F/gas mark 5.
3. Brush the fish inside and out with olive oil and season.
4. Fill the body cavity with fresh herbs.
5. Place the fish on a sheet of foil. Start to wrap up the
fish and just before closing, pour in the glass of white wine.
Seal the parcel well. Bake for 30 to 45 minutes.

Grilled Fish Steaks with Lemon and Herbs

Serves 4 at approx 150 kcals each if using white fish, 200
kcals with oily fish.
4 x 150g white fish steaks (e.g. cod) *or*
4 x 100g oily fish (e.g. mackerel, salmon)
1 tbsp extra virgin olive oil
4 tbsp freshly squeezed lemon juice
2 spring onions, finely chopped
2 cloves garlic, crushed
4 tbsp chopped fresh herbs (e.g. parsley, dill, rosemary,
thyme)
Freshly ground black pepper

1. Mix together the olive oil, lemon juice, spring onions,
garlic and fresh herbs. Marinate the fish fillets in this mixture for at least one hour. Season well with black pepper.

2. Cook under a hot grill until the flesh is just set, basting with any left-over marinade during cooking.

Bouillabaisse

Bouillabaisse is a classic Marseilles dish, made from a variety of small rock fish (e.g. rascasse which is difficult to obtain in Britain). It can be made with any variety of non-oily fish – preferably a mix of at least five different types. Serves 4 well, at approx 375 kcals each.

  1 large onion, chopped
  1 leek, chopped
  1 baby bulb Florence fennel, quartered
  3 cloves garlic, crushed
  2 tbsp extra virgin olive oil
  2 beef tomatoes, chopped
  1 tsp saffron
  1 sprig fresh thyme
  1 sprig fennel leaf
  1 bay leaf
  1 sprig fresh rosemary
  300ml dry white wine
  Zest of one orange
  1kg mixed non-oily fish fillets (e.g. dogfish, John Dory, red bream, grey mullet, monkfish, cod, gurnard)
  450g mussels, cleaned and bearded
  225g shell-on prawns
  Rock salt and freshly ground black pepper

  Garnish: garlic croûtons, rouille (see sauces), aïoli (see sauces)

1. Fry the onion, leek, fennel and garlic in olive oil in a large saucepan until turning golden.
2. Add the tomatoes, saffron, thyme, fennel leaf, bay leaf

and rosemary and cook for five minutes. Meanwhile boil 1.2 litres water.

3. Pour the boiling water over the vegetables and add the wine and orange zest. Drop in the fish fillets, larger pieces first, and simmer for 5 minutes.

5. Add the mussels and shell–on prawns and continue simmering until the mussels open.

6. Strain the soup and place all the fish and vegetables in a large dish. Keep warm.

7. Bring the strained liquor to the boil and whisk continuously for one minute to aid the emulsion of water and oil. When the soup has thickened, season to taste.

8. Pour the thickened liquor over the fish and serve. Accompany with rouille, aïoli and hot crusty bread.

Mixed Seafood in Tomato, Fennel and Chilli Sauce

A dish commonly encountered along the Mediterranean coast. Serves 4 at approx 380 kcals each.

250ml dry white wine
1kg fresh mussels, cleaned and bearded
1 bay leaf
1 large onion, chopped
2 tbsp extra virgin olive oil or herb-flavoured olive oil
2 cloves garlic, crushed
1 fennel bulb, chopped
1 small, red chilli pepper, seeded and chopped
400g beef tomatoes, chopped
30g sun-dried tomatoes
450g cod, haddock or monkfish, or a mix of all three
100g peeled prawns
Freshly ground black pepper
Juice of half a lemon (optional)

Garnish: freshly chopped parsley and fennel leaves

1. Put the wine, mussels and bay leaf in a large saucepan with a little of the chopped onion. Bring to boil and simmer until the mussels have all opened.
2. Remove the mussels from the pan with a slotted spoon. Continue boiling the liquor until reduced to about 100ml. Remove the mussels from their shells.
3. Fry the remaining chopped onion in olive oil until soft. Add the garlic and chopped fennel and fry for five minutes.
4. Add the chilli and tomatoes and continue to simmer, stirring well, for 10 to 15 minutes.
5. Bone and skin the fish. Cut into 2.5cm (1 inch) cubes.
6. When the tomato sauce has thickened, add the fish cubes, gently pressing them beneath the surface of the sauce. Cook for five minutes, or until opaque.
7. Add the mussels, prawns and mussel cooking liquor to the tomato and fish mixture. Simmer gently for 2 to 3 minutes. Check the seasoning and add lemon juice if necessary. Serve with fresh pasta, garnished with parsley.

Fish in Filo Parcels

An impressive dish for a dinner party. Serves 4 at approx 330 kcals each.

   4 fillets of salmon, sole or other firm fish – 100g each if oily fish, 150g if white fish
   150ml low-fat natural yogurt
   2 tbsp fresh dill weed, chopped
   1 packet filo pastry
   1 tbsp extra virgin olive oil
   Rock salt and freshly ground black pepper

1. Skin and bone the fish and roll or shape into tidy fillets.
2. Mix the yogurt and dill together. Season to taste.
3. Unroll the filo pastry and lay it out, if possible on a

marble or slate top. Cover with a damp cloth to keep from drying out.

4. Take a sheet of filo and brush lightly with olive oil. Place another sheet on top and brush this with oil too. Fold the layered pastry in half to form a four layered sheet measuring about 20 × 25cm (8 × 10 inches).

5. Place one fillet of fish on one side of the pastry. Spread with a generous tablespoon of yogurt and dill sauce. Wrap the fillet in the pastry, making a neat parcel. All ends should be tucked underneath. Place on a baking sheet and brush with olive oil.

6. Repeat with all the fish fillets, keeping unused filo pastry covered with a damp cloth at all times.

7. Bake the filo fish parcels in a hot oven at 220°C/425°F/gas mark 7 for 20 minutes, until golden brown. Serve with salad and boiled new potatoes.

Soused Gravadlax Mackerel

The vinegar cuts the oiliness of the mackerel in this dish, whilst dill and green peppercorns infuse an aromatic flavour. Soused gravadlax mackerel will keep well in the fridge for several days. Cut into strips or thin slices and serve with salad and crusty bread. Serves 4 at approx 340 kcals each.

  4 x 225g mackerel
  Rock salt
  1 onion, finely sliced
  300ml white wine vinegar
  2 tbsp dry white wine
  1 tbsp acacia honey
  1 tbsp wholegrain mustard
  1 tsp green peppercorns, crushed
  4 tbsp freshly chopped dill weed

1. Fillet the mackerel and rub well with coarse salt. Lay in a shallow dish, skin side down.
2. Layer the onion over the fish.
3. Combine the remaining ingredients in a large screw-top jar and shake well. Pour over the fish, completely immersing them. Add more vinegar if necessary.
4. Leave in the fridge to marinate for at least 3 days before serving.

Mackerel with Mustard and Herbs

A fish dish with its own bite. Serves 4 at approx 370 kcals each.

4 x 225g mackerel, cleaned but left whole
6 tbsp wholegrain mustard
1 tbsp fresh lemon thyme, chopped
1 tbsp fresh parsley, chopped
1 tbsp fresh chives, chopped
1 tbsp fresh basil, chopped
Freshly squeezed juice of 1 lemon
100ml dry white wine

Garnish: freshly chopped parsley

1. Cut several slashes at 2.5cm (1 inch) intervals down each side of the mackerel.
2. Mix together the mustard, lemon juice and finely chopped herbs. Rub well into the cuts in the mackerel flesh.
3. Arrange the fish in a shallow dish and pour over the white wine. Leave to marinate for at least one hour, turning occasionally.
4. Grill the mackerel for 5 to 8 minutes per side, depending on size. Serve with crusty bread and a large green salad.

Sicilian Mackerel

This dish contains a spicy version of ratatouille with which to stuff the grilled mackerel. Ideally, the fish should be grilled over a charcoal barbecue on a warm, balmy night. A green salad tossed simply in a lemon juice and walnut oil dressing, plus hot garlic bread are ideal accompaniments. The ratatouille stuffing can be made the day before if necessary. Serves 4 at approx 435 kcals each.

1 stick celery, chopped
1 large onion, chopped
1 clove garlic, chopped
2 tbsp extra virgin olive oil
225g aubergine, cut into 2.5cm (1 inch) cubes
1 beef tomato, chopped
1 tbsp tomato purée
1 tbsp red wine vinegar
1 tbsp capers
8 black olives, pitted
8 green olives, pitted
4 anchovy fillets
4 x 225g mackerel, cleaned and heads removed
1 tsp acacia honey
Freshly ground black pepper
1 tbsp fresh parsley, chopped

1. Fry the celery, onion and garlic in olive oil until the onion becomes transparent.
2. Add the aubergine and continue cooking until the aubergine begins to colour.
3. Add the tomato, tomato purée, vinegar, capers, olives and honey and cook slowly for ten minutes.
4. Meanwhile, pound the anchovies to form a paste. Add to the vegetable mixture. Cook slowly for a further 50 minutes.
5. Meanwhile, brush the mackerel lightly with olive oil. Score both sides. Ten minutes before the vegetables are

ready, grill the mackerel under a hot grill for 5 minutes per side.
6. Stuff the mackerel with ratatouille, or serve it as a side dish. Garnish with parsley.

Mackerel with Ginger and Fennel

Another classic Mediterranean combination of ingredients. Serves 4 at approx 370 kcals each.
    225g onion, thinly sliced
    2 cloves garlic, crushed
    1 tbsp extra virgin olive oil
    1 tbsp root ginger, freshly grated
    A handful of freshly chopped fennel leaves
    4 x 225g mackerel, cleaned
    Freshly ground black pepper

1. Sauté the onion and garlic in olive oil until soft. Add the ginger and fennel. Stir-fry for 1 minute.
2. Cut deep slits diagonally across each side of the mackerel, about 2.5cm (1 inch) apart and season with black pepper.
3. Stuff the fish with the onion and herb mixture.
4. Grill for 5 to 10 minutes per side until the flesh is cooked and sizzling. Serve with garlic bread and a green salad.

Sardines from Crete

I first ate these sardines in a waterside cafe, watching eels darting through the oily Cretan waters. Even now, the evocative smell of sardines, Parmesan and tomatoes gets my juices flowing. Serves 4 like kings for approx 500 kcals each.
    4 large, fresh sardines, cleaned and scaled (about 1kg)

2 tbsp extra virgin olive oil
1 large onion, chopped
2 cloves garlic, crushed
1 courgette, chopped
1 leek, chopped
150ml dry white wine
225g beef tomato, sliced
1 tbsp fresh parsley, chopped
1 tbsp fresh basil or thyme, chopped
50g wholemeal breadcrumbs
50g Parmesan cheese, freshly grated
4 anchovy fillets (optional)
Freshly ground black pepper

1. Fry the sardines in olive oil until nicely browned. Remove and set aside, keeping warm.
2. Add the onion, garlic, courgette and leek to the pan and fry until softened. Pour in the wine and simmer until the liquid is reduced by half.
3. Add the tomatoes and herbs and simmer for a further minute. Season generously with black pepper.
4. Line an ovenproof dish with the vegetable mix and lay the sardines on top. Sprinkle with breadcrumbs and Parmesan and season further with black pepper.
5. Flash under the grill until the cheese is browned and the breadcrumbs toasted. Decorate with anchovy fillets and serve. Your mouth will now be watering from the delicious aromas, too.

Sardines with Wine and Parsley

Slightly kinder on the calories, this dish serves 4 at approx 400 kcals each.

    4–8 fresh sardines (1kg) cleaned
    1 tbsp extra virgin olive oil
    3 cloves garlic, crushed

1 tbsp lemon juice plus some zest
150ml dry white wine
4 tbsp fresh parsley, chopped
1 tbsp fresh chives, chopped
Freshly ground black pepper

1. Brush the sardines with olive oil and season well with black pepper. Dry fry with garlic until starting to turn golden.
2. Add the lemon juice, white wine, parsley and chives and simmer for 5 minutes or until cooked. Serve with hot, crusty bread and a simple green salad.

Trout Almondine

Serves 4 at approx 240 kcals each.
4 x 225g rainbow trout
4 tbsp toasted flaked almonds
4 tbsp fresh parsley, chopped
100g Florence fennel, chopped into matchsticks
4 tbsp freshly squeezed lemon juice
2 cloves garlic, crushed
Freshly ground black pepper

1. Clean the trout and remove heads, fins and tails. Using your fingers, remove the ribs and back bone and discard.
2. Stuff each trout with almonds, parsley and fennel.
3. Sprinkle with lemon juice and garlic and season well with black pepper.
4. Cook under a hot grill until the flesh is just set or wrap in foil and bake in an oven pre-heated to 190°C/375°F/gas mark 5 for 20 to 30 minutes.

Grilled Trout with Walnuts and Dill

Serves 4 at approx 290 kcals each.
    4 x 225g salmon trout
    8 tbsp light fromage frais
    2 spring onions, finely chopped
    4 tbsp walnuts, chopped
    4 tbsp fresh dill weed, chopped
    Freshly ground black pepper
    4 beef tomatoes, cut in half

Garnish: lemon slices and freshly chopped dill or parsley.

1. Clean the trout and remove heads, tails and fins. Using your fingers, remove the ribs and backbone and discard.
2. Mix together the fromage frais, spring onions, walnuts and dill and stuff the cavity of each trout. Season well with pepper.
3. Cook the trout and beef tomatoes under a hot grill until the trout flesh is just set.

Baked Orange and Rosemary Trout

Serves 4 at approx 225 kcals each.
    4 x 225g rainbow trout
    2 medium oranges (blood oranges if possible)
    4 sprigs fresh rosemary
    A few coriander seeds, crushed
    Freshly ground black pepper

Garnish: parsley and coriander leaves

1. Preheat the oven to 190°C/375°F/gas mark 5.
2. Clean the trout and remove heads, fins and tails. Using your fingers, remove the ribs and backbone and discard.
3. Peel the oranges and slice the flesh.
4. Stuff the trout with sliced orange, rosemary sprigs and the coriander seeds. Season well with pepper.

5. Wrap in foil and bake for 20 minutes.

Salmon in Dill Sauce

Serves 4 at approx 240 kcals each.
    4 x 120g salmon fillets
    150ml light fromage frais
    2 tbsp freshly squeezed lemon juice
    4 tbsp fresh dill weed, chopped
    Freshly ground black pepper

    Garnish: lemon wedges; chopped parsley

1. Preheat the oven to 190°C/375°F/gas mark 5.
2. Mix together the fromage frais, lemon juice and dill to make the sauce.
3. Place the salmon fillets on a sheet of foil. Top the fish with dill sauce and season well.
4. Wrap up the fish in foil to make a parcel. (Make four individual parcels if you wish.) Bake for 15 to 20 minutes.

Mediterranean-style Cod

Serves 4 at approx 160 kcals each.
    4 x 150g cod steaks
    2 beef tomatoes, chopped
    4 small bay leaves
    4 tbsp fresh parsley, chopped
    1 lemon, cut into wedges
    200ml dry white wine
    Freshly ground black pepper

1. Preheat the oven to 190°C/375°F/gas mark 5.
2. Arrange the cod steaks in the base of a small casserole.
3. Top with the tomato, bay leaves, parsley and lemon

wedges. Season well with black pepper. Pour over the white wine.

4. Bake for 15 to 20 minutes, until the flesh has set.

Cod in Yogurt, Tomato and Basil Sauce

Serves 4 at approx 170 kcals each. The yogurt may clot but this does not affect the flavour (see note at beginning of recipe section). You may prefer to use fromage frais instead.

    150ml Greek strained yogurt
    150ml passata or 2 beef tomatoes, finely chopped
    4 tbsp fresh basil, chopped
    4 x 150g cod steaks
    Freshly ground black pepper

1. Preheat the oven to 190°C/375°F/gas mark 5.
2. Mix together the yogurt, passata (or tomatoes) and basil. Season well.
3. Place the cod pieces on a piece of foil and top the fish with the yogurt and tomato mixture. Make four individual parcels if you prefer.
4. Wrap up the cod steaks and bake for 20 minutes.

Cod in Green Sauce

A classier version of cod in parsley sauce. Serves 4 at approx 240 kcals each.

    4 cloves garlic, sliced
    1 tbsp extra virgin olive oil
    4 x 150g cod steaks (or other white fish)
    Juice of 1 lemon
    4 tbsp fresh parsley, chopped
    1 bay leaf
    1 sprig fresh rosemary

1 tbsp cornflour
120ml fish stock/water
120ml dry white wine
4 medium potatoes, sliced and boiled
Rock salt and freshly ground black pepper

1. Preheat the oven to 180°C/350°F/gas mark 4.
2. Sweat the garlic in olive oil until starting to colour. Remove with a slotted spoon and reserve both the garlic and the oil separately.
3. Season the fish steaks and arrange in an ovenproof dish. Sprinkle with lemon juice, add the fried garlic and the herbs.
4. Blend the cornflour with the fish stock and wine. Pour over the fish.
5. Top with slices of potato and brush well with the reserved garlic oil. Bake for 20 to 30 minutes until the potatoes are golden.

Grilled Lemon Sole with Coriander and Green Pepper

Serves 4 at approx 160 kcals each.
    4 slip sole, cleaned
    4 tbsp fresh coriander leaves, chopped
    A few coriander seeds, crushed
    2 green peppers, cut in half and seeded
    200ml dry white wine
    Freshly ground black pepper

1. Marinate the sole in wine and coriander leaves and seeds for at least 1 hour. Season.
2. Grill the sole and the green pepper under high heat until the fish flesh is set and the pepper skin is beginning to char.
3. Serve garnished with coriander leaves.

Sole in Red Grape Sauce

Serves 4 at approx 220 kcals each.
    4 x 150g fillets of sole, skinned
    150ml light red wine (e.g. Beaujolais)
    1 bay leaf
    1 spring onion, sliced
    1 tbsp cornflour
    150ml Greek strained yogurt
    100g seedless black grapes
    Rock salt and freshly ground black pepper

1. Preheat the oven to 160°C/325°F/gas mark 3.
2. Roll up the fillets and place in an ovenproof dish.
3. Pour over the wine and 4 tbsp water and add the bay leaf and onion. Season well with black pepper.
4. Cover with foil and place in the hot oven for 10 minutes only.
5. Remove the fish from the cooking liquor and keep warm. Strain the liquor into a saucepan and heat.
6. Mix the cornflour with a little water and add to the liquor, stirring until the mix comes to the boil. Stir until the mix thickens, then remove from the heat and allow to cool slightly.
7. Carefully stir in the yogurt and grapes and allow to heat through. Do not boil. Adjust seasoning.
8. Pour the sauce over the fillets and serve.

Sea Bass with Fennel

This classic Marseilles dish brings out the delicate flavour of 'sea wolf' – the French name for sea bass (*loup de mer*). The skin is edible and extremely tasty. Serves 4 at approx 250 kcals each.
    1kg sea bass (scaled, gutted and head removed)
    4 baby bulbs Florence fennel

1 tbsp extra virgin olive oil or herb-flavoured olive oil
50g fresh fennel leaves, finely chopped
300ml fish stock
1 tbsp Pernod or pastis
Rock salt and freshly ground black pepper

1. Pre-heat the oven to 200°C/400°F/gas mark 6.
2. Rub the bass well with salt and black pepper. Cut slits at 2.5cm (1 inch) intervals across the skin on each side.
3. Blanch the fennel bulbs in boiling water for one minute. Cut into quarters. Slide slices of fennel into each slit in the bass.
4. Brush both sides of the fish with olive oil. Stuff the cavity with chopped fennel leaves.
5. Lay the sea bass in an ovenproof dish. Arrange any remaining pieces of fennel bulb around it. Pour over the fish stock and Pernod. Cook in a hot oven for 20 minutes.

Sea Bass with Spring Onion and Ginger

This dish is classically Chinese but fulfils all the criteria for the Body Awareness Programme. Serves 4 at approx 260 kcals each.

1 kg sea bass, descaled and gutted

Marinade
2 tbsp light soy sauce
2 tbsp white wine
1 tbsp freshly squeezed lemon juice
2.5cm (1 inch) length of fresh root ginger, peeled and finely chopped
1 tsp acacia honey
2 tbsp extra virgin olive oil
4 spring onions, finely chopped
Rock salt and freshly ground black pepper

318

1. Make slits across each side of the bass at 2.5cm (1 inch) intervals.

2. Rub the fish well with rock salt and freshly ground black pepper. Lay in a shallow earthenware dish.

3. Mix together all the ingredients for the marinade. Pour over the marinade, making sure it enters the slits in the skin and the body cavity.

4. Leave to marinate for an hour, turning frequently.

5. Either wrap the fish in foil and bake in a hot oven (200°C/400°F/gas mark 6) for 20 minutes, or grill for 10 minutes both sides. Serve with a simple green salad and crusty bread.

Pickled Peppered Herrings

This Scandinavian dish is delicious served with warm, walnut bread, fresh cucumber and a yogurt-dill dressing (see below). Unfortunately, it takes three to four days before the herrings are fully cured and ready to eat. (See Marinated Herring Salad, page 278, also.) 230 kcals per 100g herring fillet.

    4 fresh herrings, filleted
    1 tsp green peppercorns
    1 tsp pink peppercorns
    ½ tsp black peppercorns
    300ml herb vinegar, e.g. dill
    2 tbsp acacia honey
    2 bay leaves
    1 tbsp fresh dill weed, chopped
    1 tsp mustard seed
    1 tsp fennel seed
    Rock salt

1. Sprinkle the herrings with crushed rock salt and leave for 30 minutes to dehydrate.

2. Crush together the peppercorns with a pestle and mortar (or in a coffee grinder).

3. Mix together the vinegar, honey, 4 tbsp water, peppercorns, bay leaves, dill, mustard and fennel seeds.

4. Dry the herring fillets on absorbent paper. Place the fish in an earthenware bowl and pour over the vinegar mixture.

5. Cover and place in the fridge. Leave to marinate for 3 to 4 days before eating.

Dressings for the marinated herrings

Yogurt and dill: This is simply made by mixing together two finely chopped spring onions with Greek strained (or low-fat) yogurt, dill weed and black pepper according to taste.

Honey and mustard: Mix together equal quantities of wholegrain mustard and honey. Flavour with chopped dill weed and a drop of wine vinegar to taste. Season with black pepper. Use sparingly.

Swordfish Steaks with Pink Grapefruit

If you manage to find fresh swordfish steaks (as opposed to frozen which are very different) they can be grilled with olive oil, lemon juice and herbs or prepared in this interesting way with sweet, pink grapefruit. Serves 4 at approx 290 kcals each.

  4 x 175g swordfish steaks
  2 tbsp extra virgin olive oil
  2 tsp green and pink peppercorns, crushed
  2 small, pink grapefruit
  1 tbsp acacia honey

  Garnish: sprigs of watercress

1. Brush the swordfish with olive oil, then press the crushed peppercorns well into the flesh.
2. Peel one grapefruit and separate into segments, removing the pith and membranes. Cut the remaining pink grapefruit into thin slices.
3. Brush the grapefruit slices with half the honey and flash brown under the grill. Put to one side and keep warm.
4. Grill the steaks for 5 minutes on one side, then turn and brush with oil. Grill for 3 minutes.
5. Place the grapefruit segments on top of the partially grilled steaks and brush with remaining honey.
6. Grill for a further 1 to 2 minutes until the meat is cooked through. Serve the steaks on a bed of grilled grapefruit slices.

Mediterranean-style Monkfish

A filling, aromatic meal. Serves 4 at approx 250 kcals each.
   2 onions, chopped
   3 cloves garlic
   2 tbsp extra virgin olive oil
   3 peppers (yellow, red and green), seeded and cut into strips
   225g beef tomatoes, chopped
   2 bay leaves
   1 sprig fresh rosemary
   1 sprig fresh thyme
   100ml white wine
   700g monkfish, cut into bite-sized chunks
   Rock salt and freshly ground black pepper

   Garnish: Freshly chopped herbs

1. Pre-heat the oven to 180°C/350°F/gas mark 4.
2. Fry the onion and garlic in the oil until soft.
3. Add the strips of pepper, chopped tomato, herbs and

wine and simmer until the liquid has reduced and the sauce is fairly thick. Season to taste.

4. Line the base of an ovenproof dish with the monkfish chunks. Spoon over the sauce and cook for 15 minutes. Serve with crusty bread and a green salad.

Monkfish and Herb Kebabs

Serves 4 at approx 200 kcals each.
  700g monkfish, cut into bite-sized pieces.
  16 button chestnut mushrooms
  12 small bay leaves

Marinade
  4 tbsp freshly squeezed lemon juice
  2 tbsp extra virgin olive oil
  4 tsp mixed fresh herbs, chopped
  2 spring onions, finely chopped
  2 cloves garlic, crushed
  Freshly ground black pepper

1. Mix together the marinade ingredients and pour over the fish and chestnut mushrooms. Allow to marinate for at least 1 hour.
2. Thread the monkfish, mushrooms and bay leaves onto kebab skewers.
3. Barbecue or grill until the fish flesh is just set.

Paella

Any kind of fish or shellfish can be used for this classic dish. Traditionally, paella contains chicken as well. Serves 4 generously at approx 600 kcals each, or 6 as a lighter meal at 400 kcals each.
  1 onion, chopped

2 cloves garlic, crushed
2 tbsp extra virgin olive oil
225g monkfish, cut into bite-sized cubes
1 red pepper, seeded and cut into strips
2 beef tomatoes, sliced
350g short-grain rice
Pinch of saffron, infused in 2 tbsp hot water
4 baby squid, cleaned and cut into rings
225g shell-on prawns
4–6 tiger prawns
450g mussels, scrubbed
100g fresh, young garden peas
1 tbsp fresh dill weed, chopped
1 tbsp fresh parsley, chopped
Rock salt and freshly ground black pepper

1. In a large pan, sweat the onion and garlic in olive oil until soft. Add the monkfish and cook until the flesh is just set, then remove the fish and set aside.

2. Add the red pepper and tomatoes to the pan and fry for a few minutes.

3. Add the rice, stirring well and fry to cook off any starch. Add the saffron and 1 litre water. Bring to the boil. Simmer for 20 minutes.

4. Add the squid, prawns, mussels and garden peas and continue cooking for 10 minutes or until the water has been absorbed and the rice is fluffy. If necessary, add more water, or boil off excess.

5. Add the monkfish and chopped herbs, stir through gently and serve with a green salad.

Drunken Sea Bream with Fennel

I first tasted this dish – an interesting and attractive variation on the fish with fennel theme – in Marseilles. Serves 4 at approx 250 kcals each.

4 small or 2 larger sea bream (approx 1kg), cleaned
1 tbsp extra virgin olive oil
Several sprigs of fresh fennel
Several sprigs of fresh thyme
220ml dry white wine
1 beef tomato, sliced
1 lemon, thinly sliced
Freshly ground black pepper

1. Make diagonal scores across both sides of the fish about 2.5cm (1 inch) apart.
2. Brush the fish with olive oil and season with black pepper.
3. Insert fennel sprigs into the slits down the fish and place the thyme in the fish body cavities.
4. Pour over the white wine and leave to marinate for at least 1 hour.
5. Pre-heat the oven to 180°C/350°F/gas mark 4.
6. Brush a roasting pan with olive oil and arrange the sliced tomatoes in the base. Lay the marinated sea bream on the tomatoes and arrange the lemon slices on top. Pour over any remaining wine marinade. Season.
7. Bake for 15 to 20 minutes until the fish is cooked through. Serve with steamed vegetables and rice to soak up the juices.

Mediterranean-style Red Mullet

The olives complement the red mullet well. Serves 4 at approx 350 kcals each.

1 onion, chopped
2 cloves garlic, crushed
2 tbsp extra virgin olive oil
2 tbsp fresh parsley, chopped
1 sprig fresh rosemary
1 bay leaf

1 sprig fresh thyme
1 beef tomato, chopped
1 tsp tomato purée
100ml dry white wine
8–16 black olives, stoned
4 medium-sized red mullet, cleaned and scaled

Garnish: lemon slices

1. In a large pan, sweat the onion and garlic in olive oil until soft.
2. Add the herbs, tomatoes and tomato purée and cook for 15 minutes.
3. Add white wine, olives and mullet. Cover and simmer gently for 15 minutes until the fish are cooked.
3. Remove the herb sprigs and serve the fish garnished with lemon wedges.

Grey Mullet with Herbs and Cheese

The combination of fish and cheese always works well. Poaching the fish first moistens and aromatizes the flesh. This dish can be made with any white fish, but not with oily fish. Serves 4 at approx 300 kcals each.

4 grey mullet (approx 1kg), cleaned and heads removed
4 cloves garlic, crushed
2 tbsp fresh parsley, chopped
1 tbsp tomato purée
1 tbsp extra virgin olive oil
2 tbsp fresh basil, chopped
2 beef tomatoes, chopped
Rock salt and freshly ground black pepper
100ml dry white wine
2 tbsp Parmesan cheese, freshly grated

Court bouillon
1 sprig fresh thyme

1 bay leaf
4 peppercorns
1 large onion, sliced

1. Bring the ingredients for the court bouillon and 1 litre water to the boil. Add the mullet and poach gently for 8 to 10 minutes. Remove fish and leave to drain.
2. Pre-heat the oven to 180°C/350°F/gas mark 4.
3. Pound together the garlic, parsley, tomato purée, olive oil and the basil.
4. Arrange the chopped tomatoes in the base of an oven-proof dish. Season well.
5. Stuff each fish with the garlic, herb and tomato paste and lay on top of the chopped tomatoes. Pour over the wine, sprinkle with Parmesan cheese and bake for 15 minutes.

Gurnard with Walnut Sauce

An unusual combination of fish and sweet nuts. Serves 4 at approx 500 kcals each.
    1 gurnard, weighing 1.5kg, cleaned
    100g fresh walnuts
    1 slice crustless white bread soaked in milk
    2 tbsp extra virgin olive oil
    1 tbsp freshly squeezed lemon juice
    1 tbsp fresh coriander, chopped

    Court bouillon
    1 sprig fresh thyme
    1 bay leaf
    4 peppercorns
    1 stalk celery
    1 carrot, grated
    1 large onion, sliced

1. Bring the ingredients for the court bouillon and 1 litre

water to the boil. Add the gurnard and poach gently for 30 minutes. If the court bouillon does not cover the fish, add more water. Remove fish and leave to drain.

2. Pound together the walnuts, bread, olive oil, lemon juice and coriander until the sauce is the consistency of paste. Add a little more milk if necessary.

3. Arrange the fish on a plate. Spoon over the walnut sauce and garnish with sprigs of coriander and lemon wedges. Eat hot or cold with salad and boiled potatoes.

John Dory in Orange and Cointreau Sauce

A favourite dinner party dish. Serves 4 at approx 210 kcals each.

   2 spring onions, chopped
   2 cloves garlic, chopped
   1 tbsp extra virgin olive oil
   2 tbsp Cointreau
   120ml freshly squeezed orange juice and zest of two oranges
   1 tsp fresh lemon balm, chopped
   4 x 150g fillets of John Dory
   2 tbsp dry white wine
   1–2 tsp cornflour

1. Sweat the onion and garlic in olive oil until soft.

2. Pour over the Cointreau and flambé.

3. Add the orange juice, lemon balm and fillets. Cover and poach gently for 5 to 10 minutes until the fish is cooked. Remove the fillets and keep warm.

4. Blend a little cornflour with the white wine and stir into the orange sauce until thickened.

5. Serve the John Dory garnished with lemon balm and a little orange sauce poured over.

John Dory in Marsala

Marsala is a wine frequently used in Sicilian cooking.
Serves 4 at approx 260 kcals each.

    4 x 150g fillets of John Dory
    1 tbsp cornflour
    1 tbsp extra virgin olive oil
    200ml Marsala
    200ml fish/vegetable stock or water

1. Coat the fish fillets with a light dusting of flour.
2. Fry in the olive oil until slightly coloured on both sides.
3. Add the Marsala and stock and continue cooking
gently until the amount of liquid is reduced by half. Serve
with broccoli and boiled new potatoes plus a side salad.

Poached Turbot with Wine and Lime

This dish has appeared on several English restaurant
menus. Turbot can be expensive or difficult to obtain –
try using John Dory or fillets of sole instead. Serves 4 at
approx 160 kcals each.

    1 tbsp extra virgin olive oil
    4 x 150g fillets of turbot
    ½ tsp fresh root ginger, crushed
    1 tbsp fresh coriander, chopped
    Juice and zest of 1 lime
    120ml dry white wine
    Freshly ground black pepper

1. Brush the base of a warm, heavy pan with olive oil and
arrange the turbot fillets on top.
2. Sprinkle on the ginger, coriander, lime juice and zest.
Season with black pepper. Pour over the white wine.
3. Cover and simmer gently for 15 minutes.

4. Remove the fish and keep warm. Reduce the cooking juices until slightly thickened to form a sauce.

Mussels

Rules for eating mussels

1. Never pick mussels from the seashore and use them in home cooking. The chances are you will spend the next 24 hours incarcerated in the bathroom with food poisoning. Commercial mussels are cleansed and purified to remove virulent bacteria.
2. Wash mussels well under cold, running water. Scrub their shells with a stiff nailbrush kept specifically for this use.
3. Scrape off barnacles and calcified worm casts using a small, sharp knife. Pull out the beards before cooking.
4. Discard any uncooked mussels that do not close when tapped.
5. After cooking, discard any mussels that refuse to open.

Moules Marinières

Moules Marinières is a classic Mediterranean soup. Some chefs prepare it with double cream and others thicken the sauce with flour or, horror of horrors, dilute the wine and juices with water. The simplest versions are by far the best. Use a decent white wine, preferably one you enjoy drinking. Moules Marinières made with cheap plonk tastes exactly as you might expect it to. Serves 4 as a main course (320 kcals each) or 6 as a starter (215 kcals each).

  1 medium onion, finely chopped
  3 cloves garlic, crushed
  2 tbsp extra virgin olive oil
  1 bottle dry white wine

4 tbsp fresh parsley, chopped
1 sprig fresh thyme and 1 stem fresh tarragon or rosemary
tied together
2kg fresh mussels, cleaned
Freshly ground black pepper

Garnish: freshly chopped parsley

1. Fry the onion and garlic in the oil in a saucepan until soft.
2. Add the wine and herbs. Bring to the boil and simmer for two minutes.
3. Add the cleansed mussels and plenty of freshly ground black pepper.
4. Cover and simmer for 8 to 10 minutes, or until all the mussels have opened. Don't overcook or the mussels will shrivel and become rubbery. They should remain plump with their flesh just set.
5. Remove the bouquet garni and garnish with freshly chopped parsley. Serve immediately with hot, crusty bread.

Mussels with Cider, Saffron and Leeks

Mussels and the sweetness of leeks go well together. Use a light, dry cider or alternatively, substitute the cider with dry white wine. Serve 4 as a main course (250 kcals each) or 6 as a starter (170 kcals each).

2kg fresh mussels, cleaned
400ml dry, light cider (or white wine)
250g leeks
1 small onion, finely sliced
2 cloves garlic, crushed
2 tbsp extra virgin olive oil
A large pinch of saffron
1 tbsp cornflour

Garnish: chopped parsley

1. Place the mussels and cider in a saucepan, cover and bring to the boil. Steam for five minutes, shaking the pan until all the mussels are open. Discard any mussels which do not open. Strain, reserving the liquor. Put the mussels to one side to cool.
2. Fry the leeks, onion and garlic in olive oil until starting to turn golden.
3. Add the mussel liquor, 200ml water and saffron and cook for 15 minutes.
4. Mix the cornflour with a little water (or extra cider) and add to the liquor. Thicken for five minutes.
5. Meanwhile discard the empty top mussel shells and any remaining beards.
6. Place the mussels in a serving bowl, pour over the leek, cider and saffron liquor and serve immediately with hot, crusty bread.

Greek Mussels

A common dish in Mediterranean cafés. Serves 4 as a starter at approx 190 kcals each.

1kg mussels, cleaned
150ml dry white wine
1 tbsp freshly squeezed lemon juice
2 tbsp extra virgin olive oil
1 large onion, chopped
1 tbsp coriander seeds, crushed
½ red pepper, seeded and chopped
3 cloves garlic, crushed
700g beef tomatoes, chopped
2 bay leaves
1 tbsp fresh basil leaves, chopped
2 tbsp mixed fresh herbs, chopped (e.g. oregano, thyme, parsley)

331

Freshly ground black pepper

Garnish: freshly chopped parsley

1. Place the mussels, wine and lemon juice in a large pan. Cover and steam until the mussels open – don't overcook. They should be plump and juicy.

2. Strain and reserve the liquor. Remove the mussel meat from their shells. Discard any that have not opened. Leave to cool.

3. Fry the onion, coriander seeds, pepper and garlic in olive oil until starting to colour.

4. Add the chopped tomatoes, herbs and cooking liquor from the mussels and bring to the boil.

5. Boil rapidly until the sauce is reduced and thickened.

6. Remove from the heat and cool slightly before stirring in the cooked mussels. Serve with crusty bread and green salad.

Mussels in Spiced Cream (Mouclade)

Mussels are eaten all over the Mediterranean in this delicious, curried cream sauce that has many variations. Serves 4 as a light meal at approx 440 kcals or 6 as a starter at approx 290 kcals.

    500ml dry white wine
    4 cloves garlic, crushed
    1 nutmeg
    1 clove
    1 bay leaf
    1 sprig fresh thyme
    1 handful fresh parsley, chopped
    2kg mussels, cleaned
    2 large onions, finely chopped
    4 tbsp extra virgin olive oil
    1–3 tsp curry powder depending on strength required
    2 tbsp plain flour

3 egg yolks
150ml Greek strained yogurt

1. Place the white wine, half the garlic, nutmeg, clove, bay leaf, thyme and some parsley in a saucepan and bring to the boil.

2. Add the mussels and cover. Cook for 5 minutes, shaking the pan until all the mussels have opened. Strain, reserving the liquor. Discard the nutmeg and clove, and any mussels that have not opened.

3. Discard the top shell from each mussel and any remaining beards.

4. Fry the remaining garlic and onion in olive oil until soft. Add the curry powder and cook, stirring well for 2 minutes. Add the flour and cook, still stirring well, for 1 minute.

5. Slowly pour on the strained liquor, stirring continuously to make a thin cream. Simmer this sauce until reduced by one third, thickened and smooth.

6. Beat the egg yolks and strained yogurt together and whisk into the sauce. Add the half mussel shells and garnish with the remaining parsley. Heat through but do not boil. Serve with hot, crusty bread.

Mussels in Lemon Cream

An unusual starter for 6 at 210 kcals or a light meal for 4 people at 315 kcals.

　　1 onion, finely chopped
　　1 clove garlic, crushed
　　1 tbsp extra virgin olive oil
　　100ml dry white wine
　　Grated zest and juice of 3 lemons
　　1 stalk lemon grass (optional)
　　1 tsp fresh lemon balm, chopped (optional)
　　2 tbsp fresh chives, chopped

2kg mussels, cleaned
450ml Greek strained yogurt
Freshly ground black pepper

Garnish: freshly chopped parsley

1. Fry the onion and garlic in olive oil until soft.
2. Add the wine, lemon zest and juice, herbs and mussels and cover. Cook, shaking the pan until the mussels open.
3. Remove the mussels, reserving the liquor. Discard any that have not opened. If wished, discard one shell from each mussel. Keep warm.
4. Bring the reserved liquor to the boil. Remove pan from the heat and add the yogurt. Heat slowly until just under boiling point, so the yogurt doesn't clot.
5. Pour the lemon cream over the mussels, sprinkle with chopped parsley and serve.

Stuffed Mussels with Coriander, Walnuts and Cheese

These *Moules farcies* are delicious served as a hot hors d'oeuvre with aperitifs or as a starter. The French serve this dish in style – on earthenware plates with twelve mussel-shaped hollows so the shells don't rock and spill their delicious stuffing. This meal is high in calories at approx 65 kcals per mussel, but as an occasional treat, it's worth it.

48 large mussels
60ml dry white wine
2 cloves garlic, crushed
100g walnuts, crushed
4 tbsp fresh coriander, chopped
120ml (8 tbsp) walnut oil
30g dried breadcrumbs
50g Parmesan cheese, freshly grated

Freshly ground black pepper

1. Place the cleaned mussels and white wine in a covered saucepan and steam over a strong heat for five minutes. Shake the pan frequently until all mussels are opened. Strain, reserving the liquor as stock for another recipe.

2. When the mussels are cool enough to handle, discard the empty top shell and any remaining beards. Discard any mussels that have not opened.

3. Mix together the crushed garlic, crushed walnuts, coriander and walnut oil. Season well with freshly ground black pepper.

4. Arrange the half mussel shells on a grilling pan. Divide the walnut mixture between them.

5. Mix together the breadcrumbs and Parmesan cheese and sprinkle over each shell.

6. When ready to serve, flash under the grill.

Stuffed mussels with garlic and parsley

An alternative, less calorific 'traditional' *Moules farcies* stuffing can be made by:

1. Omitting the crushed walnuts.
2. Substituting extra virgin olive oil for walnut oil.
3. Substituting chopped, fresh parsley for the coriander.
   These mussels work out at approx 50 kcals each.

Genoese Mussels

A similar dish using basil instead of coriander and much less stuffing works out at even less calories. Serve as a starter or an aperitif with a dry white wine. Approx 30 kcals per mussel.

1 small onion, finely chopped
60ml (4tbsp) dry white wine
48 large mussels, cleaned
Handful of fresh basil leaves, chopped

Handful of fresh parsley, chopped
2 cloves garlic
30g walnuts, finely chopped
4 tbsp walnut oil
50g Parmesan cheese, freshly grated
Freshly ground black pepper

1. Put the onion and wine in a large pan and cook until softened.
2. Add the mussels, cover and steam shaking the pan gently until the shells have opened. Remove the mussels, discarding any that have not opened, and reserving the cooking liquor.
3. Discard the upper half of each shell, plus any remaining beards. Arrange the mussels on a serving dish and keep warm.
4. Place the herbs, garlic, walnuts, walnut oil and half the Parmesan in a blender. Process until a smooth paste is obtained. If mix is too dry, add some of the reserved cooking liquor.
5. Spoon some of the Genoese mixture into each mussel and sprinkle the top with pepper and the remaining Parmesan cheese.
6. Flash under the grill to melt the cheese and reheat.

Mussels Stuffed with Basil and Tomato

Another recipe for *Moules farcies* with an aroma typical of the Mediterranean diet. Serves 4 at approx 20 kcals per mussel (240 kcals per person).

48 large mussels
60ml (4 tbsp) dry white wine
4 spring onions, finely chopped
3 cloves garlic, crushed
30ml (2 tbsp) extra virgin olive oil
175g tomatoes, peeled, seeded (if preferred) and chopped

Handful fresh basil leaves, chopped
Freshly ground black pepper

Garnish: basil sprigs

1. Place the cleaned mussels and wine in a saucepan and steam for 5 minutes, shaking the pan until all the mussels are opened. Strain, reserving the liquor.
2. Discard the upper half of each shell, plus any remaining beards and any mussels that have not opened. Arrange the mussels on a serving dish and keep warm.
3. Fry the spring onion and garlic in olive oil until soft. Add 100ml liquor, keeping the rest for another recipe.
4. Reduce the mussel liquor until almost totally evaporated, then add the tomato flesh and cook, stirring frequently, for 2 minutes.
5. Add the basil leaves and season with pepper.
6. Spoon the sauce into the mussel shells and serve immediately with hot, crusty bread.

Crispy Mussels

This recipe produces the most delicious, crispy tidbits. They are ideal as an aperitif at a cocktail party – or as a rare treat. Mussels cooked as in *Moules marinières* are perfect for this dish on those rare occasions when any are left over. Approx 35 kcals per mussel.

1 egg, separated
1 tbsp extra virgin olive oil
1 tbsp red wine
1 tbsp fresh parsley, finely chopped
80g plain flour, sifted
250g shelled, cooked mussels
Rock salt and freshly ground black pepper
Olive oil for deep frying

Garnish: freshly chopped parsley

1. Make the batter by beating the egg yolk with the tablespoon of extra virgin olive oil.
2. Add the red wine, parsley, 50ml water and the flour, plus a pinch of salt and plenty of pepper.
3. Whip the egg white until frothy but not too firm. Fold it into the batter.
4. Heat the olive oil for frying. Coat the mussels well with the batter and drop them into the hot oil. They should be crisp and golden in around 3 minutes.
5. Drain the mussels on absorbent paper. Serve sprinkled with salt, pepper and chopped parsley.

Lobster

Baby Lobster Salad

Around my home town of Padstow, Cornwall, the most delicious concoctions are invented to use sweet and tender lobster too small to sell, but too big to throw back. As a starter for 4 this provides approx 110 kcals. As a light meal for 2, 220 kcals.

  150ml Greek strained yogurt
  Fresh squeezed juice of half a lemon
  1 tbsp fresh basil leaves, chopped
  1 tbsp fresh chives, chopped
  ½ tsp fresh lemon balm, chopped
  ½ tsp fresh mint, chopped
  225g lightly poached lobster meat, chilled
  225g mixed salad leaves
  Freshly ground black pepper

1. Combine the yogurt, lemon juice and chopped herbs. Season well.
2. Roughly chop the lobster meat, removing any black veins.
3. Combine the meat and yogurt dressing and arrange on

338

a bed of salad leaves. Serve garnished with basil leaves or parsley, with boiled new potatoes.

Lobster Salad with Basil and Strawberries

This recipe makes a colourful salad for lunch on a hot summer's day. Approx 120 kcals if divided between 4 as a starter or 240 kcals as a light meal for 2.

    1 beef tomato, chopped
    1 tsp acacia honey
    100ml Greek strained yogurt
    1 tbsp freshly squeezed lemon juice
    Handful of fresh basil leaves, chopped
    1 tsp fresh chives, chopped
    225g lightly poached lobster meat, chilled
    100g ripe strawberries
    225g mixed red salad leaves (e.g. lollo rosso)
    4 fronds fresh coriander leaf
    Freshly ground black pepper

1. Place the tomato in a small saucepan with the honey and 1 tbsp water. Cook gently until most of the liquid has evaporated. Pass through a sieve, reserving the skins and pips for a soup recipe.
2. When cooled, add the sweetened tomato pulp to the yogurt. Mix in the lemon juice, basil and chives. Season.
3. Roughly chop the lobster meat, removing any black veins.
4. Combine the basil yogurt sauce and the lobster meat. Mix in any scarlet roes.
5. Thinly slice the strawberries. Season with pepper.
6. Serve the lobster mixture on a bed of mixed lettuce leaves. Garnish with slices of peppered strawberry and coriander fronds.

Tarragon Lobster with Madeira

Serves 4 as a starter at 200 kcals each or 2 as a light meal at 400 kcals per portion.

    225g lightly poached lobster meat, chilled
    Handful of fresh tarragon, chopped
    1 tbsp fresh chives, chopped
    1 tbsp walnut oil
    1 tbsp freshly squeezed lemon juice
    75ml (5 tbsp) Madeira (or dry sherry)
    300ml Greek strained yogurt
    Freshly ground black pepper

1. Roughly chop the lobster meat, removing any black veins.
2. Sauté the lobster meat, tarragon and chives in walnut oil until warmed through. Add the lemon juice, season and stir well.
3. Flame the Madeira and pour over the lobster meat, shaking the pan until the flames die down.
4. Pour over the yogurt and stir continuously until the sauce is heated through. Don't allow to boil or the yogurt will clot.
5. Serve immediately either on rice with salad, or with broccoli and new boiled potatoes.

Chicken

Chicken with Tomato and Basil Sauce

This deliciously fragrant, creamy sauce tastes unbelievably decadent, yet is an excellent example of healthy eating. Serves 4 at approx 300 kcals each.

    4 chicken breasts, skinned and boned
    4 spring onions, finely chopped
    2 cloves garlic, crushed

1 tbsp extra virgin olive oil
240ml white wine
2 tbsp tomato paste
2 beef tomatoes, skinned and coarsely chopped
20 fresh basil leaves, finely chopped
120ml (8 tbsp) Greek strained yogurt
Rock salt and freshly ground black pepper

1. Preheat the oven to 180°C/350°F/gas mark 4.
2. Fry the chicken breasts, spring onions and garlic in olive oil until slightly golden and cooked most of the way through. Place in a casserole dish and keep warm.
3. De-glaze the frying pan with white wine. Add the tomato paste and stir, cooking lightly for a few minutes.
4. Add the tomato and basil and cook until the mixture has reduced and started to thicken.
5. Pour the tomato and basil sauce over the chicken breasts. Cook in the oven for 15 minutes.
6. Remove the chicken breasts and arrange on a plate, keeping warm. Stir the yogurt into the tomato sauce and heat, but do not boil as the yogurt may clot.
7. Pour the tomato and basil cream sauce over the chicken breasts and garnish with sprigs of basil and slices of tomato. Serve with baked potatoes or rice and boiled spinach.

Tarragon Chicken

A classic dish serving 4 at approx 215 kcals each. Now that tarragon is regularly seen in supermarkets, this is a more accessible dish.

4 chicken pieces, skinned and boned
1 tbsp extra virgin olive oil
1 onion, finely chopped
1 clove garlic, crushed
1 tbsp flour

150ml white wine
300ml chicken stock (made from the bones, without the skin) or water
A handful of fresh tarragon leaves, finely chopped
Rock salt and freshly ground black pepper

Garnish: tarragon leaves

1. Sauté the chicken pieces in oil until beginning to colour. Remove and keep warm.
2. Fry the chopped onion and garlic until softened. Sprinkle over the flour and cook, stirring until all the oil is absorbed.
3. Slowly add the wine and chicken stock or water, and bring to the boil, stirring continuously so no lumps form.
4. Add the tarragon leaves. Simmer to reduce slightly.
5. Return the chicken pieces to the pan. Cover and cook gently for 20 minutes.

Chicken Marengo

A dish invented for Napoleon after the battle of Marengo in 1800. All ingredients were obtained from a local farmer and a neighbouring stream. The original dish was garnished with fried eggs and boiled crayfish. These are usually omitted now and replaced with less adventurous onion and a glass of brandy. Serves 4 at approx 255 kcals each.

4 chicken breasts, skinned and boned
8 baby onions (or shallots), peeled
1 clove garlic, crushed
1 tbsp extra virgin olive oil
1 tbsp plain flour
300ml dry white wine
2 beef tomatoes, chopped
225g button mushrooms, halved
½ white truffle, finely chopped (optional)

25ml (1 spirit measure) brandy
Rock salt and freshly ground black pepper

Garnish: chopped fresh parsley, garlic croûtons.

1. Sauté the chicken pieces, onion and garlic in olive oil for 10 minutes or until turning golden.
2. Sprinkle over the flour and cook, stirring, until all the oil is absorbed.
3. Slowly add the wine and bring the mixture to the boil. Simmer on a gentle heat for ten minutes.
4. Add the tomatoes, mushrooms and truffle. Season to taste.
5. Cover and cook over a low heat for 15 minutes, stirring occasionally to prevent burning.
6. Stir the brandy into the sauce and cook for another five minutes. Serve with boiled, new potatoes and salad.

Coq au Vin Rouge

A classic French dish that is best made with a fine Burgundy wine. It may be tempting to add a cheap cooking wine, but your meal will then taste of . . . cheap cooking wine. Only half a bottle is used here, leaving the rest to be enjoyed as cook's perks. Serves 4 at approx 260 kcals.

4 chicken breasts, skinned and boned
1 clove garlic, crushed
8 button onions, peeled
6 button mushrooms, sliced
1 tbsp extra virgin olive oil
25ml (1 spirit measure) brandy
375ml red Burgundy wine
1 bouquet garni (bayleaf, sprig of fresh thyme and sprig of fresh rosemary tied together with thread)
Rock salt and freshly ground black pepper

Garnish: French toast, chopped parsley

1. Sauté the chicken, garlic, onions and mushrooms in the olive oil until turning golden.

2. Pour over the brandy and set alight to flambé. As the flames die, add the burgundy and bouquet garni.

3. Cover and cook for 30 minutes. Thicken with corn-flour if desired.

4. Remove the bouquet garni, season to taste and serve garnished with crisp French toast and parsley.

Chicken with Lemon and Olives

This dish originated on the Moroccan side of the Mediterranean. It is full of fragrance, improved by mari-nating the chicken overnight before cooking. Serves 4 at approx 240 kcals each.

  2 tbsp extra virgin olive oil
  1 clove garlic, crushed
  1 tsp fresh ginger root, chopped
  1 red chilli pepper, seeded and finely chopped
  ¼ tsp cumin seed, freshly ground
  ½ tsp coriander seeds, freshly ground
  4 large chicken breasts, skinned and boned
  1 onion, finely chopped
  3 tbsp fresh parsley, chopped
  3 tbsp fresh coriander, chopped
  A pinch of saffron (or ½ tsp turmeric root, powdered)
  30g green olives, stoned and halved
  100ml dry white wine
  200ml chicken stock or water
  1 lemon, sliced
  Rock salt and freshly ground black pepper

1. Mix together the olive oil, garlic, ginger, chilli, cumin and coriander seeds. Rub well into the chicken breasts.

2. Place the chicken pieces in an earthenware dish. Cover and marinate overnight in the fridge.

3. When ready to cook, place the chicken pieces, onion, parsley, coriander and saffron (or turmeric) in a saucepan. Pour on the wine and stock or water and bring to the boil. Simmer gently for 20 minutes.

4. Add the olives and lemon slices. Cook gently for a further 10 minutes.

5. Remove the chicken pieces, lemons and olives with a slotted spoon. Place in a serving dish and keep warm.

6. Reduce the sauce and season to taste. Pour the sauce over the chicken and serve with couscous or rice.

Orange Chicken with Herbs

This fragrant boiled chicken is a healthy alternative to roast chicken. Serve with salad and boiled rice to soak up the delicious sauce. Traditionally, a handful of walnuts is added to this dish during cooking. As 100g chopped walnuts contains 688 kcals, only add these if you are not counting calories strictly. Serves 6 at approx 400 kcals each.

1 large onion, chopped
2 cloves garlic, crushed
2 tbsp extra virgin olive oil
1.5kg boiling chicken, preferably skinned
300ml chicken or vegetable stock
120ml dry white wine
1 bunch fresh parsley, chopped
1 bunch fresh chives, chopped
6 tbsp fresh coriander, chopped
4 tbsp mint, freshly chopped
175ml freshly squeezed orange juice
Grated zest of two oranges
Rock salt and freshly ground black pepper

Garnish: walnut halves

1. In a large pan, sweat the onion and garlic in olive oil until soft.

2. Add the chicken and stock and season well with black pepper. Bring to the boil, cover and simmer for 1 hour, basting regularly.

3. Add the chopped fresh herbs, orange juice and zest. Continue simmering for a further 30 minutes.

Lamb

Lamb is a well-recognized component of the Mediterranean diet. It contains saturated fat and should therefore be eaten in moderation, i.e. no more than once a week.

Lamb Shish Kebabs

A popular meal for summer barbecues. Serves 4 at approx 330 kcals each.

    500g lean fillet of lamb
    1 red pepper
    1 yellow pepper
    1 large onion
    8 button mushrooms

Marinade
Freshly squeezed juice of one lemon
4 tbsp extra virgin olive oil
2 cloves garlic, crushed
1 spring onion, finely chopped
1 tsp fresh oregano, chopped
1 tsp fresh parsley, chopped
1 tsp fresh rosemary, chopped
Rock salt and freshly ground black pepper

1. Cut the lamb into 2.5cm (1 inch) cubes. Discard all visible fat.

2. Mix the marinade ingredients together. Place the lamb cubes in a bowl and pour on the marinade. Mix well. Leave to infuse for at least 1 hour, preferably overnight. Turn occasionally.

3. Seed the peppers and cut into pieces approx 3cm (1¼ inch) square.

4. Peel the onion, cut into quarters and separate the layers.

5. Thread the lamb, pepper, onion squares and the button mushrooms onto skewers in an attractive alternating pattern.

6. Brush with any remaining marinade mixture, or with extra virgin olive oil.

7. Barbecue or grill under a high heat for several minutes to seal the meat and char the edges of the peppers. Then remove (or turn down) to a medium heat and cook for 10 to 20 minutes, or until the lamb is cooked to your preference. Turn and baste frequently during cooking. Traditionally served with rice, Greek salad and warm pitta bread.

Lamb and Aubergine Kebabs

A classic Mediterranean char-grill recipe. I had these delicious kebabs on a cruiser whilst crossing from Greece to Turkey by sea. Serves 4 at approx 330 kcals each.

500g lean fillet of lamb
1 aubergine

Marinade
4 tbsp extra virgin olive oil
Freshly squeezed juice of one lemon
2 cloves garlic, crushed
1 tsp fresh rosemary, chopped
1 tsp fresh thyme, chopped

Rock salt and freshly ground black pepper

1. Cut the lamb fillet into 2.5cm (1 inch) cubes, discarding all visible fat.
2. Mix together the marinade ingredients and pour over the lamb cubes. Marinade for at least 1 hour, preferably overnight. Turn occasionally.
3. When ready to cook, peel the aubergine and cut into 2.5cm (1 inch) cubes.
4. Thread the marinated lamb and the aubergine cubes alternately onto skewers. Brush with any remaining marinade mixture or extra virgin olive oil.
5. Barbecue, or grill, over high heat for several minutes to seal the meat. Then turn down to moderate heat and cook for 10 to 20 minutes or until the lamb is cooked according to preference. Baste and turn frequently. Serve with rice, Greek salad and warm pitta bread.

Spicy Lamb Kebabs with Lemon Balm

Wonderfully aromatic spears of meat. Serves 4 at approx 300 kcals each.

500g lean fillet of lamb
1 large onion, cut into quarters and separated into chunks

Marinade
2 tbsp extra virgin olive oil
2 tbsp balsamic or wine vinegar
2 cloves garlic, crushed
1 tsp coriander seeds, crushed
½ tsp cumin seed, crushed
1 small chilli pepper, chopped
1 tsp ground turmeric root
2 tsp acacia honey
4 bay leaves
1 handful young lemon balm leaves, chopped
1 tbsp mango or other chutney

Rock salt and freshly ground black pepper

1. Cut the lamb fillet into 2.5cm (1 inch) cubes, discarding all visible fat.
2. Combine all the marinade ingredients and add the cubed lamb and onion chunks. Marinade for several hours, or overnight if possible.
3. Thread the lamb, onion and bay leaves onto skewers.
4. Barbecue or grill for 15 to 20 minutes until brown and sizzling, basting with extra marinade throughout the cooking period. Serve with hot, garlic bread or rice plus salad.

Roast Rosemary and Garlic Lamb with Cannellini Beans

My favourite Sunday roast. Serves 6 at approx 460 kcals each.

225g dried cannellini beans, soaked overnight
1 bouquet garni (1 bay leaf, 1 sprig rosemary, 1 sprig thyme tied together)
6 juniper berries
6 peppercorns
2 cloves garlic, crushed
1 onion
1 beef tomato, chopped
1 tbsp tomato purée
2 tbsp fresh parsley, chopped
1 tbsp fresh sage (or thyme), chopped
1 tbsp fresh coriander leaves, chopped

Lamb
1 kg lamb, lean fillet of leg, boned
4–6 sprigs fresh rosemary
4 cloves garlic, sliced

3 tbsp extra virgin olive oil
Rock salt and freshly ground black pepper

Garnish: chopped fresh parsley

1. Cover the soaked cannellini beans with water, add the bouquet garni, juniper berries, peppercorns and crushed garlic. Bring to the boil and simmer for 1¼ hours whilst preparing the meat. Top up with water as necessary to prevent boiling dry. (Then continue cooking beans as in step 6 below, after meat starts cooking.)
2. Heat the oven to 180°C/350°F/gas mark 4. Make holes from one end of the lamb joint to the other with a skewer. Using the skewer, thread the rosemary sprigs through the centre of the meat.
3. Make little pockets all over the meat with a sharp knife and insert slices of garlic.
4. Brush the joint with olive oil. Season well.
5. After the beans have been cooking for 1¼ hours, place the lamb joint in the oven and roast for 45 minutes, basting occasionally with olive oil.
6. Add the onion, chopped tomato and purée to the beans. Continue cooking until the meat is ready, allowing the bean mixture to boil fairly dry at the end but without burning.
7. Drain the beans and discard the bouquet garni. Stir in the chopped herbs and season well. Place the lamb joint in the middle of a serving plate and surround with the beans. Garnish.

Serve with boiled potatoes and salad. If you want roast potatoes, parboil peeled potatoes. Brush lightly with olive oil and place around the roasting meat. Do not allow the potatoes to sit in a puddle of oil and fat.

Lamb Lasagna

Lasagna made with lamb is much tastier than that made with beef. Serves 4 at approx 575 kcals each.

1 large onion, chopped
2 cloves garlic, crushed
1 tbsp extra virgin olive oil
450g lean minced lamb
1 carrot, grated
400g fresh tomatoes, all chopped except one
30g sun-dried tomato (optional)
2 tbsp tomato purée
150ml light red wine
1 tsp fresh rosemary, chopped
2 tbsp fresh parsley, chopped
12 sheets easy-cook spinach lasagna
250g low-fat natural yogurt
50g Parmesan cheese, freshly grated
Rock salt and freshly ground black pepper

1. Fry the onion and garlic in oil for 5 minutes. Add the minced lamb and fry for a further 5 minutes.
2. Add the grated carrot, tomatoes, tomato purée, wine, 150ml water and herbs. Cover and simmer for 30 minutes, stirring occasionally.
3. Preheat the oven to 180°C/350°F/gas mark 4.
4. Brush an ovenproof dish with olive oil and line the base with four sheets of oven–ready lasagna.
5. Top with half the lamb sauce, then spread with one third of the yogurt.
6. Repeat the pasta, meat and yogurt layers and top with remaining pasta and yogurt. Thinly slice the remaining whole tomato. Decorate the top of the lasagna with tomato slices, then sprinkle with Parmesan cheese. Bake for 45 minutes.

Mediterranean Moussaka

Moussaka made traditionally can be brimming with saturated fat. As it is too delicious to be excluded from this book, I have perfected a healthier version to include as part of your Mediterranean-style diet. Serves 4 at approx 300 kcals each.

1 onion, chopped
1 leek, chopped
2 cloves garlic, crushed
1 tbsp extra virgin olive oil
350g lean, minced lamb
120g potatoes, sliced
225g tomatoes, chopped
2 tbsp tomato purée, *or* 2 sun-dried tomatoes, chopped
1 small carrot, grated
½ small Florence fennel bulb, chopped
75ml red wine
1 tbsp fresh parsley, chopped
1 small sprig fresh rosemary
1 bay leaf
1 medium aubergine, sliced
Rock salt and freshly ground black pepper

Sauce
2 tsp cornflour
300ml low-fat natural yogurt
2 eggs, size 4, lightly whisked
¼ tsp nutmeg, freshly ground
1 tbsp fresh parsley, chopped
Freshly ground black pepper

Topping
30g Parmesan cheese, freshly grated

1. Heat the oven to 180°C/350°F/gas mark 4.
2. Fry the onion, leek and garlic in the oil until beginning

to colour. Add the minced lamb and fry for 5 minutes. Season well.

3. Bring a pan of water to the boil and add the sliced potato. Cook for five minutes.

4. Drain excess fat from the lamb. Then add the tomatoes, tomato purée, carrot, fennel, red wine and herbs. Simmer for 15 minutes.

5. Add the sliced aubergine to the potatoes and continue boiling for a further five minutes.

6. Blend the cornflour and yogurt together. Add the remaining sauce ingredients and lightly whisk. Season to taste.

7. Place a thin layer of potato and aubergine in the base of an ovenproof casserole dish. Top with the lamb mixture and repeat, finishing with a layer of potato and aubergine. Press down well.

8. Pour the sauce on top. Scatter with grated Parmesan and pepper.

9. Bake for 30 minutes, or until the topping is golden. Serve with a green salad and hot, crusty bread.

Lamb with Herbs, Lemon and Black Olives

The ingredients of this dish impart a delicious fragrance to the lamb. Serve accompanied with brown rice and a watercress salad, or with plenty of vegetables and crusty bread. Serves 4 at approx 450 kcals each.

    700g lean lamb, cubed and trimmed of all visible fat
    2 tbsp extra virgin olive oil
    1 medium onion, sliced
    2 cloves garlic, crushed
    100ml dry white wine
    Juice and zest of half a lemon
    1 tbsp fresh parsley, chopped

1 tbsp fresh mint, chopped
1 tbsp fresh chives, chopped
12 stoned black olives, chopped
1 red chilli pepper, seeded and finely chopped
Rock salt and freshly ground black pepper

Garnish: chopped parsley, lemon wedges and black olives

1. Fry the lamb in hot oil over high heat to seal it.
2. Add the onions and garlic and continue frying for 5 minutes.
3. Pour over the white wine, then add the lemon juice, zest and herbs. Season well.
4. Cover and simmer for 20 minutes, then add the olives and chilli pepper.
5. Reduce the heat and simmer gently for a further 30 minutes.

Lamb Alla Romana

This lamb is typical of southern Italy – strong, spicy and drenched with flavour. Serves 4 at approx 450 kcals each.

1kg lamb on the bone, cut into four chunks
3 tbsp extra virgin olive oil
2 sprigs fresh rosemary
4 large anchovy filets, drained
6 large fresh basil leaves, chopped
4 cloves garlic, crushed
4 tbsp red wine vinegar
Rock salt and freshly ground black pepper

1. Grind equal amounts of salt and black pepper onto a plate and roll the meat to coat and season well.
2. Heat the olive oil over a high heat and fry the lamb for 10 minutes until browned.
3. Add one rosemary sprig and 125ml water, lower the heat, and continue to cook for 20 minutes.

4. Strip the leaves from the remaining rosemary sprig and pound together with the anchovies, basil and garlic. Add the red wine vinegar.

5. Pour the anchovy and vinegar mix over the meat and continue to cook for a further 5 minutes. Add extra water if necessary to prevent the meat drying out. Serve with boiled potatoes and salad.

Lamb Curry

A good lamb curry made with yogurt, fresh home-mixed whole spices and handfuls of shredded coriander leaves is difficult to beat. I often add two whole bunches of coriander leaves to one curry. Serves 4 at approx 525 kcals each. Best with basmati rice and lime pickle.

225ml Greek strained yogurt
1kg joint lamb, boned and cubed
1 large onion, sliced
4 cloves garlic, crushed
2 tbsp extra virgin olive oil
2.5cm (1 inch) piece ginger root, finely chopped
1–4 chilli peppers (depending on desired heat), seeded and chopped
2 beef tomatoes, chopped
450g vegetables (optional), e.g. cubed potatoes, okra, spinach
1 tbsp ground amchoor (mango) powder
1 large bunch of fresh coriander, chopped

Curry powder
Coarsely grind together the following:
1 tbsp coriander seeds
1 tsp cumin seeds
1 tsp fenugreek
1 tsp mustard seeds
6 green cardamoms

2 cloves
2.5cm (1 inch) cinnamon bark
1 tsp powdered turmeric
1 bay leaf
1 tsp rock salt

1. Mix together the freshly ground curry powder, half the garlic and the yogurt. Pour onto the lamb and marinate for at least 4 hours or overnight.
2. Fry the onion and garlic in olive oil until starting to colour.
3. Add the curried lamb and yogurt mix and cook, stirring gently, for 10 minutes.
4. Add the chopped ginger root, chilli, tomatoes, additional vegetables (if used) and enough water to just cover. Cover and simmer gently for 30 minutes.
5. Add the amchoor powder and chopped coriander and cook for a further 10 minutes, reducing the liquid to the consistency of a thick sauce. Serve garnished with fresh coriander.

Vegetarian Main Courses

Green Herbed Omelette

This baked French omelette is ideal for a light lunch when served with hot crusty bread or baked potatoes and salad. Serves 4 at approx 225 kcals each.

6–8 eggs, depending on size
1 leek, chopped
4 spring onions, chopped
100g spinach, freshly chopped
2 tbsp fresh parsley, chopped
1 tbsp fresh tarragon, chopped
1 tbsp fresh coriander leaves, chopped
1 tbsp fresh basil, chopped

1 tbsp walnuts, chopped
1 tbsp extra virgin olive oil
2 tbsp Parmesan cheese, freshly grated (optional)
Rock salt and freshly ground black pepper

1. Preheat the oven to 180°C/350°F/gas mark 4.
2. Beat the eggs together in a large bowl and add the chopped vegetables, herbs and walnuts. Season well.
3. Oil an ovenproof dish and pour in the mixture. Sprinkle with Parmesan cheese.
4. Cover and bake for 20 minutes. Then uncover and brown for a further 15 minutes until the top is golden.

Ratatouille

This French gypsy dish from Provence is an old favourite. Jazzed up with the addition of freshly chopped herbs and white wine, it makes an excellent main course. Serve with brown rice, pasta, crusty bread or baked potatoes and a mixed leaf salad. Serves 4 at approx 120 kcals each.

1 large onion, sliced
2 cloves garlic, crushed
1 tbsp extra virgin olive oil
1 large red pepper, seeded and sliced lengthways
1 tbsp coriander seeds, crushed
1 large aubergine, chopped
1 large courgette, chopped
4 beef tomatoes, chopped
150ml white wine
1 tbsp fresh parsley, chopped
1 tbsp fresh basil, chopped
1 tbsp fresh coriander leaves, chopped
1 tsp fresh thyme, chopped
Rock salt and freshly ground black pepper

1. Sweat the onion and garlic in olive oil in a large saucepan until translucent.
2. Add the pepper, coriander seeds and aubergine and stir-fry for 5 minutes.
3. Add all the remaining ingredients, cover and simmer with the lid on for 30 minutes. Stir occasionally.
4. Season to taste, then serve immediately.

Roasted Red Pepper Devils

These delicious, roasted red peppers serve 4 at approx 150 kcals each. I have cut down the amount of olive oil classically used in this dish. You may want to increase this by drizzling 1 tbsp extra virgin olive oil into each pepper half – but remember the additional calories this entails of 120 kcals per scant tablespoon of oil.

  4 large red peppers
  2 tbsp extra virgin olive oil
  2 cloves garlic, crushed
  Freshly squeezed juice of one lemon
  2 tbsp fresh basil, chopped
  2 tbsp fresh coriander, chopped
  2 beef tomatoes, cut into eighths
  16 anchovy fillets
  2 tbsp capers
  1 red chilli pepper, seeded and finely chopped
  Cayenne pepper
  Freshly ground black pepper

1. Preheat oven to 180°C/350°F/gas mark 4.
2. Cut the red pepper and stalk in half lengthways and remove seeds.
3. Lightly brush the pepper inside and out with olive oil and lemon juice. Place on a baking sheet or in a shallow tray.
4. Place the crushed garlic and half the chopped basil and

coriander inside the pepper halves. Season with black pepper.

5. Place 2 pieces of beef tomato inside each pepper half.

6. Divide the anchovies, capers and chilli pepper between the pepper halves and sprinkle with cayenne pepper. Curl the anchovy fillet round each piece of tomato.

7. Place the peppers in the oven and roast for 45 to 50 minutes, until the skins start to char. Garnish with the remaining basil and coriander leaves.

Aubergines Parmesan

This dish is one of my favourites – rich, aromatic and meaty, despite being vegetarian. It is excellent served with brown rice, a mixed green salad and a light, fruity red wine. Serves 4 at approx 400 kcals each.

    1 large onion, sliced
    4 cloves garlic, crushed
    4 tbsp extra virgin olive oil
    700g beef tomatoes
    2 tbsp tomato purée
    120ml dry white wine
    2 tbsp fresh basil, chopped
    1 tbsp fresh oregano, chopped
    1 tbsp fresh parsley, chopped
    2 large aubergines, sliced lengthways
    225g Mozzarella, sliced *or* low-fat Cheddar cheese, grated

Topping
50g Parmesan cheese, freshly grated
1 beef tomato, sliced

Garnish: freshly chopped basil

1. Preheat oven to 180°C/350°F/gas mark 4.

2. Fry the onion and garlic in 1 tbsp olive oil for 5 minutes until just beginning to colour.

3. Add the tomatoes, tomato purée, wine and herbs. Cover and simmer for 30 minutes, stirring occasionally. Season to taste.

4. Brush the pan with some of the remaining olive oil and lightly fry the aubergine slices in batches until soft and beginning to colour. Re-brush the pan between batches, trying to keep the absorption of oil to a minimum. Drain the aubergine slices on absorbent paper.

5. Layer the tomato sauce, aubergine slices and cheese in a casserole dish, starting and finishing with tomato sauce.

6. Top with a layer of sliced beef tomato and sprinkle with Parmesan cheese.

7. Bake for 30 minutes or until nicely browned. Serve garnished with chopped basil.

Stuffed Cinnamon Aubergines (Imam Bayildi)

This is a classic aubergine dish from Turkey. It is named after the Muslim holy man – the Imam – who fainted from sheer pleasure when first tasting this exquisite meal. Make sure the cinnamon is freshly ground. Stale cinnamon loses its piquant flavour and will produce an inferior dish. Serve hot or cold with salad, warm walnut bread or with roast meat. Serves 4 at approx 160 kcals each.

> 2 large aubergines
> 3 tbsp extra virgin olive oil
> 2 large onions
> 2 cloves garlic
> 2 beef tomatoes, chopped
> ½ tsp acacia honey
> 1 tbsp fresh parsley, chopped
> 1 tbsp fresh coriander, chopped
> ½ tsp cinnamon, freshly ground
> ½ tsp coriander seeds, freshly ground

1 tbsp pine kernels (or chopped walnuts)
Rock salt and freshly ground black pepper

1. Preheat the oven to 180°C/350°F/gas mark 4.
2. Cut the leaf base from the aubergines, cover with boiling water and boil for 10 minutes. Drain, then plunge into cold water until cool enough to handle.
3. Cut the aubergines in half lengthways. Scoop out and reserve most of the flesh, leaving a 1 cm (½ inch) thick shell.
4. Lightly oil the insides of the hollowed aubergine shells and season well. Place on a greased oven tray and bake for 30 minutes. Meanwhile, chop the reserved flesh.
5. Fry the onion and garlic in 1 tbsp olive oil for 5 minutes or until beginning to colour.
6. Add the tomatoes, honey, herbs and spices. Simmer for 15 minutes.
7. Add the chopped aubergine flesh and pine kernels to the mixture and continue cooking for 10 minutes. Season to taste.
8. Remove the aubergine shells from the oven. Stuff them with the spiced tomato and aubergine mixture and serve immediately.

Aubergine and Spinach Bake

A layered dish that reheats well. Serves 4 at approx 485 kcals each.

2 tbsp extra virgin olive oil
450g aubergines, sliced lengthways
450g baby spinach leaves, chopped
120g Mozzarella (or Cheddar) cheese, grated
30g Parmesan cheese, freshly grated

Sauce
450g beef tomatoes, chopped
1 onion, chopped

2 cloves garlic, crushed
1 tbsp extra virgin olive oil
1 tbsp tomato purée
1 tbsp fresh basil, chopped
1 tbsp fresh oregano, chopped
1 tbsp fresh parsley, chopped
100ml dry white wine
1 red pepper, seeded and cut into strips
100g mushrooms, sliced
100g walnuts, coarsely chopped
Rock salt and freshly ground black pepper

1. Lightly brush a heavy pan with olive oil and fry the aubergine slices until starting to colour. Drain on absorbent paper.

2. Place the spinach leaves in a saucepan with a few tablespoons of water. Cover and steam until tender.

3. Pre-heat the oven to 190°C/375°F/gas mark 5.

4. To make the sauce, purée the tomatoes in a blender.

5. Fry the onion and garlic in the oil until beginning to colour. Add the blended tomatoes, tomato purée, herbs and white wine. Bring to the boil and cook, stirring, until starting to thicken.

6. Add the red pepper and mushrooms and simmer for 5 minutes. Add a little water or more wine if the sauce becomes too thick.

7. Remove from heat and season. Stir in the walnuts.

8. Place alternating layers of aubergine slices, sauce and spinach in an ovenproof dish. Top with the grated cheese and bake for 30 minutes. Serve with pasta or hot, crusty bread and salad.

Italian Pepper Salad (Peperonata)

This Italian salad is served hot with grilled meat and fish, or cold with black olives, hard-boiled eggs, anchovies and crusty bread. With Parma ham and figs, it makes an excellent light lunch. Serves 4 at approx 250 kcals each.

    4 mixed red, yellow, orange and green sweet peppers
    900g mixed yellow and red tomatoes
    4 tbsp extra virgin olive oil
    1 large onion, peeled and chopped
    3 cloves garlic, crushed
    1 chilli pepper, seeded and finely chopped (optional)
    Freshly squeezed juice of half a lemon
    1 tsp acacia honey (optional)
    Rock salt and freshly ground black pepper

1. Grill the peppers until their skins blister and blacken. Wrap in a damp cloth for 30 minutes. The skins are then easily removed by rubbing under cold running water.
2. Cut the pepper flesh into strips and roughly chop the tomatoes. Some cooks prefer to skin and seed the tomatoes first, but this lowers the fibre and vitamin value of the meal.
3. Fry the pepper, onion and garlic in oil until soft but not browning.
4. Add the tomatoes, chilli and lemon juice and season well with black pepper. Glaze with honey if desired.
5. Cook over a low heat for 25 minutes or until the juice from the tomatoes has evaporated.
6. Adjust seasoning and serve hot or cold.

Peppery Scrambled Eggs (Piperade)

A lingering memory from Southern France is eating this delicious red pepper and scrambled egg dish in a little village café. It is particularly effective at curing a wine-taster's hangover. Serve with garlic bread or wholemeal toast and mixed leaf salad. It goes particularly well with char-grilled sardines. Serves 4 at approx 250 kcals each.

    1 onion, finely chopped

2 cloves garlic, crushed
2 tbsp extra virgin olive oil
450g red peppers, seeded and cut into strips
2 beef tomatoes, chopped
6 eggs, size 1
2 tbsp fresh parsley or basil, chopped
1 tbsp fresh chives, chopped
½ tsp cayenne pepper
1 tbsp Greek strained yogurt (optional)
Rock salt and freshly ground black pepper
Garnish: chopped parsley or basil

1. Fry the onion and garlic in oil for 5 minutes.
2. Add the peppers and tomatoes and fry for a further 5 minutes. Make sure most of the liquid has evaporated.
3. Beat the eggs together lightly. Add herbs, cayenne pepper and yogurt, if used. Season well.
4. Pour the eggs over the vegetable mix and cook, stirring constantly until the eggs are lightly scrambled. Serve immediately, garnished with chopped fresh herbs.

Cheese and Lentil Herb Loaf

Lentils and cheese combine well to make a classic vegetarian dish. This is delicious served hot or cold with warm, crusty bread, watercress and a green side salad. Serves 4 at approx 330 kcals each.

175g red lentils
100g low-fat hard cheese (e.g. reduced-fat Cheddar), grated
2 tbsp walnuts, chopped
1 onion, chopped
1 tbsp fresh parsley, chopped
1 tbsp fresh chives, chopped
1 tbsp fresh basil, chopped
½ tsp cayenne pepper

1 egg, size 1
1 tbsp freshly squeezed lemon juice
3 tbsp Greek strained yogurt
1 tbsp tomato purée
2 beef tomatoes, thinly sliced
Rock salt and freshly ground black pepper
A little olive oil

1. Pre-heat the oven to 190°C/375°F/gas mark 5.
2. Rinse the lentils. Place in a tightly covered pan with 350ml water. Simmer for 10 to 15 minutes. The lentils should reduce to a stiff purée. Moisten with a little more water if necessary.
3. Remove from the heat and mix in the grated cheese, walnuts, onion, chopped herbs and cayenne pepper.
4. Beat the egg lightly and stir in the yogurt, lemon juice and tomato purée.
5. Add the egg mixture to the lentil mix and combine thoroughly.
6. Brush the inside of a 450g loaf tin with olive oil. Line with one third of the sliced tomatoes. Add one third of the lentil mixture and press down well. Top with half the remaining beef tomato slices.
7. Add half the remaining lentil mix and press down well. Top with the remaining tomato slices. Finally, add the remaining lentil mix and press down.
8. Bake for 45 to 50 minutes until the top is golden brown. Leave to stand in the tin for 10 minutes before turning out.

Asparagus, Walnut and Mushroom Roast

Nut roasts provide a delicious and popular alternative to meat. When layered with asparagus stalks, this loaf is attractive on cutting. Serve hot with warm, crusty bread, watercress and a mixed leaf salad. Serves 6 at approx 390 kcals each.

1 onion, finely chopped
120g chestnut or brown cap mushrooms, chopped
2 cloves garlic
1 tbsp extra virgin olive oil
3 medium parsnips, boiled
3 tbsp Greek strained yogurt
1 tsp fresh rosemary, chopped
1 tsp fresh thyme, chopped
1 tbsp fresh parsley, chopped
1 egg, size 1
225g walnuts, ground
120g fresh wholemeal breadcrumbs
150ml hot water or stock
1 tsp yeast extract (if not using stock)
4 walnut halves
2 small bay leaves
½ red pepper, cut into strips lengthways
8 long asparagus stalks, lightly steamed
Rock salt and freshly ground black pepper
Olive oil for greasing

1. Pre-heat the oven to 180°C/350°F/gas mark 4.
2. Fry the onion, mushrooms and garlic in oil until beginning to brown.
3. Mash the parsnips with the yogurt and fresh herbs. Season well.
4. Beat the egg and add to the ground walnuts and breadcrumbs. Fold into the parsnip mix with the fried onion, mushrooms and garlic.
5. Add the stock or yeast extract dissolved in hot water to the nut roast mix. Combine well and season to taste.
6. Lightly brush a 900g loaf tin with olive oil. Arrange the four walnut halves and 2 bay leaves in the base so they form a pattern when the loaf is turned out.
7. Layer a third of the nut roast mix in the bottom of the

loaf tin. Arrange half the red pepper strips and asparagus stalks lengthways on top. Add half the remaining mix and top with the remaining pepper strips and asparagus. Finally, top with the remaining nut roast mix.

8. Cover with foil and bake for 50 minutes. Leave to stand for 10 minutes before turning out.

Mediterranean Fennel Bake

Italy is world famous for Florence fennel – the vegetable with the wonderful, aniseed-like flavour. When baked with other staples from the Mediterranean area, fennel makes an excellent light dinner served with wholemeal bread and salad. It is best accompanied by a robust red wine. Serves 4 at approx 180 kcals each.

1 large onion, chopped
3 cloves garlic, crushed
1 tbsp extra virgin olive oil
1lb Florence fennel bulbs, thinly sliced
3 beef tomatoes, sliced
100ml red wine
1 tbsp fresh parsley, chopped
1 tbsp fresh basil, chopped
50g fresh wholemeal breadcrumbs
50g Parmesan cheese, freshly grated
Rock salt and freshly ground black pepper

Garnish: feathery green fennel leaves

1. Fry the onion and garlic in oil until beginning to colour. Add the sliced fennel and stir-fry for five minutes.
2. Add the tomatoes, red wine and herbs. Cover and simmer gently for 30 minutes.
3. Pour into an earthenware serving dish. Top with the breadcrumbs and grated Parmesan cheese. Grill until crisp

and golden. Serve immediately. Garnish with fine, feath-ered fennel leaves.

Baked Potatoes Stuffed with Herbs, Spinach and Cheese

Stuffed baked potatoes are a firm British favourite. This version has a Mediterranean air to it. Serves 4 at approx 330 kcals each.

 4 x 200g baking potatoes
 350g baby spinach, chopped
 4 spring onions, finely chopped
 150ml Greek strained yogurt
 1 tbsp fresh parsley, chopped
 1 tbsp fresh coriander, chopped
 1 tbsp fresh basil or oregano, chopped
 100g Mozzarella (or Cheddar) cheese, sliced
 Rock salt and freshly ground black pepper

1. Preheat the oven to 200°C/400°F/gas mark 6.
2. Prick the potato skins and bake for 1 hour. Leave to cool.
3. Place the spinach in a saucepan with a few tablespoons of water and steam until tender.
4. Cut cooked potatoes in half lengthways and scoop out the flesh. Reserve the skins.
5. Mash the potato flesh until smooth, then add the spinach, spring onions, yogurt and herbs. Mix well, seasoning to taste.
6. Spoon the mixture back into the potato skins. Top with the grated cheese and bake for 20 minutes until golden. Serve with salad as a tasty, light but filling meal.

Avocado, Herb and Vegetable Bake

Avocado takes on a different, vegetable-like flavour when baked. It combines especially well with tomatoes and cheese in this vegetable bake. Serves 4 at approx 350 kcals each.

1 onion, chopped
1 leek, chopped
2 cloves garlic, crushed
2 tbsp extra virgin olive oil
120g mushrooms, sliced
1 red pepper, seeded and cut into strips
1 courgette, sliced
1 carrot, grated
1 tbsp fresh parsley, chopped
1 tbsp fresh basil, chopped
1 tbsp fresh coriander, chopped
1 sprig fresh rosemary
1 tbsp pine kernels
120g broccoli, chopped
100ml dry white wine
1 avocado, peeled, stoned and sliced
1 beef tomato, sliced
120g Mozzarella (or Cheddar), grated
Rock salt and freshly ground black pepper

1. Pre-heat the oven to 180°C/350°F/gas mark 4.
2. Fry the onion, leek and garlic in olive oil until beginning to colour. Add the mushrooms, pepper, courgette and carrot and continue stir-frying for 5 minutes.
3. Add the stir-fry mixture, herbs, pine kernels and chopped broccoli to an ovenproof dish and mix together. Pour over the glass of wine and season well.
4. Top with the sliced avocado and tomato. Sprinkle on the cheese and bake for 30 minutes.

Mediterranean Chickpeas

This dish resembles a coarse, more meaty version of hummus. The herbs and spices can be varied according to taste and availability. Serves 4 at approx 400 kcals each.

225g chickpeas, soaked overnight
1 onion, chopped
3 cloves garlic, crushed
2 tbsp extra virgin olive oil
1 tsp cumin seeds, freshly ground
1 tbsp coriander seeds, freshly ground
225g spinach, chopped
450g beef tomatoes, chopped
2 tbsp fresh coriander, chopped
1 tbsp fresh parsley, chopped
1 tbsp fresh oregano, chopped
100g Mozzarella (or Cheddar) cheese, grated
1 tbsp Parmesan cheese, freshly grated
4 tbsp Greek strained yogurt
Rock salt and freshly ground black pepper

1. Simmer the soaked chickpeas in water for 45 minutes until tender. Drain, reserving the cooking liquor.
2. Liquidize one quarter of the chickpeas with a little cooking liquor to make a smooth paste.
3. Fry the onion and garlic in olive oil until beginning to colour.
4. Add the ground seeds and the remaining whole chickpeas. Cook, stirring, for 5 minutes.
5. Stir in the spinach, tomatoes and herbs. Add 200ml cooking liquor and bring to the boil. Simmer for 5 minutes.
6. Remove from the heat. Season to taste. Add the grated cheese and yogurt and stir until the cheese has melted.

Pasta

Pasta is relatively high in calories at 320–390 kcal/100g according to type. Eaten plain, however, pasta is highly filling and an excellent source of carbohydrate. At around 75% carbohydrate, it is an excellent fuel for working muscles.

By the time you've added a sauce containing olive oil, the calorie cost will soar but you can still eat and enjoy pasta on a diet. Just keep an eye on your total calorie intake and ensure you take plenty of exercise to help burn it up.

I've kept the olive oil content of these recipes to a minimum – classic Italian recipes would contain more. Do add more extra virgin olive oil if you are at your ideal weight; if you are counting calories make the appropriate adjustment. One scant tablespoon of olive oil is approx 120 kcals.

A teaspoon of olive oil added to the water when cooking pasta helps stop it sticking together. Pasta is ready to eat when it is *al dente* which means it is sticky to the teeth. The traditional way of checking this with spaghetti is to throw a strand at a wall. If it sticks, the pasta is ready to eat.

When draining pasta, leave a little water clinging to the strands. This helps a sauce to coat the pasta more easily.

Pasta with Pesto

Tagliatelle or fettuccine are ideal for this recipe. This sauce is bound to feature regularly in your new eating plan once you've converted those excess pounds to muscle. Serves 4 at approx 600 kcals each.

    50ml extra virgin olive oil
    50ml walnut oil (or more olive oil)
    2 tbsp pine nuts, lightly toasted
    2 cloves garlic, crushed

50g fresh basil leaves
50g Parmesan cheese, freshly grated
450g fresh pasta *or* 350g dried pasta
Rock salt and freshly ground black pepper

1. Blend or pound the olive oil, walnut oil, nuts, garlic and basil into a smooth paste. Stir in the cheese. Season to taste.
2. Meanwhile, cook the pasta in plenty of boiling water until *al dente*. Drain but leave moist so the sauce will coat the pasta well.
3. Mix the pasta and pesto sauce together. Toss well and serve with a green salad.

Pasta with Walnuts and Coriander

Another favourite, this recipe serves 4 at approx 575 kcals each.
50ml walnut oil
25ml extra virgin olive oil
50g walnuts, crushed
2 cloves garlic, crushed
2 tbsp fresh coriander, chopped
1 tbsp fresh parsley, chopped
1 tsp fresh oregano/marjoram, chopped
1 tsp coriander seeds, crushed
30g Parmesan cheese, freshly grated
450g fresh pasta *or* 350g dried pasta
Rock salt and freshly ground black pepper

1. Blend or pound the oil, nuts, garlic, herbs and seeds into a smooth paste. Stir in the cheese. Season to taste.
2. Meanwhile, cook the pasta in plenty of boiling water until *al dente*. Drain but leave moist so the sauce will coat the pasta well.

3. Mix the pasta and coriander walnut sauce together. Toss well and serve with a green salad.

Pasta with Fennel and Mixed Mediterranean Herbs

Serves 4 at approx 435 kcals each.
  1 onion, finely chopped
  1 small bulb Florence fennel, chopped into matchsticks
  2 cloves garlic, crushed
  4 tbsp extra virgin olive oil
  450g fresh pasta *or* 350g dried pasta
  1 tbsp fresh parsley, chopped
  1 tbsp fresh basil, chopped
  1 tbsp fresh oregano or marjoram, chopped
  1 tbsp fresh thyme, chopped
  1 tsp fresh rosemary, chopped
  Rock salt and freshly ground black pepper

1. Sauté the onion, fennel and garlic in olive oil until beginning to colour.
2. Meanwhile, cook the pasta in plenty of boiling water until *al dente*. Drain but leave moist so the sauce will coat the pasta well.
3. Add the freshly chopped herbs and pasta to the fennel mixture and stir-fry for one minute. Season to taste.

Pasta with Tomato and Mozzarella Sauce

A pizza-flavoured pasta meal, this dish sums up the best of Italian cooking. Serves 4 at approx 600 kcals each.
  1 onion, chopped
  2 cloves garlic, crushed
  4 tbsp extra virgin olive oil

450g beef tomatoes, skinned and chopped
1 tbsp fresh oregano or marjoram, chopped
50ml dry white wine
450g fresh pasta *or* 350g dried pasta
100g Mozzarella cheese, grated
50g Parmesan cheese, grated
Freshly ground black pepper

1. Sauté the onion and garlic in olive oil until beginning to colour.
2. Add the tomatoes, oregano and wine and cook, stirring occasionally, for 15 minutes.
3. Meanwhile, cook the pasta in plenty of boiling water until *al dente*. Drain but leave moist so the sauce will coat the pasta well.
4. Mix the pasta and sauce together and season well.
5. Top with the cheese and flash under the grill until the cheese is melted.

Pasta with Tomato, Cinnamon and Bay

This fragrant dish is full of the lovely, warm tang of cinnamon and bay leaves. I like it best made with tagliatelle but any pasta will do. Serves 4 at approx 380 kcals each.

1 tbsp extra virgin olive oil
1 onion, chopped
2 cloves garlic, crushed
900g beef tomatoes, skinned and chopped
1 tbsp fresh parsley, chopped
6 fresh bay leaves
Rock salt and freshly ground black pepper
1 stick cinnamon (or ¼ tsp ground cinnamon)
450g fresh pasta *or* 350g dried pasta

1. Sauté the onion and garlic in olive oil until beginning to colour.

2. Add the tomatoes, herbs and cinnamon. Cook for 15 minutes, stirring occasionally. Season to taste.

3. Meanwhile, cook the pasta in plenty of boiling water until *al dente*. Drain but leave slightly moist so the sauce will coat the pasta well.

4. Mix the pasta and sauce together and toss well.

Pasta with Garlic Oil and Chilli

This is one of the most popular dishes served in Italy, almost a Mediterranean equivalent to British chips as a dietary staple. It goes well with grilled fish and salad, or is enjoyed on its own if a quick snack is required. If you want a fiery taste, chop the chilli finely and leave in the seeds. If you prefer something milder, cut the chilli in half and remove the seeds. I like to add a few chopped herbs such as basil or coriander leaves to this dish too. Serves 4 at approx 425 kcals each.

> 450g fresh pasta *or* 350g dried pasta
> 4 cloves garlic, crushed
> 1 fresh or dried chilli, chopped
> 60ml (4 tbsp) extra virgin olive oil
> 2 tbsp mixed fresh herbs, chopped (optional)
> Rock salt and freshly ground black pepper

1. Cook the pasta in plenty of boiling water until *al dente*. Drain but leave moist so the sauce will coat the pasta well.

2. Sauté the garlic and chilli in olive oil until soft.

3. Add the pasta and herbs (if using) to the pan and stir-fry for 1 minute. Season to taste and then serve immediately.

Pasta Al Funghi

This dish is best made with a selection of fresh, wild

375

mushrooms, available from good delicatessens. Chestnut, oyster and shiitake mushrooms will do. Serves 4 at approx 450 kcals each.

1 onion, finely chopped
2 cloves garlic, crushed
2 tbsp extra virgin olive oil
225g mixed wild mushrooms
50ml dry white wine
1 tbsp fresh parsley, chopped
1 tbsp fresh oregano or marjoram, chopped
450g fresh pasta *or* 350g dried pasta
4 tbsp Greek strained yogurt
30g Parmesan cheese, freshly grated
Rock salt and freshly ground black pepper

1. Sauté the onion and garlic in oil until soft.
2. Add the mushrooms and stir-fry over a low heat until their liquid starts to run. Add the white wine and herbs and cook gently for ten minutes. Add a little more wine if the sauce is in danger of going dry.
3. Meanwhile, cook the pasta in plenty of boiling water until *al dente*. Drain but leave slightly moist so the sauce will coat the pasta well.
4. Remove the mushrooms from the heat and stir in the yogurt. Season well.
5. Combine the pasta and mushroom sauce and toss well. Sprinkle with Parmesan cheese and serve with a green salad.

Pasta with Mixed Vegetables

Char-grilled vegetables marinated in herbs, garlic and olive oil are a favourite side dish in Italy. Here, I've combined them with pasta to make a delicious vegetarian dish. This recipe is best made using a char-grill or barbecue. It can be made under a hot domestic grill, but you will lose some of the lovely char-grilled flavour. Serves 4 at approx 475 kcals each.

    2 small aubergines
    4 small courgettes
    1 large yellow pepper (or two small ones)
    1 large red pepper (or two small ones)
    2 beef tomatoes, cut in half
    450g fresh pasta *or* 350g dried pasta
    60ml (4 tbsp) extra virgin olive oil
    Juice and zest of one lemon
    2 cloves garlic, crushed
    1 tsp acacia honey
    2 tbsp fresh basil, chopped
    1 tbsp fresh oregano or marjoram, chopped
    Parmesan cheese (optional)
    Rock salt and freshly ground black pepper

1. Cut the aubergines in half lengthways, then into eighths.

2. Cut the courgettes in half lengthways, and then into quarters.

3. Place the whole peppers on the char-grill and turn frequently until their skins are blackened on all sides. Put the peppers in a plastic bag and seal until cool. The steam released will loosen the skins and allow easy peeling.

4. When cool, peel off the black skin and seed. Divide the peppers into segments.

5. Place the tomato halves, aubergine and courgette slices on the char-grill until cooked and coloured on one side. Turn the vegetables and repeat. Season whilst grilling.

6. Meanwhile, cook the pasta in plenty of boiling water until *al dente*. Drain.

7. Place the olive oil, lemon juice, garlic, honey and herbs in a screw-top jar. Season well and shake thoroughly.

8. Place the pasta on a large serving plate. Arrange the grilled vegetables on top and pour over the dressing. Top with grated Parmesan cheese if desired.

Pasta with Lemon Cream

An unusual, fresh-flavoured pasta which goes well with lamb kebabs. Also delicious served on its own as a light lunch with green salad. Serves 4 at approx 400 kcals each.

    450g fresh pasta *or* 350g dried pasta
    1 tbsp extra virgin olive oil
    75ml (5 tbsp) freshly squeezed lemon juice plus zest of one lemon
    50ml dry white wine
    1 tsp fresh lemon balm, chopped
    1 tbsp fresh parsley, chopped
    200ml low-fat, natural bio yogurt
    30g Parmesan cheese, freshly grated
    Rock salt and freshly ground black pepper

1. Cook the pasta in plenty of boiling water until *al dente*. Drain but leave moist so the sauce will coat the pasta well.
2. Meanwhile, heat the olive oil, lemon juice and zest, wine and herbs in a heavy based pan.
3. Add the yogurt and stir until hot but do not boil or the yogurt will clot. Season well with plenty of black pepper.
4. Combine the pasta and lemon sauce and toss well. Sprinkle over Parmesan cheese.

Pasta with Anchovies

A hot, spicy meal with loads of character and an assortment of textures. Dried, salted anchovies are best for this recipe, but drained canned ones will do. Although Parmesan cheese is not traditionally served with fish pasta dishes, I include it here as I can't resist it. Serves 4 at approx 600 kcals each.

    60ml (4 tbsp) extra virgin olive oil
    120g ciabatta, made into coarse breadcrumbs
    4 cloves garlic, crushed

200g salted anchovies, rinsed to remove salt
Juice and zest of half a lemon
1 tbsp wholegrain mustard
450g fresh pasta *or* 350g dried pasta
3 tbsp fresh parsley, chopped
2 dried chillies, chopped, *or* one large fresh one, chopped
50g Parmesan cheese, freshly grated (optional)
Freshly ground black pepper

1. Heat the olive oil and fry the breadcrumbs and 2 crushed garlic cloves until golden and crisp (about 5 minutes). Remove with a slotted spoon and drain on absorbent paper.

2. Add the anchovy fillets to the hot oil and mash with a wooden spatula into a paste. Stir in the lemon juice and zest, mustard and remaining garlic. Season well with black pepper and stir-fry for 1 minute.

3. Meanwhile, cook the pasta in plenty of boiling water until *al dente*. Drain but leave moist so the sauce will coat the pasta well.

4. Add the pasta to the anchovy paste and stir-fry for one minute. Serve sprinkled with parsley, chillies, lemon zest, Parmesan and plenty of crunchy, golden breadcrumbs.

Pasta with Smoked Salmon and Fennel

An elegant meal. Serves 4 at approx 450 kcals each.

2 cloves garlic, crushed
1 small bulb Florence fennel, chopped into matchsticks
1 tbsp extra virgin olive oil
1 tbsp fennel leaves, chopped
1 tbsp freshly squeezed lemon juice
zest of half a lemon
300ml low-fat fromage frais
450g fresh pasta *or* 350g dried pasta
175g smoked salmon, cut into thin strips

Rock salt and freshly ground black pepper

Garnish: Fennel leaves

1. Sauté the garlic and Florence fennel in oil until beginning to colour. Season well.
2. Add the herbs, lemon juice, zest and fromage frais. Heat through, stirring continuously. Do not allow to boil or the fromage frais may clot.
3. Meanwhile, cook the pasta in plenty of boiling water until *al dente*. Drain but leave moist so the sauce will coat the pasta well.
4. Combine the pasta and fennel sauce. Toss well then add the smoked salmon strips. Garnish with fennel leaves. Serve immediately with crusty bread and salad.

Pasta with Mussels, Tomato and Garlic

Serves 4 at approx 450 kcals each.
    32 mussels, scrubbed and de-bearded
    100ml dry white wine
    1 small onion, finely chopped
    4 cloves garlic, crushed
    1 tbsp extra virgin olive oil
    2 beef tomatoes, skinned and chopped
    2 tbsp fresh parsley, chopped
    1 bay leaf
    450g fresh pasta *or* 350g dried pasta
    Freshly ground black pepper

    Garnish: chopped parsley

1. Put the mussels and wine in a large saucepan. Cover and steam until all the mussels are open. Strain, reserving the cooking liquor. When they are cool enough to handle, remove the mussels from their shells and keep warm. Discard any mussels that have not opened.
2. Sauté the onion and garlic in oil until soft.

3. Add the tomato, parsley, bay leaf and liquor from the mussels and cook for 5 minutes. Season well.

4. Meanwhile, cook the pasta in plenty of boiling water until *al dente*. Drain but leave moist so the sauce will coat the pasta well.

5. Combine the pasta, mussels and tomato sauce. Garnish with fresh parsley and serve immediately.

Pasta Alla Puttanesca

A hot, spicy pasta dish with a gutsy kick. I remember first eating *penne alla puttanesca* as a medical student at Cambridge. I swooned with delight and pestered my Italian colleague for the recipe. Only later did he tell me the real meaning of the name – *puttana* is an Italian prostitute. Serves 4 at approx 520 kcals each.

  2 spring onions, finely chopped
  3 cloves garlic, crushed
  1 fresh or dried chilli, chopped
  3 salted anchovies, rinsed and chopped *or* 1 x 50g tin of anchovy fillets, drained
  60ml (4 tbsp) extra virgin olive oil
  700g beef tomatoes, chopped
  450g fresh pasta *or* 350g dried pasta
  100g black olives, stoned
  1 tbsp capers
  2 tbsp fresh parsley, chopped
  Rock salt and freshly ground black pepper

  Garnish: chopped parsley

1. Sauté the spring onions, garlic, chilli and anchovies in the oil, stirring frequently and pounding the anchovies until they disintegrate.

2. Add the chopped tomatoes and simmer for 10 minutes, stirring occasionally.

3. Meanwhile, cook the pasta in plenty of boiling water until *al dente*. Drain but leave moist so the sauce will coat the pasta well.

4. Add the black olives, capers and parsley to the tomato sauce and cook gently for a further 2 minutes. Season to taste.

5. Add the pasta to the pan and stir-fry for 1 minute. Garnish with plenty of parsley and serve immediately with hot, crusty bread and salad.

Pasta with Tomato, Tuna and Parsley Sauce

This was the first dish I ever cooked as an impoverished student. It still graces the dining table, especially when a hot, nourishing and tasty meal is required at short notice. Serves 4 at approx 460 kcals each.

1 onion, chopped
2 cloves garlic, crushed
2 tbsp extra virgin olive oil
350g beef tomatoes, chopped
1 chilli, fresh or dried, chopped
50ml dry white wine
200g tuna fish (fresh or drained from brine), flaked
1 tbsp wholegrain mustard
12 black olives, stoned and chopped
2 tbsp fresh parsley, chopped
450g fresh pasta *or* 350g dried pasta
Freshly ground black pepper

Garnish: chopped parsley

1. Sauté the onion and garlic in olive oil until beginning to colour.

2. Add the chopped tomatoes, chilli and wine and simmer gently for 10 minutes, stirring occasionally.

3. Add the tuna, mustard, olives and parsley and simmer gently for 10 minutes. Season well.

4. Meanwhile, cook the pasta in plenty of boiling water until *al dente*. Drain but leave slightly moist so the sauce will coat the pasta well.

5. Toss the pasta and sauce together and garnish with parsley. Although Parmesan cheese is not traditionally served with fish and pasta dishes, I find it complements this dish very well if you can spare the calories.

Pizza

Pizza is a traditional and wholesome Italian staple. It combines carbohydrate with fibre, vitamins and protein and doesn't have to be high in fats. Try the following mix–and–match recipes, combining the dough and toppings of your choice. Serve with mixed or green salads and plenty of fresh herbs.

All ingredients given are for four pizzas. Bake individual pizzas at 240°C/475°F/gas mark 9 for about 10 minutes until the crust around the edge of the pizza is crisp and the dough cooked through.

Dough Mixes

Traditional White Luxury Egg Dough

Makes 4 pizza bases at approx 530 kcals each. Reserve for special treats when you have budgeted for the calories. Allow at least 4 hours for rising and proving.

   400g plain strong white flour
   ½ tsp ground rock salt
   2 tbsp extra virgin olive oil
   ½ sachet easy blend dried yeast

300ml warm water
2 eggs, lightly beaten
100g strong white flour for final kneading
Extra flour and water for rolling dough, correcting consistency, etc.

1. Sieve the flour into a large bowl. Add the salt, 1 tbsp olive oil and dried yeast. Blend well.

2. Add enough warm water to make a dough. Knead for 15 to 20 minutes. Place in an oiled bowl and cover with a damp cloth. Leave in a warm place for 2½ hours or until doubled in size.

3. Remove dough from bowl. Knock back and replace in bowl. Cover and leave to prove in a warm place for another hour.

4. Remove the dough and knock back again. Make a hollow in the centre and add the eggs and the remaining 1 tbsp olive oil. Add as much of the extra flour as necessary to maintain a good dough consistency. Knead thoroughly for 10 minutes.

5. Divide and roll out into four large individual pizza bases. Place on an oiled baking tray and cover with a damp cloth. Leave to rise for 1 hour.

6. Carefully add tomato sauce and selected topping and bake individual pizzas at 240°C/475°F/gas mark 9 for about 10 minutes until the crust around the edge of the pizza is crisp and the dough cooked through.

Variations
At the final kneading stage try adding one of the following:
- 4 tbsp chopped fresh coriander
- 1 clove crushed garlic
- 2 tbsp fresh grated Parmesan cheese
- 4 tbsp chopped walnuts
- 4 tbsp chopped black olives

Basic Pizza Dough

Makes 4 pizzas at approx 400 kcals each.
  400g plain strong white flour
  ½ tsp ground rock salt
  2 tbsp extra virgin olive oil
  ½ sachet easy blend dried yeast
  2 tbsp warm semi-skimmed milk
  Approx 150ml warm water

1. Sieve the flour into a large bowl.
2. Make a well in the centre and add the salt, olive oil, dried yeast and milk. Mix thoroughly, adding enough warm water to make a smooth, non-tacky dough. Add extra flour if necessary. Knead for 15 minutes.
3. Place the dough in an oiled bowl and cover with a damp cloth. Leave in the warmth to rise for 1 hour.
4. Remove dough and divide into four. Shape into pizza bases and add toppings as required.
5. Bake individual pizzas at 240°C/475°F/gas mark 9 for about 10 minutes until the crust around the edge of the pizza is crisp and the dough cooked through.

Wholemeal Pizza Dough

Makes 4 pizza bases at approx 320 kcals each.
  400g wholemeal flour
  1 tsp ground rock salt
  15g fresh yeast plus 1 tsp brown sugar or ½ sachet easy blend dried yeast
  300ml warm water

1. Mix together the flour and salt.
2. If using fresh yeast, mix the sugar and fresh yeast with 150ml warm water and leave to froth for 10 minutes.
3. Add the fresh yeast mix to the flour or add the half

sachet of easy blend dried yeast to the flour, then add the sugar and 150ml water.

4. Mix well, adding enough extra water to make a smooth, non-tacky dough. Knead lightly for 5 minutes.

5. Divide into four and roll out into individual pizzas. Leave to prove for 10 to 15 minutes before adding the topping.

Variations

Try adding the following to the wholemeal dough to make a flavoured pizza base:

- 1 small egg (size 4) plus 110g grated low-fat hard cheese plus 1 clove garlic, crushed.
- 3 cloves garlic, crushed, plus 1 tbsp chopped fresh parsley and 1 tbsp chopped fresh chives.

Toppings

Original Cheese and Herb La Marinara

Makes 4 pizza toppings, adding approx 55 kcals to each pizza base calorie value.

> 12 tbsp passata
> 1 beef tomato, sliced
> 2 cloves garlic
> 1 tbsp fresh oregano, chopped
> 1 tbsp fresh basil, chopped
> 1 tbsp fresh parsley, chopped
> 1 tbsp extra virgin olive oil (optional)
> Rock salt and freshly ground black pepper

Spread the passata over the pizza bases. Arrange the beef tomato slices on top and sprinkle with garlic and fresh herbs and season well. Drizzle with olive oil. Flash under the grill.

Original Cheese and Tomato La Margherita

Invented for Queen Margherita of Savoy whilst she was staying in Naples, this soon became a national favourite as its colours – red, white and green – were those of the Italian flag. Enough for 4 toppings, adding approx 125 kcals to each pizza base.

    12 tbsp passata
    120g Mozzarella cheese, coarsely chopped
    1 tbsp fresh oregano, chopped
    1 tbsp fresh basil, chopped
    1 tbsp extra virgin olive oil (optional)
    Rock salt and freshly ground black pepper

Spread the passata over the pizza. Scatter with the Mozzarella, oregano and basil and season well. Drizzle with olive oil if using.

Original Anchovy La Napoletana

The spicy topping reminiscent of *pasta alla puttanesca* – spicy, salty and fishy. Enough for 4 toppings, adding approx 180 kcals to each pizza base.

    12 tbsp passata
    120g Mozzarella cheese, coarsely chopped
    1 small can anchovy fillets, drained and chopped
    1 tbsp extra virgin olive oil
    1 tbsp black olives, stoned and chopped
    1 tbsp capers
    Cayenne pepper
    Freshly ground black pepper

Spread the passata over the pizza base. Scatter with Mozzarella, anchovies, black olives, capers. Drizzle with olive oil and sprinkle on cayenne pepper and black pepper. Flash under the grill.

Original Mushroom Pizza Al Funghi

Enough for 4 toppings, adding approx 140 kcals to each pizza base.

12 tbsp passata
120g button chestnut or brown cap mushrooms, finely sliced
1 tbsp fresh oregano, chopped
120g Mozzarella cheese, coarsely chopped
1 tbsp extra virgin olive oil (optional)

Spread the passata over the pizza dough. Scatter with mushrooms, oregano and cheese. Drizzle with olive oil, if using, and season well.

Original Four Seasons Pizza

Use the dough recipes to make one giant pizza. Mark into four quarters and decorate with a different topping on each quarter. Adds approx 680 kcals (170 kcals each for four) to the pizza dough base.

1st Quarter
3 tbsp passata
60g Mozzarella cheese
2 thin slices prosciutto *or* lean smoked ham, cut into strips
1 tbsp fresh basil, chopped

2nd Quarter
3 tbsp passata
1 clove garlic, chopped
1 tbsp fresh oregano, chopped
4 anchovy fillets, chopped
1 tbsp capers

1 tbsp black olives, chopped

3rd Quarter
3 tbsp passata
2 tbsp prawns
1 tbsp fresh parsley, chopped

4th Quarter
2 tbsp passata
60g button mushrooms, sliced
60g mozzarella, chopped
1 tbsp fresh chives, chopped

Season the entire pizza with freshly ground black pepper. Drizzle with extra virgin olive oil if desired for authenticity, but beware of the extra calories. Flash under the grill.

Bread

The following recipes can be made in a food processor fitted with a dough hook as described, or kneaded by hand in a large bowl. Kneading by hand takes twice as long to produce a nice, elastic dough – but is a more satisfying achievement!

Coriander and Garlic Pitta Breads

Pitta breads are ideal for making sandwiches with a difference. They can be cut in half and stuffed with salads, or can be dipped into steaming hot soups. They are popular as an accompaniment to kebabs in Mediterranean countries. Makes 12 pitta breads at approx 220 kcals each.
700g strong white flour
1 sachet easy blend dried yeast (e.g. Harvest Gold)
2 tsp salt

1 tsp garlic, crushed (optional)
2 tbsp coriander, finely chopped (optional)
2 tbsp extra virgin olive oil
400ml warm water

1. Place the flour in a food processor fitted with a dough hook and stir in the yeast, salt, garlic and coriander.
2. Switch on the processor and add the olive oil. Slowly dribble in most of the warm water until you have a soft but non-sticky dough.
3. Place the dough in a lightly oiled bowl and cover with a moist cloth. Leave in a warm place for about an hour until doubled in size.
4. Preheat the oven to its maximum setting. Oil two baking sheets.
5. Divide the pitta dough into twelve. Knead each lump into a smooth ball and roll out into an oval about the size of the palm of your hand. Place on lightly floured trays and cover with a damp cloth. Leave to prove for 30 minutes.
6. When the oven is at its maximum temperature, quickly put in the oiled baking sheets to heat up. Remove them and put 3 pitta breads on each. Sprinkle with water and place in the oven.
7. After a few minutes, the pitta breads will puff up and start to brown. Watch carefully and remove them from the oven after about 4 minutes, before they become too hard. You will need to experiment depending on your oven.
8. Cover the pitta with a damp cloth and bake the next batch.

Olive Bread

3170 kcals per large loaf.
700g strong white flour
1 sachet easy blend dried yeast (e.g. Harvest Gold)

2 tsp salt
4 tbsp extra virgin olive oil
400ml warm water
1 onion, peeled and finely chopped
1 clove garlic, crushed
2 tbsp fresh parsley, finely chopped (optional)
250g ripe black olives, pitted and roughly chopped
Freshly ground black pepper

1. Place the flour in a food processor fitted with a dough hook and stir in the yeast and salt.

2. Switch on the processor and add half the olive oil (2 tbsp). Slowly dribble in most of the warm water until you have a soft but non-sticky dough.

3. Place the dough in a lightly oiled bowl and cover with a moist cloth. Leave in a warm place for about an hour until doubled in size.

4. Fry the onion and garlic in 1 tbsp olive oil until just beginning to colour.

5. When the dough has risen for the first time, knock it back and fold in the fried onion and garlic. Add the remaining olive oil, parsley and olives. Season with pepper, then knead well.

6. Shape into a loaf and place in an oiled tin. Cover with a damp cloth or place the tin in a large plastic bag. Leave to rise for 40 minutes. Heat the oven to 180°C/350°F/gas mark 4.

7. Bake for 45 minutes. The base of the tin should sound hollow when tapped. Good served with a simple cottage cheese and watercress salad or with avocado and prawns.

Walnut Bread

This bread accompanies salads and fish well. For variation, 100g chopped dried apricots may be added to make apricot and walnut bread. A large loaf equals 2850 kcals, and with added apricots 3010 kcals.

700g wholewheat flour
1 sachet dried yeast
30g ground rock salt
30ml (2 tbsp) walnut oil
600ml warm water
50g walnuts, chopped

1. Place the flour in a food processor fitted with a dough hook and stir in the yeast and salt.
2. Switch on the processor and add the walnut oil. Slowly dribble in most of the warm water until you have a soft but non-sticky dough.
3. Knead for 3 minutes, adding the walnuts at the end and mix in.
4. Shape into a loaf and place in a large, oiled tin. Cover with a damp cloth or place the tin in a large plastic bag. Leave to rise until doubled in size. Heat the oven to 230°C/450°F/gas mark 8.
5. Bake for 35 minutes. Then remove from the tin and bake for a further 5 minutes. The base of the loaf should sound hollow when tapped.

Olive and Coriander Focaccia

This traditional Italian dough makes one large flat bread (1689 kcals), or two smaller ones (845 kcals per loaf). Various flavourings can be added instead of the olives and coriander. Traditionally, flavourings are added as a topping and pushed into the risen loaf before baking. I add my herbs into the dough as this disperses their flavour more satisfyingly.

350g plain white flour
½ sachet easy blend dried yeast (e.g. Harvest Gold)
1 tsp ground rock salt

3 tbsp extra virgin olive oil
200ml warm water
120g black olives, stoned
2 tbsp fresh coriander, coarsely shredded
1 tsp coriander seeds, crushed

1. Place the flour in a food processor fitted with a dough hook and stir in the yeast and half the salt.
2. Switch on the processor and add 2 tbsp olive oil. Slowly dribble in the warm water until you have a soft but non-sticky dough. If necessary, add a little more water.
3. Knead for 5 minutes. Then add the olives, coriander leaves and seeds and incorporate.
4. Shape into a loaf and place in a large, oiled tin. Drizzle the remaining 1 tbsp olive oil over the top of the loaf and sprinkle on the remaining ½ tsp salt.
5. Cover with a damp cloth or place the tin in a large plastic bag and leave to rise until doubled in size. Heat the oven to 190°C/375°F/gas mark 5.
6. Bake for 15 to 20 minutes until golden on the outside and cooked in the centre. The bread should sound hollow when the base is tapped. Serve warm.

Other flavourings you could add to your focaccia include:
• rosemary, onion and sun-dried tomatoes
• sage and onion
• onion, garlic and chives
• coriander, garlic and walnut

Appendix 1: Understanding Calories

The calorie is a standard unit for measuring heat energy. One calorie is the amount of heat energy needed to raise the temperature of 1g of water by 1° from 15°C to 16°C. This is also called the standard calorie (cal), spelt with a small 'c'.

The unit commonly used in both slimming and medicine is the kilocalorie or kcal. This is also known as the Calorie spelt with a big 'C' and equals 1000 cals.

This can lead to confusion. In this book, whenever we talk about calories, we mean multiples of the kilocalorie (kcal).

Measuring the Calorie Value of Foods

How do we know how much energy each food contains? How can we say with confidence that 28g of olive oil contains 255 kcals, or that one large eating apple contains 70 kcals?

The amount of energy freed by the breakdown (catabolism) of food in the body is the same as that released when the food is burned outside the body.

If you incinerate a slice of toast under the grill, the heat given out by the flames contains an amount of energy closely related to that which would be liberated if the toast were eaten and metabolized inside you.

Nutritionists calculate that:

- dietary carbohydrates provide 4 kcals per gram
- dietary proteins 4 kcals per gram
- dietary fats 9 kcals per gram

Specific Dynamic Actions of Food

Proteins, fats and carbohydrates in the diet use up different amounts of energy just to break them down and liberate the energy they contain. This is called their Specific Dynamic Action and results in our metabolic rate being increased.

Digestion of 100 kcal-worth of protein increases the metabolic rate by a total of 30 kcal; a similar amount of carbohydrate increases it by 6 kcal and dietary fat by only 4 kcal.

This means that the amount of calories available from each of the three food types is reduced by this amount as the energy used up in assimilating the foods must come either from the food itself or from the body's energy stores.

The specific dynamic action of food is not yet fully understood. It can last for up to six hours and probably involves the activation of brown fat cells.

Complex carbohydrates in the diet are quickly and easily broken down into glucose and burned to liberate energy. This process starts as soon as carbohydrate is in the mouth by the action of salivary gland enzymes.

In contrast, dietary fat is not readily metabolized but is easily converted into body fat without too much processing. Both food types therefore require the expenditure of relatively little energy to process them.

The metabolism of dietary protein is a complex procedure requiring lots of energy to drive it. Eating protein therefore uses up more calories than when eating either carbohydrate or fat.

The products of protein metabolism tend to be poisonous. The body converts these to urea and uric acid which are then excreted. If too much protein is ingested, toxins build up in the body. The most famous example is **gout**, where uric acid crystals are deposited in joints and tissues to cause painful inflammation.

Today's healthy eating recommendations are that we obtain:

- at least 50–60 per cent of our daily calories in the form of natural-source, unrefined, complex carbohydrates
- 15–20 per cent from protein
- less than 30 per cent from dietary fats.

When wanting to lose weight, a low-fat diet providing only 20 per cent of energy in the form of fat is ideal.

The Body Awareness Mediterranean Slim Diet provides

- 55–60 per cent of energy as carbohydrate (+ or – 5 per cent as wine)
- 20 per cent as protein
- 20 per cent as fat.

Appendix 2:
Metabolism and Fat

The term **'metabolism'** literally means 'change'. It describes all the chemical and energy transformations that occur in the body, including those converting food into available body energy and energy stores. These metabolic processes are regulated by the nervous system and **hormones**.

Hormones are chemical messengers secreted by ductless glands (e.g. pituitary, thyroid, adrenals) and transported in the blood stream to their target cells (e.g. liver, ovaries, fat storage cells).

Unlike plants, which derive energy from sunlight during photosynthesis, animals (including humans) obtain energy by burning carbohydrates, proteins and fats which they seek out and eat.

Energy Balance

The first law of thermodynamics suggests that **energy can neither be created nor destroyed**. Apart from the realms of science fiction, it is difficult to break this principle. Equally, the human being who can photosynthesize (convert light energy into food) has not been genetically engineered. If you are overweight, it is because you have eaten more food energy than your body needs.

However, when fat people say they 'hardly eat anything' and miserably swear they survive on lettuce leaves and little else, they are not necessarily telling lies. Their problem is that they have a very efficient metabolism. Overweight people also tend to be inactive and do not generate enough muscle work to burn up the little food energy they do eat. Research has shown that overweight people are capable of maintaining their excess fat, even when food intake is strictly controlled and limited. The rate at which they burn food energy is optimized and little is wasted as heat.

In contrast, when some normal weight individuals are fed thousands of extra calories per day, their weight may increase only a little and then level off. The rate at which they burn food energy is increased and the extra energy is given out as heat.

The key to both observations is the body's metabolism and the metabolic rate we have each individually inherited.

Burning Food

Essentially, our body is a giant chemical reactor. Under normal circumstances, when food is plentiful, 40 per cent of dietary energy is stored as chemical energy and used to fuel exercise and metabolism. The remaining 60 per cent is dissipated as heat.

The process of oxidizing food is not a rapid, one-step, explosive reaction but a complex, slow, multi-step process which liberates energy in small, usable parcels.

Enzymes (complex molecules consisting of proteins, minerals and vitamins) are essential for controlling these metabolic reactions. They work as catalysts to trigger chemical interactions which would otherwise not occur, or would only happen slowly in their absence.

During digestion, dietary proteins are broken down into smaller units called amino acids, fats to fatty acids and carbohydrates to glucose.

These smaller units are then oxidized (combined with oxygen) to release carbon dioxide, water and energy. Some are recombined to make new complex proteins (e.g. enzymes), carbohydrates (e.g. glycogen) and fats (e.g. cholesterol) that are needed for the body to work properly.

The energy released from food during oxidation is stored in the form of energy-rich molecules containing phosphates and complex proteins, fats or carbohydrates synthesized from simpler chemicals. These energy storing compounds are generated in a process called **anabolism**.

Anabolism is the reverse of **catabolism** – the breaking down of body energy stores which occurs during fasting, anorexia, starvation and, of course, in a controlled manner during the slimming process.

Our overall body size is a balance between anabolic building-up processes of metabolism and catabolic breaking down reactions.

The Weight-loss Process

Anabolism and catabolism are continual processes. When we put on weight, anabolic pathways are more active than catabolic ones. When we want to lose weight, we must ensure that catabolic pathways are more active than the anabolic ones. Our percentage of body fat will then fall as our energy stores are used up.

In a male weighing 70kg (11 stone) around 2500 kcals are stored as carbohydrate and 112,000 kcals (about 80 per cent of body fuel supplies) are stored as fat. The remaining fuel is stored as protein (e.g. muscle). If we want to lose weight, we must encourage our body to burn fat.

Most of our energy output is concerned with keeping metabolic reactions ticking away hour after hour. For the average person, metabolism uses up almost 1500 kcals per day. Surprisingly, this is only equivalent to the energy used by leaving a 75 watt light bulb on for 24 hours.

When food is plentiful, the metabolic pathways used to digest food tend to be wasteful of calories. Under these ideal circumstances, the body finds it easiest to burn dietary carbohydrate to provide energy and to convert dietary fat into adipose storage tissue (flab).

When food is scarce, as on a strict diet, the body recognizes the threat of starvation and our metabolic rate slows by at least 30 per cent. It becomes ultra-efficient to make the available energy sources stretch as far as possible. Every calorie eaten will stick. As a result, we can eat fewer calories than before but, because they aren't being wasted as heat and are converted into energy-rich molecules with the greatest efficiency, we won't lose very much weight.

The body can easily convert protein to carbohydrate (glucose) for instant energy but cannot convert fat into glucose. Fat stores have to be mobilized and broken down into fatty acids to be oxidized by the muscles. This takes time and, in the emergency situation of a crash diet, the body resorts to burning extra protein as this is easier.

In addition, the body finds it difficult to mobilize the energy from fat molecules without a plentiful supply of chemicals resulting from the break down of dietary carbohydrate. To use a common analogy, if we think of our excess fat stores as **logs** we want to burn in the **fire** of our metabolism, we need carbohydrate **kindling** to get the flames going.

Very low calorie diets delivering under 800 kcals per day are a bad idea. They:

- initially encourage the breakdown of lean, muscle protein and can place dangerous stress on the heart
- they often fail to provide all the nutrients the body requires
- deficiencies of essential fats may lead to depression, premenstrual syndrome, cyclical breast pain, eczema, irregular or absent periods

As a result, you will feel tired, listless and lacking in energy. Fat stores will not be broken down to any great extent (as carbohydrate intake to kindle this is restricted) and little energy is expended on burning the relatively small amounts of food available.

In addition, very low calorie diets change our metabolic processes so they become ultra-efficient. This effect will continue after eating returns to normal and weight will pile back on with frightening ease.

By eating more of the right sorts of food, you would actually speed up the rate at which your body burns fat and waste more calories as heat. You would end up losing more weight – despite eating more calories overall.

Small amounts of dietary glucose significantly counteract the breakdown of protein as an emergency energy source. This is called the **protein–sparing effect** of glucose. By eating enough complex carbohydrate, which is broken down into glucose, you are less likely to burn lean body tissue, such as muscle, and more likely to mobilize those mountains of excess fat.

World Health Organization guidelines recommend that we eat at least 50 per cent of our daily calorie intake as carbohydrate. This complements the aims of the Body Awareness diets.

Latest research suggests that every individual has a unique personal ratio of body fat to lean muscle. As we lose weight, we will lose some lean tissue as well as fat tissue to maintain this personal ratio.

By eating plentiful carbohydrate, we no longer have to worry that by losing weight too quickly, we will end up losing excessive amounts of lean tissue.

Why Some People Put on Weight Easily

Some bodies have very efficient anabolic pathways and convert food energy to body stores with exemplary efficiency. These people (endomorphs) will always have to struggle to maintain a healthy weight and will need to control their diet for the rest of their lives. For them, slimming is not a temporary process – it must permeate their life for ever and they need to be **body aware**.

Other people have less efficient anabolic pathways. Their oxidation of food energy is uncoupled from the processes generating energy storage molecules. They waste food energy by dissipating more as heat and converting less to storage molecules such as fatty tissue.

These people (ectomorphs) rarely have a serious weight problem and can lose a few extra pounds with nauseating ease. Chemical processes occurring in so-called **brown fat** are involved.

Types of Body Fat Stores

The fats found in cells are of two main types:
- structural lipids (e.g. cell membranes)
- neutral fat (fatty acids combined with glycerol) which are excess energy stores in the adipose cells of our fat depots.

In fit, normal-weight males, neutral fat makes up about 12–18 per cent of body weight depending on age. In fit, normal-weight women, the percentage of adipose fat is higher at 18–24 per cent. During slimming, it is the adipose depot fat that is mobilized whilst the structural fat is preserved.

Adipose fat is not the inert lump it was once thought to be. It is a dynamic tissue, undergoing constant breakdown (catabolism) and re-synthesis (anabolism). In these tissues, glucose is metabolized and converted into fatty acids and neutral fats are constantly broken down into free fatty acids that are released into the circulation.

Brown Fat

A third, special type of fatty tissue is brown fat. This makes up only a small percentage of total body fat and is more abundant in infants than adults. It is located:

- between the shoulder blades (scapulae)
- at the nape of the neck
- along the large arteries and veins in the chest and abdomen

and is scattered in other, variable locations around the body.

Brown fat cells are interesting because, unlike normal white adipose fat cells which contain neutral fat, they receive an extensive nerve supply. Also, ordinary white fat cells contain only a single large droplet of fat, whereas brown fat cells contain several small droplets of fat.

The metabolic reactions inside cells occur in small structures (organelles) known as **mitochondria**. These are literally the cell power houses. Interestingly, a sustained exercise programme increases both the number and size of mitochondria found within our body cells.

Brown fat cells contain many more mitochondria than white fat cells. These mitochondria are also of a different type. They are able to short circuit certain chemical reactions so that instead of generating energy-rich storage molecules during metabolism, food energy is mostly converted to heat.

This process is stimulated by nerve impulses coming directly into the cells during eating and provides a mechanism for varying the amount of weight gained per unit of food ingested.

Needless to say, people with a weight problem tend to have less brown fat than people who can eat as much as they want and never put on any weight.

There is a strong genetic component to overweight and obesity. The quantity of brown fat we inherit and the efficiency of our metabolism is mainly to blame. It is now thought that the increased risks associated with an apple-shaped fat distribution over those with a pear-shaped fat distribution (high blood cholesterol levels, high blood pressure, glucose intolerance, diabetes, coronary heart disease) are related to altered metabolism of intra-abdominal brown fat.

Faulty Metabolism, Hormones and Glands

The overweight often worry that their glands are at fault. If you are significantly overweight, or have great difficulty in losing weight by normal means, it's worth asking your doctor whether a blood test to assess the function of your thyroid gland is necessary.

The thyroid gland is situated at the front of the neck. It secretes two hormones: thyroxine and triiodothyronine, which help to determine your metabolic rate.

The symptoms of an underactive thyroid include: lethargy, tiredness, increased weight, feeling the cold, dry skin, brittle hair, thickening of the ankles and legs (brawny oedema), slow pulse and, if severe, a coarsening of facial features, decreased body hair and deepening of the voice. A goitre may be present. Symptoms usually creep up on you, so it's a disease which can be difficult to spot.

The good news is that an underactive thyroid (hypothyroidism) is diagnosed with a blood test and easily treated with daily thyroxine hormone replacement tablets. Your body will soon recover and most changes are reversible. You will still need to eat healthily to improve your general fitness after the insult of a major disease.

The Metabolic Rate

The amount of energy liberated in our body per unit of time is our basal metabolic rate. This is affected by many factors including:
- muscular exertion (exercise)

- specific dynamic action of recently ingested food
- high or low environmental temperature
- body temperature
- age
- our height
- weight and surface area
- whether we are male or female
- our emotional state
- circulating thyroid hormone levels
- circulating adrenaline and ACTH hormone levels
- the time of day or night
- medications

Muscular exertion increases the metabolic rate. This is discussed later in this section.

Specific dynamic action of food increases the metabolic rate.

Temperature Most chemical reactions occur at a faster rate as the temperature increases. Our metabolic rate is faster the hotter we are, e.g. when we have a fever. In hot weather, however, we burn up less calories than when we are cold. This is because the body has to burn up extra energy reserves to maintain our body heat and the muscle shivering that occurs. In hypothermia, the metabolic rate slows significantly to the extent that some unconscious, live patients have occasionally been certified dead.

Age As we get older, our metabolic rate naturally declines. It is at its highest around the age of 27 years and then slows by up to 3 per cent per year. Between the ages of 27 and 47, the metabolic rate has often fallen by as much as 12 per cent. If exercise levels remain the same, calorie intake must also drop to avoid putting on weight.

Between the ages of 25 and 70, the following average changes occur across the population:
- Body fat increases from 20 per cent to 30 per cent of body weight in men and from 27 per cent to 40 per cent in women.

405

- Lean body mass declines from 60kg to 50kg in men and from 40kg to 35kg in women.
- Muscle mass declines from about 450 g/kg to 300 g/kg.
- Body density goes down from 1.072 to 1.041 in men and from 1.040 to 1.016 in women.
- Height and bone density fall, particularly in post-menopausal women not taking hormone replacement therapy.

Despite the significant increase in ratio of total body fat to muscle, average body weight surprisingly goes down after middle age. **This is because selective death among the obese plays a significant role.**

Over the age of 75 years, women need approximately 130 calories per day less than when they were aged 49. Men need 440 calories less per day on average. Levels of exercise decrease and, if calorie intake stays the same (in practice, it often goes up), a woman could expect to ingest an excess $130 \times 365 = 47,450$ kcals per year. The equivalent figure for men is $440 \times 365 = 160,600$.

One kilogram of fat is equivalent to 7,000 kcal. Therefore, a woman may put on an additional 6.78kg per year from not decreasing her food intake or increasing her exercise levels to match her declining metabolism. A male can put on as much as 22.9kg per year.

Although this argument is simplistic, it does illustrate the possible significance of decreasing metabolic rate on our health as we get older. As a rough rule of thumb, for every five years after the age of 27, you will need 50 less calories per day. This explains that insidious middle-aged spread.

Height The taller you are, the higher your metabolic rate will be. Ectomorphs who are long and thin have a higher metabolic rate than endomorphs who are shorter and more rounded. Mesomorphs have a high metabolic rate, partly due to their well developed musculature.

Weight Surprisingly, the overweight have a higher metabolic rate than those who are slim. It takes many more calories to maintain and move 95kg (15 stone) in weight than it does to mobilize a body only weighing 57kg (9 stone).

Studies comparing the rates at which both fat and thin people burn up calories have consistently shown that the overweight need several hundred calories per day more than a slim person to maintain their weight. If they diet, they can lose weight on many more calories than a slim person would. As a fat person becomes slim however, their metabolic rate will slowly fall in line with the weight they have lost.

Once they are slim, their metabolic rate will be lower than it was when they were fat, but it will not be significantly lower than a person of similar age, height, weight and build who has never been overweight. What will differ is the efficiency with which their metabolism converts calories to fat stores rather than wasting them as heat.

Sex Males tend to have a faster metabolic rate than females of the same height and weight. This is partly to do with their increased muscle:fat ratio. They also tend to be ectomorphic or mesomorphic rather than endomorphic.

Emotional state Very anxious people expend a lot of energy through nerves. They fidget, are constantly on the move and have high levels of circulating stress hormones (e.g. adrenaline) that speed up the metabolism. Anger and fear have similar effects. During periods of relaxation, calm or depression, the metabolic rate will slow.

The thyroid gland helps to regulate the metabolic rate through secretion of the hormone, thyroxine. (See above.)

If the thyroid gland is overactive, weight loss will occur. If it is underactive, weight gain is inevitable. In extreme cases, a condition called myxoedema occurs where the sufferer slows right down in thought as well as deed. Replacement therapy with thyroxine tablets will correct this condition and allow the metabolic rate to rise to normal.

A single dose of thyroxine hormone increases the metabolic rate for six days or more. Large doses cause enough extra heat production to raise body temperature.

A few cowboy diet clinics were known in the past to prescribe thyroxine tablets to speed weight loss in exchange for fat fees. This practice is dangerous.

Adrenaline hormone is secreted by the adrenal glands. In times of stress, it is secreted in high quantities to prepare us for the **'fight or flight'** reaction.

The nervous diarrhoea, sweating and constant need to spend a penny before a driving test or an interview are good examples. Adrenaline increases the metabolic rate, raises blood sugar levels, increases the rate at which protein is broken down and also mobilizes free fatty acids from fat stores. These actions are all important in providing emergency energy supplies.

The adrenal gland is stimulated by a hormone (ACTH) secreted by the pituitary gland in the brain. ACTH secretion shows a diurnal rhythm, which means it is secreted in more frequent bursts in the morning (starting before we wake up) and less frequently in the evening. Our metabolic rate is therefore highest in the morning and lowest at night. That's why calories eaten late at night are more likely to be converted into fat than immediately burned for energy.

Some prescription drugs are able to affect the metabolism. Beta-blockers, used to treat a number of conditions (especially high blood pressure, angina, heart attack, anxiety and migraine), slow the metabolism down. Others that can slow the metabolism, encourage weight gain or stimulate the appetite include oral steroids, insulin, the contraceptive pill, progestogen-only methods of contraception, pizotifen, tricyclic antidepressants, beta-adrenergic drugs and probably many more.

If you are on the Pill and find it difficult to lose weight, it may be worth requesting a change to a brand with a lower overall dose of hormones.

Measuring the Metabolic Rate

Our basal metabolic rate can be estimated by measuring the amount of oxygen consumed to oxidize our food. This is measured in a process known as **indirect calorimetry**.

It is relatively simple to assess the amount of oxygen used by the human body as oxygen is not stored and consumption usually keeps pace with immediate metabolic needs. The amount of oxygen used per unit of time is therefore proportionate to the total energy liberated during catabolism.

Oxygen consumption varies slightly depending on whether fat, protein or carbohydrate is being oxidized. Scientists know that approximately 4.82 kcal of energy is liberated for every litre of oxygen we consume.

The most important factor affecting our metabolic rate is exercise. Our metabolic rate is elevated during exercise and for a significant amount of time afterwards. Combining a healthy slimming diet with a regular exercise regime will boost the metabolism and speed up the rate at which we burn fat energy stores.

Resting muscle uses fatty acids for its metabolism. During exercise, the energy needs of muscle are initially met by breaking down glycogen stores in the muscle itself and by increased uptake of circulating glucose in the blood. After exercise, the muscle glycogen stores are replenished either from carbohydrate in the diet or by breaking down protein from lean tissues if food supplies are scarce (e.g. during a crash diet).

The glycogen stores in our muscles are expandable. Someone who leads a sedentary lifestyle will have around

1g of glycogen per 100g of muscle. A trained athlete may have as much as 4g glycogen per 100g of muscle weight. Muscles well supplied with glycogen are able to exercise more easily and for longer. In turn, this increases muscle bulk and increases the amount of glucose you burn. In addition, your basal metabolic rate will raise as the majority of energy expended is utilized by our muscles.

When glycogen stores run out, muscles rapidly tire. When stores are plentiful, you can exercise longer without feeling tired.

Muscle Energy Sources

Muscular activity is the biggest contributor to our basal metabolic rate. When we exercise, blood vessels in our muscles dilate and blood flow is significantly increased to bring extra oxygen in. This accounts for the rapid pumping up effect observed in body-builders.

Muscular contraction during exercise requires energy which comes from energy-rich organic phosphate derivatives such as the molecule ATP (adenosine triphosphate).

The ultimate sources of this energy are carbohydrates and fats in our diet. These energy producing reactions occur mainly in the mitochondria of our cells (see Brown Fat). Regular, sustained exercise increases the number and size of mitochondria in our muscle cells – so more energy producing and oxygen using reactions can occur.

When the molecular bonds in ATP are broken down by enzyme reactions, energy is released to fuel muscle contraction, and a molecule called ADP (adenosine diphosphate) is formed.

Usually, ADP is immediately converted back into the energy store, ATP, to provide muscle cells with fresh energy stores for the next contraction. The fuel for

410

this chemical conversion is blood glucose and oxygen. Exercise is then said to be *aerobic*.

If oxygen is used up so fast that insufficient is brought in by the blood, the muscle energy source (ATP) would rapidly deplete. Muscles would then tire and lose the ability to contract any further.

A back-up molecule (phosphorylcreatine) is present in small amounts and can be used as a rich source of energy when oxygen availability is compromised. This molecule can be broken down to provide energy for the refor- mation of ATP from ADP without the need for oxygen. Exercise is then said to be *anaerobic*.

We cannot exercise anaerobically for long, as a waste product of metabolism, lactic acid, builds up within the muscle. As conditions become more and more acidic, muscles rapidly tire and painful cramping results.

Anaerobic metabolism in muscles is useful for provid- ing an additional 'spurt' of strength in times of danger, stress or when quick responses are required.

The Oxygen Debt

Usually, the increased amount of oxygen consumed by muscles is proportionate to the amount of energy ex- pended (i.e. 4.82 kcal energy per litre oxygen) and all energy needs are met by aerobic processes.

When muscle exertion is very great the anaerobic processes within muscle cells provide an emergency, though self-limiting, supply of energy. After this exertion is over, extra oxygen is still needed to :
- remove the built up lactic acid
- replenish stores of energy rich molecules used in aerobic metabolism (ATP)
- replenish the emergency stores of phosphorylcreatine molecules.

411

The amount of extra oxygen needed is proportionate to the oxygen deficiency encountered during the period of intense exercise. An **oxygen debt** has been incurred. Experimental measurements show that by forming an oxygen debt which can be repaid later, the human body is capable of **six times** the exertion that would have been possible without this mechanism.

There is a limit to the oxygen debt we can build up. Violent exertion is possible only for short periods of time, though with less strenuous forms of exercise, the debt can be incurred over longer periods.

You will notice as your fitness level improves, you will tire less easily and soon you will be exercising with much less effort.

Ketosis

Many slimming diets result in the build up of ketones in the blood. These result from the breakdown of fat stores and are metabolized with difficulty in the liver. They are normally rapidly metabolized in tissues but require products of glucose metabolism for this.

If too many ketones are formed in conditions where carbohydrate intake is depressed (e.g. crash diets, high fat-low carbohydrate diets) they cannot be mopped up and spill over into the circulation.

Ketones are an important source of energy in some emergency situations, such as temporary starvation or after prolonged vomiting. If they build up in the body however, they can be dangerous and cause cell damage.

Ketones can also affect the brain, leading to confusion. Diets that claim to function via the production of ketosis are therefore not a good idea.

Appendix 3: Carbohydrates

Carbohydrates supply us with our main source of energy and should make up at least 55–60 per cent of daily calories.

Monosaccharides are the simplest carbohydrates and consist of a single sugar molecule – a saccharide. The most important monosaccharide is glucose.

Disaccharides consist of two saccharide molecules linked together. The best known example is sucrose – ordinary table sugar – consisting of a glucose molecule linked to a fructose molecule. Unhappily, 17 per cent of calories in a typical Western diet are derived from sucrose.

Polysaccharides are long chains of saccharides linked together, of which the most important is starch.

Monosaccharides	glucose (grape sugar), galactose (milk sugar), fructose (fruit sugar)
Disaccharides	sucrose (table sugar), lactose (milk sugar), maltose
Polysaccharides	starch, cellulose

The carbohydrates that the human body can utilize include starches (complex carbohydrates) and sugars (simple carbohydrates). These are found in cereals, root vegetables and fruits. The refined carbohydrates (e.g. sucrose and cornflour) are highly processed pure products consisting of pure sugar or pure starch with no additional nutrients.

Unavailable carbohydrates (e.g. cellulose) pass through us virtually unchanged and make up the bulk of dietary fibre, also known as roughage.

How Our Body Uses Carbohydrate

The simple sugars (monosaccharides) are absorbed into the blood stream unchanged. The body can use monosaccharides as instant energy and they are often referred to by slimming specialists as 'empty' calories with no nutritional value. They do have a nutritional value as a pure energy source but provide nothing in the way of vitamins or trace minerals and consist of pure calories.

The disaccharides and starches must be broken down into monosaccharides before they can be used as sources of energy. Enzymes that do this are found in the saliva and gut.

Table sugar (sucrose) is broken down relatively easily and the monosaccharides released quickly increase blood sugar levels.

Starch digestion takes longer and a steady stream of sugars enters the blood. This is why eating complex carbohydrate is less likely to cause blood sugar swings and trigger the release of excess insulin. In addition, unrefined complex carbohydrates usually contain many other valuable substances such as vitamins, trace elements and dietary fibre.

Once carbohydrates are broken down into their constituent monosaccharides (mostly glucose), they are absorbed through the gut wall into the blood for distribution to the tissues. Galactose and fructose cannot be used directly by the cells and are converted into glucose in the liver before they are used.

All cells in the body, but especially brain cells and red blood cells, need a constant supply of glucose to survive. Glucose molecules are 'burned' by metabolic process in cells to generate energy. Any excess glucose is carried to the liver, muscles and fatty tissues for conversion to glycogen (a starch storage compound) and fat. When energy is required quickly, glycogen is rapidly broken down into glucose. It is an important source of energy for muscles.

It is not possible to convert fat back into glucose, but fat can be burned to spare glucose. Blood sugar levels are controlled by two pancreatic hormones, insulin and glucagon, and by the liver. When blood glucose levels are high, the liver generates stores of glycogen. When blood sugar levels are low, glycogen is broken down and glucose molecules released.

Carbohydrate and Our Metabolism

Many miracle diets are based on low carbohydrate regimes which rapidly deplete muscle glycogen stores. They leave you feeling lethargic and de-energized. The Body Awareness Diet supplies 55–60 per cent of your energy intake as carbohydrate to boost your metabolism, provide kindling to burn those excess fat stores and provide you with plenty of energy.

Carbohydrate and the Brain

When we eat carbohydrate, something extraordinary happens in our brain. Tiny puffs of a special chemical are released in an area known as the hypothalamus. This chemical, **serotonin**, is a neurotransmitter. It helps to relay messages across important nerve connections (synapses) in the brain.

One of the functions of serotonin is to influence appetite and food selection. It regulates satiety (that feeling of having eaten enough) and therefore controls our eating behaviour. Serotonin gives us a little **high**. One of the reasons we crave chocolate when we feel low or depressed is because chocolate contains substances converted into serotonin in our brain.

When we eat carbohydrate, serotonin is released, the

brain realizes food has been eaten and starts to signal 'enough'. Carbohydrate therefore makes you feel more full, more quickly, and for longer than any other dietary source of energy.

Low levels of serotonin in the hypothalamus have been linked experimentally with over-eating and carbohydrate-craving.

What usually happens in the overweight is that they snack on foods high in carbohydrate – but also high in fat (e.g. doughnuts, sausage rolls, cream cakes).

Carbohydrates in this diet also boost your metabolic rate and make you feel energized.

The Body Awareness diet utilizes the biochemistry of the brain to make your food work for you. Carbohydrate snacks are eaten regularly throughout the day to sate your appetite, boost your energy levels and boost your metabolism. Don't cheat by being too strict. If you miss your snack, you might eat something you regret later.

Beating the Snack Attack

- One of the best foods to eat during a snack attack is a banana. This fruit contains just enough simple sugar to raise your blood sugar level without inducing a sudden increase in insulin secretion. Bananas are rich in complex carbohydrates. These are slowly broken down to simpler forms and continue to release sugar into the blood stream over an extended period of time. In addition, the fibre content of bananas helps to make you feel full and satisfied.
- Eat a small apple (or a large beef tomato) and a slice of wholemeal bread. The same principles apply to this combination as eating a banana.
- Drink a large glass of sparkling mineral water to which the juice of ½–1 lemon has been added. This will fill you up quickly and take the edge off your appetite.

- Take some exercise. Go for a long walk or a workout at the gym. During exercise, body energy stores are mobilized to raise the blood sugar levels. These will be burned off as energy rather than being deposited on your hips or tummy!
- Drink a large mug of your favourite herbal or fruit tea (unsweetened).
- If you are feeling stressed, make a conscious effort to relax. Remove yourself from the stressful situation or person. Have a relaxing aromatherapy bath. Give yourself a face mask. Go for a float. Stress results in the release of several body hormones which are likely to magnify your blood sugar level swings.
- Whatever you do, don't take the easy way out. Don't drink a sugary drink, indulge in sweets, chocolate, cakes and biscuits. This will result in blood sugar level swings and only prolong your agony – and the damage to your diet.

Blood sugar level swings may also contribute to hardening of the arteries and in the long term lead to serious conditions such as high blood pressure, heart disease or strokes. There is also thought to be a link with the development of diabetes.

How to Prevent Sugar Swings Occurring

Blood sugar levels can be kept relatively constant by eating regular, healthy meals spaced throughout the day. When you are not trying to lose weight, meals can be taken three or four times per day. Snacking between meals is fine as long as you don't eat snacks high in simple, refined carbohydrates.

When you are trying to lose weight, your calorie intake is obviously restricted. This means that hypoglycaemia is more likely purely from the fact that you are eating less dietary forms of energy. The body needs to be trained to maintain its blood sugar levels by constantly burning fat. This is where the Body Awareness Diet comes in. By eating foods:

- that are high in complex carbohydrates
- low in simple sugars
- spread little and often during the day
- high in fibre
- high in natural vitamins essential for keeping the metabolism ticking over

You will lose weight easily, healthily and safely without the swinging blood sugar levels that are detrimental to both your long-term health and your slimming plans.

After a week on the Body Awareness Food Exchange or Mediterranean Slim diets, your blood sugar level controls should be back to normal. You are unlikely to feel hungry between meals and you will not develop hypoglycaemic swings.

It is important to follow the diet closely however. Missing a meal in an attempt to lose weight more quickly may have the opposite effect. Your metabolism will not be working at an optimum tick-over rate to burn up your fat stores and you will risk your blood sugar running low. When this happens, a snack attack is likely to follow.

- Always eat breakfast
- Always eat your planned diet meals
- Always take your exercise or relaxation periods

Appendix 4: Fibre

Why High Fibre?

The Body Awareness diet has a high fibre content and provides at least 30g fibre per day. This roughage is essential. Whilst it provides little nutritional value, it aids the digestion and absorption of other foods.

Fibre encourages peristalsis (the muscular, wave-like motion which transports digested food through the intestines), helps regulate bowel voiding and absorbs water, toxins and bacteria.

Dietary fibre is important in keeping the bowel motions smooth and regular. A high-fibre diet helps prevent constipation, diverticular disease, irritable bowel syndrome and some bowel tumours. Recent evidence suggests that dietary fibre absorbs fats and sugars in the bowel and can significantly lower our blood glucose and cholesterol levels too. This is because more dietary fat is excreted rather than absorbed.

Dietary fibre is a broad term describing those parts of carbohydrate foods which are indigestible. Fibre is an essential component of all plant cell structures. The main components are chemicals called cellulose, hemicellulose, lignin, pectins and gums.

We lack the enzymes necessary to break these down and release their energy values but bacteria in our gut can break them down in a process known as fermentation, which produces acids and gases.

Chemical analysis of dietary fibre shows there are two main types: soluble and insoluble.

Soluble fibre is important in the stomach and upper intestines, where it slows down the processes of digestion and absorption. This ensures blood sugar and fat levels rise slowly rather than rapidly — and our metabolism can handle nutrient fluctuations more easily.

Insoluble fibre is most important in the large bowel. It bulks up the faeces, absorbs water and hastens stool excretion. In general, soluble fibre is totally broken down in the large bowel, whilst insoluble fibre is passed out in the motions.

All plant foods contain both soluble and insoluble fibre, though some sources are richer in one type than another. The following table gives some common examples of foods rich in dietary fibre:

Sources of Soluble and Insoluble Dietary Fibre

CLASSIFICATION	PLANT SOURCE	EXAMPLES
Soluble	Oats	Porridge, muesli
	Barley	Pearl barley
	Rye	Rye bread, crispbread
	Fruit	Figs, apricots, tomatoes, apples
	Vegetables	Carrots, potatoes, courgettes
	Pulses	Cannellini beans, kidney beans
Insoluble	Wheat	Wholemeal bread, cereals
	Maize	Sweetcorn, corn bread
	Rice	Brown rice
	Pasta	Wholemeal pasta, spinach pasta
	Fruit	Rhubarb, blackberries, strawberries
	Leaf vegetables	Cabbage, spinach, lettuce
	Pulses	Peas, lentils, chickpeas

The easiest way to increase the amount of fibre in our diet is to eat more unrefined complex carbohydrates, such as wholemeal bread, cereals, nuts, grains, root vegetables and fruits.

The recommended daily intake is at least 25–30g per day. As a rough idea:

- bran provides 40g fibre per 100g portion
- dried apricots 18g per 100g
- peas 5g per 100g
- prunes 13g per 100g
- cooked brown rice 4g per 100g
- cooked wholemeal spaghetti 4g per 100g
- brown bread 6g per 100g
- walnuts 6g per 100g

Each gram of fibre eaten daily adds approximately 5g to the daily weight of excreted stool. The additional weight comes from absorbed water and other substances plus the additional bulk of bacteria that multiply from the energy they derive by fermenting insoluble fibre.

Appendix 5:
Low-fat Diets

Why Low-fat?

Low-fat diets are the modern answer to healthy eating and a healthy heart. From a slimming point of view, limiting fat intake makes good dietary sense. At 9 calories per gram, fats yield more than twice the calories of either protein or carbohydrate (4 calories per gram) and, to make things worse, usually occur in a concentrated form.

When dieting and restricting lipid intake, it is important that those fats you do consume are chosen wisely to provide the greatest nutritional contribution.

The Body Awareness Diet places heavy emphasis on the types of fat we consume in our diet. Specifically, it recommends:

- Eicosapentanoic acid (EPA) – derived from marine oils. (An Omega 3 series fatty acid – polyunsaturated)
- Gamma-linolenic acid (GLA) – derived from evening primrose oil, borage oil or starflower oil. (An Omega 6 series fatty acid – polyunsaturated)
- Oleic acid – derived from olive oil (A monounsaturated fat)

Why We Need Fats at All

The lipid fraction of our diet supplies us with :
- building blocks for cell membranes
- fatty acids necessary for the central nervous system
- precursors for important hormone-like chemicals called prostaglandins
- substrates for hormone production
- molecules from which to make bile salts
- fat-soluble vitamins A, D, E

Symptoms of Fat Deficiency

A diet deficient in fats, or providing fats of the wrong sort, can produce symptoms such as:

- dry, scaly, itching skin
- thickened, coarse skin
- dehydrated skin from increased permeability to water
- eczema
- psoriasis
- acne
- brittle hair and nails
- hair loss
- slower than normal growth rate in children
- slow wound healing
- breast pain – especially cyclical, before a period
- painful and heavy periods
- pre-menstrual syndrome

Deficiencies can also result from following long-term low-fat slimming diets.

The Body Awareness Diet takes the nutritional needs of your metabolism into account and includes a healthy mix of dietary fats including oil of evening primrose (or starflower), eiscosapentanoic acid and olive oil.

The fats and oils we are familiar with in cooking do not exist in an isolated form. They are refined from other sources, e.g. butter and cream from milk, lard and suet from animal fat, vegetable oils from seeds, nuts or fruits either by pressing or by chemical solution.

Fats can be classified into saturated, monounsaturated and polyunsaturated.

Saturated fats (hydrogenated) tend to be solid at room temperature whilst monounsaturated and polyunsaturated fats are liquid, i.e. oils.

Most fats contain a blend of saturates, monounsaturates and polyunsaturates in varying proportions. Olive oil is the richest source of monounsaturated fat available. It's these monunsaturates that are now known to be associated with long-term health benefits.

Some polyunsaturates are now viewed with suspicion. They are highly reactive and rapidly oxidize to form carcinogenic (cancer-forming) chemicals. They also affect cell membranes, interfering with cellular transport and possibly promoting early ageing.

When polyunsaturates are partially hydrogenated, trans-fatty acids are produced. These are associated with an increased occurrence of coronary heart disease and may be an even greater health hazard than dairy products and natural saturated fats. They may also interfere with the way our body handles other essential fatty acids and eicosapentanoic acid (from fish oil), so their beneficial effects are not fully realized.

The amount of trans-fatty acids in our diet varies but average consumption is around 5–7g per day. Some people eat as much as 25–30g of trans-fatty acids per day, particularly if they use cheap margarines and lots of processed foods.

Trans-fatty acid content of some foods

Food	Total trans-fatty acids as a percentage total of fatty acids
Bread	10–28%
Cake	10–24%
Crackers	3–31%
French fries	5–35%
Instant puddings	30–36%
Hard margarine	18–36%
Soft margarine	11–21%
Olive oil based spread	<8%
Crisps	14–33%
Butter	<1%

Fats and Slimming

Successful slimmers who are losing weight are burning fat stores. If they have previously followed a normal Western diet, their fat stores contain large amounts of trans-fatty acids and another fat called arachidonic acid. These are released into the circulation as fat stores are broken down.

As a result, slimmers have an increased need for dietary essential fatty acids to balance these out and prevent the blood suddenly becoming more sticky and prone to clot formation.

Most diets promote the use of margarines – full of polyunsaturated fats – and lean red meat, both of which add to the already high trans-fatty acids in the blood. Most slimming diets therefore aggravate matters and cause a potentially harmful situation. This is why many experts are now very anti-dieting.

The strength of the Body Awareness Diet is that it is full of fish oils and monunsaturated fats that are actively working to thin the blood and overcome the adverse effects of the fats released from the fat stores of dieters.

Just by altering the types of fat in our diet, we can significantly manipulate our body chemistry. This was demonstrated very convincingly in the 1970s, after it was noticed that heart disease is almost non-existent amongst Greenland Eskimos, despite having the highest consumption of fats in the world. In addition, their chance of developing debilitating Western diseases such as cancer, diabetes, gall stones, diverticulitis, ulcerative colitis, and even constipation and acne, is also very low.

Fats and the Blood

In 1979 Dr Hugh Sinclair arranged for a deep frozen seal to be delivered to the Institute of Human Nutrition in Oxfordshire. For three months, he followed a pure Eskimo diet untainted by Western foods – no alcohol, chips or even chocolate! Nothing but seal flesh, fish, crustaceans and water for 100 days. His only food supplement was Vitamin E, taken to protect the marine oils in his diet from oxidation in our warmer climes. His willpower was remarkable.

During the experiment, Dr Sinclair lost 12kg in weight and his body showed a number of physiological changes:

- the number of platelets (clotting particles) in his blood fell dramatically
- the length of time it took for his blood to clot was prolonged to over eight minutes
- the number of low density fats (LDLs) in his blood was greatly reduced
- the high density fat fraction (HDLs) increased
- his overall blood cholesterol rose from 4.55mmol/1 to 4.81mmol/1 – but in a desirable HDL/LDL ratio
- he had a tendency to nose bleeds and bruised easily
- his sperm production almost stopped

All this from altering the types of fat in his diet.

As a result of this pioneering work, a number of modern day dietary concepts took root, the most important being:

- Blood cholesterol is made up of two fractions – high density beneficial lipids (HDLs) and low density harmful lipids (LDLs).
- Blood cholesterol is not directly related to pre-formed cholesterol in the diet but to total fat eaten.
- A marine oil derivative exists which slows blood clotting and discourages hardening of the arteries and heart disease.

The Eskimo diet produced a higher blood cholesterol but only by increasing the protective HDLs. The harmful LDLs were lowered.

Eicosapentanoic acid (EPA) was isolated as the beneficial oil affecting clotting of the blood. It's now known that this is synthesized by minute algae called phytoplankton. These are eaten by fish and stored in concentrated form in their body oils. It can also be made in very small quantities in humans.

A typical Western diet is high in Omega 6 fats (cholesterol series) and low in Omega 3 fats (EPA series). A typical Eskimo diet contains huge quantities of Omega 3 fats and virtually no Omega 6 chains at all. Experts now advise that we include 300g of oily fish in our weekly diet for health (when not trying to lose weight). Those who do not like fish should seriously consider adding food supplements such as Efamol Marine or Maxepa to their diet.

Appendix 6:
Flotation Therapy

Why Relaxation?

Stress is a major component of the twentieth century lifestyle. It is also a risk factor for sudden cardiac death. Relaxation makes us feel calm and encourages release of brain chemicals associated with euphoria. It enhances our self-esteem and self-confidence. One of the most effective ways of achieving profound relaxation is flotation therapy. For maximum body awareness, an hour of floating per week is ideal. Some floaters find a session in a float tank generates beneficial effects lasting for over two weeks.

Alternative ways of relaxing include meditation, yoga, breathing exercises, acupuncture and aromatherapy.

The Benefits of Flotation Therapy

Flotation therapy is an alternative technique which helps many medical conditions. It quickly and safely induces profound relaxation, reduces high blood pressure and eases chronic pain. It has also produced spectacular results in combating stress, anxiety and depression.

Even if you're fit and healthy, it's worth finding time to float. Studies have shown it can help you give up smoking, lose weight and reduce alcohol intake.

Flotation therapy takes place in a light-proof, sound-insulated tank containing a shallow, 25cm (10 inch) deep pool of warm water. 315kg of Epsom Salts (magnesium sulphate) are dissolved in this to form a super-saturated solution more buoyant than the Dead Sea.

The floater is suspended on a silky bed of minerals like

a cork on vintage champagne and a constant skin temperature of 34.5°C is maintained. Floating is totally effortless and experienced floaters who enjoy their own company stay in the tank for up to two hours or more. Beginners usually tolerate 50 minutes.

Music may be used during orientation to the tank and for those requiring it.

Why Flotation Works

A number of theories attempt to explain what happens during a course of floats.

Normally, 90 per cent of brain activity is concerned with interpreting information from outside. This includes sound, vision, smell, temperature, body posture and balance. During flotation therapy, all external stimuli are blocked and a process called REST (Restricted Environment Stimulation Therapy) occurs. Your senses are deprived of light, sound, gravity and temperature stimuli and suddenly you are on your own, with nothing but your thoughts and body sounds to entertain you for approximately one hour.

The removal of external stimuli and gravitational force is important. It has been suggested that 90 per cent of all central nervous system activity is concerned with the effects of gravitational pull on the body. By freeing large parts of the brain and musculo-skeletal system from posture calculations and balance adjustment, an enhanced awareness of internal states (homeostatic biofeedback) can occur. The shutting 'off' of external stimuli allows the brain to focus on information from the internal organs to the extent that many individuals in flotation tanks are able to increase or decrease their heart rate at will.

Floating increases right brain (minor hemisphere) function by decreasing the amount of stimuli being fed to the left hemisphere for analysis. This frees the right side of the brain for those tasks it is best at, namely pattern recognition and creative thought and it goes into super-drive.

During relaxation, alpha and theta waves are generated by the brain. Elusive theta waves are accompanied by vivid memories, creative thought and feelings of serenity. These are difficult to maintain without falling asleep and are the fruits sought by those perfecting the art of meditation. Theta waves are literally the source of good ideas or 'brain-waves'. Intuitive insights and bursts of understanding occur.

Studies at the University of Colorado have shown that floaters quickly enter the theta state whilst remaining awake. They continue to generate large amounts of creativity-promoting theta waves for up to three weeks after the therapy.

Floating significantly decreases blood pressure in both normal and hypertensive subjects. In hypertensives, this effect continues gradually across repeated sessions and the lower blood pressure is maintained after flotation therapy has ceased.

Blood levels of stress-inducing hormones (adrenaline, noradrenaline, cortisol and adrenocorticotrophic hormone) are reduced during repeated float sessions and this reduction is maintained even five days after flotation therapy has stopped.

Control studies using subjects reclining in dimly lit, quiet rooms do not show the same effects, so it is not merely the process of relaxation inducing the measured changes.

The hindbrain (cerebellum, pons and medulla), mid-brain (tectum and tegmentum) and forebrain (cerebral cortex, thalamus and limbic system) are interconnected and capable of acting synergistically – so the whole is greater than the sum of its parts.

This interaction can be diminished by background

neural noise. The flotation tank provides an environment in which neural noise is dramatically reduced due to sensory deprivation. Heightened awareness then occurs.

Most exciting of all, the levels of heroin-like chemicals in the brain (endorphins) are raised and this, together with the theta waves generated, explains the euphoria and pain relief many floaters feel.

Patients suffering from rheumatoid arthritis, osteoarthritis, migraine, back pain and sports injuries have all benefited significantly. In one study, 80 per cent of patients with chronic pain became totally free of symptoms during treatment, to the extent that many bought flotations tanks for their own home.

Stress can result in a failure of adaptation. A depressive-like state occurs with loss of appetite and libido, sleep disturbances including early-morning waking, labile emotions and lethargy. Loss of motivation is the biggest pitfall of all. A course of flotation therapy helps to reverse this trend. Constant homeostatic adjustment allows the body to focus on regeneration and restoration of the normal physical and mental state.

Using the audio-visual system built into some tanks, floaters can study languages, musical pieces or listen to self-improvement tapes.

In some cases, a form of self-hypnosis occurs which raises self-esteem. Positive thoughts and goal enhancement statements can improve motivation and performance which can have startling effects on the weight loss process.

Flotation is a complementary therapy that will benefit everyone. Healthy individuals need relaxation as well as those with hypertension or stress-related conditions.

What Floating Feels Like

Every floater experiences something different. The

first-time floater is understandably apprehensive and to help this, dreamy music is played for 15 minutes whilst you orientate to the tank. Once you get the hang of lying back and relaxing, you won't feel any part of your body – the boundary between you and the water simply disappears!

What happens next varies, but many floaters experience pleasant sensations of flying, swaying or spinning. It's as if the brain can't cope with the lack of information and invents experiences of its own. Some floaters notice exotic smells, others remember events not thought about for years. Hours after a float, you may still feel as if you're gliding on a cushion of air; colours are vivid, smells more intense and an amazing feeling of calm pervades the air.

Appendix 7:
Appetite and Food Selection

Many of us over-eat because we are attracted to certain types of food, e.g. carbohydrates, fats, spices, alcohol or sweetness. Research shows that individual appetites and tastes can contribute to excess weight but they can be altered in several ways. Once we are aware of our tastes, we can consciously make different, healthier food choices:

- by giving up certain foods (e.g. added sugar) altogether
- by recognizing what our body is craving (e.g. carbohydrate) and eating only that – not artificially sweet, fatty foods that pile on the calories and fail to satisfy
- by eating several small snacks per day
- by using a light box if suffering from Seasonal Affective Disorder (SADs)
- by changing some prescribed drugs (e.g. some contraceptive pills) to other, more appetite-friendly ones

The Control of Appetite

Appetite, or the desire for food, is a very personal phenomenon. It is influenced by sensations of hunger but can produce an insidious, niggling desire to eat even when your stomach is groaning with food.

Appetite is regulated by two areas in the brain – the **feeding centre** and the **satiety centre**. There is also a **thirst** centre which regulates our intake of fluids.

When food is present in certain parts of the gut hormones are released which help to signal fullness. The digestion and metabolism of food generates heat which also helps to switch on feelings of satiety. Some people who are overweight can eat through all these indicators of repleteness because of especially strong appetite signals or food cravings.

One theory suggests that appetite is partly controlled by the size of our fat stores. As we put on weight, we will naturally start to eat more.

Personal Tastes

When we are born, we have tastebuds all over our mouths. As we get older, they decrease in number and are eventually found only on the tongue.

Adults possess around 10,000 tastebuds which detect four food sensations: sour, sweet, salt and bitter. Even the most delicious gourmet flavours are only made up from a combination of these four basic tastes plus smell, consistency, texture . . . and pain. Pain comes from irritation by spices, such as pepper, mustard and chilli, and also from the temperature of hot foods.

These factors all play a role in our simple food preferences, such as for sweets, chocolate, fine wine and delicacies like lobster or oysters. They are also involved in our personal dislike of strong flavours, such as Brussels sprouts.

We can easily retrain our simple tastes. By going without sugar or sweetener in our tea or coffee, there will soon come a time when we can't bear these drinks if sugar has been added. It's all a matter of perseverance.

If we eat a food we have previously adored (e.g. mussels) and then suffer violent food poisoning, we often develop a strong abhorrence for the offending dish. This is nature's way of protecting us from eating tainted foods and was useful to man in the wilds to prevent eating poisonous berries or roots.

Some people who seem addicted to hot, spicy curries have irritated and inflamed their tastebuds so much that

434

they need hotter and spicier foods to stimulate them. The elderly also have a preference for strongly flavoured foods as the senses of smell and taste becomes less acute with age.

But there is a deeper, more complex level of appetite control in all of us. This is less easily overcome by simple measures such as avoidance or retraining our eating habits.

Carbohydrate and Appetite

When we eat carbohydrate, two things occur in our body:
- **insulin** is secreted by the pancreas
- tiny puffs of a chemical called **serotonin** are released in the brain

Both insulin and serotonin play a major role in controlling our eating behaviour.

Insulin is a hormone that allows blood glucose to enter cells and provide a source of energy. Without insulin, glucose would accumulate in the blood and cells would be starved of energy (e.g. diabetes). Usually, just enough insulin is secreted after eating to cope with the exact amount of carbohydrate ingested. Insulin levels then start to fall, and this triggers the release of serotonin in the brain.

Serotonin is a 'neurotransmitter'. It relays messages across important nerve connections (synapses) and has a number of different functions. These include influencing appetite, the way we select certain foods and the regulation of satiety (that feeling of having eaten enough).

Serotonin also gives us a little 'high'. It makes us feel good and is able to lift depression. One of the reasons we crave chocolate when we feel low is because chocolate (and some other foods) contains tryptophan – a chemical converted to serotonin in the body. It really is possible to guzzle our way to happiness.

When carbohydrate is eaten, serotonin is released and

the brain starts to signal 'enough'. Eating carbohydrate therefore switches off appetite and also keeps us feeling fuller for longer.

Low levels of serotonin in the hypothalamus have been linked experimentally to over-eating and carbohydrate craving.

Sometimes our desire to eat, even in the absence of hunger, can become an overwhelming craving that compels satisfaction. It can even take over our lives.

Unfortunately, what usually happens when we crave carbohydrate is that we snack on foods that are also high in fat (e.g. doughnuts, sausage rolls, cream cakes, crisps). This is why carbohydrate craving and snacking rapidly lead to excess weight.

Dieting Vicious Circles

In some people, the appetite mechanism is knocked off balance because they produce too much insulin in response to carbohydrate intake.

Blood insulin levels fail to fall quickly so serotonin is not released in the brain. Feelings of satiety remain firmly switched 'off' and the low blood sugar results in hunger and food craving. A vicious cycle results: increased carbohydrate intake → increased excess insulin secretion → lack of serotonin → more hunger → more carbohydrate intake, etc. The repetition of this cycle results in the phenomenon of carbohydrate addiction.

This fits in with the classic dieting vicious cycle suggested in the 1970s but explains it more scientifically:

Restricted eating on a slimming diet → hunger → over-eating → guilt and feeling out of control → depression → comfort over-eating → guilt → restricted eating, etc.

When Appetite Goes Wrong

Eating Disorders

Up to 2 per cent of young adult women in the UK suffer from bulimia, experiencing episodes of massive over-eating (sometimes over 15,000 kcal eaten in 1–2 hours) with a loss of control of appetite and a morbid fear of becoming fat. A few males are affected too.

Around 1 per cent of teenage girls suffer from anorexia. Food intake becomes inadequate and rapid weight loss ensues.

Evidence suggests there is an increased serotonin activity in victims of anorexia and reduced serotonin activity in bulimics.

These changes are consistent with what we already know about the regulation of appetite. In fact, bingeing on carbohydrates may be a form of self-medication for bulimics as they are biologically driven to restore their brain serotonin levels to normal.

Interestingly, bingeing is not a modern eating disorder. The Romans had feasting down to a fine art too. Some installed vomitoria near their dining rooms so they could pop out during a Bacchanalian orgy, empty their stomachs and continue to satisfy their appetites.

Seasonal Affective Disorder (SADs)

SADs was first described in 1984. It is a form of depression occurring in the winter months and characterized by:

- low mood
- anxiety and irritability
- low energy levels
- increased need for sleep

- carbohydrate craving
- increased appetite and increased weight

Once the days draw out again, symptoms improve, appetite returns to normal and the excess weight is often lost.

It is thought that SADs represents an extreme end of the normal spectrum of sensitivity to seasonal changes, perhaps a primitive preparation for hibernation, and that it affects all of us to a greater or lesser extent. SADs can usually be cured by bright, artificial light.

Drugs

Many commonly prescribed drugs can cause weight gain either by directly stimulating our appetite or by slowing down our metabolism. These include:
- hormonal methods of contraception
- tri-cyclic antidepressants
- monoamine oxidase inhibitors
- lithium
- beta-blockers
- steroids
- insulin
- pizotifen

It may be possible to change some of these but many are life-saving and it's a question of weighing up their good effects against their bad. Oral contraceptive pills that are predominantly progestogenic stimulate weight gain. Changing to a lower-dose, more oestrogenic brand may help.

Anti-obesity drugs (e.g. dexfenfluramine) are available that stimulate release of serotonin in the brain. This produces a sensation of satiety without having eaten a carbohydrate meal. They act as diet selectors and, as the brain already thinks it's had a carbohydrate snack, healthier foods such as cottage cheese salads are preferred.

These drugs can be prescribed in cases where overweight is seriously affecting health (body mass index of greater than 30kg/m^2) and where conventional dieting methods have failed. As they are only prescribable for short courses, they are effective in the long term only if given under close supervision, with specialist dietary advice and behaviour modification techniques.

Similar drugs that prolong the action of serotonin are prescribed as anti-depressants. One is indicated for the treatment of bulimia.

How to Assess Your Personal Taste in Food and the Categories You Overdo

Questionnaire

Write out a list of your five favourite foods – ones that you can remember craving in the past.
Are they predominantly:

- Complex carbohydrates (e.g. baked potato, bread, banana, muesli)?
- Fat (e.g. chocolate, cheese, pork pie, fresh cream, butter)?
- Protein (e.g. fish, cottage cheese, lean meat)?
- Fruit or vegetable (e.g. apple, peach, carrot, broccoli, pear)?
- Simple unrefined, sweet carbohydrates (e.g. sweet coffee, sweet wine, sticky puddings and buns, sweet biscuits)?

If your personal tastes err towards sweet and fatty foods, you are more likely to have a weight problem. If you prefer complex carbohydrates and eat them without additional fat, you are following a healthy diet as recommended by the World Health Organization and are likely to be slim and fit.

Food cravings for protein or vegetables and fruit are uncommon but can lead to problems. Excess protein intake is linked with the development of gout. There is evidence that the desire to eat protein is regulated independently of body weight. A cold environment stimulates protein appetite whilst a hot environment depresses it.

Carrots are the most famously addictive vegetable. One male recently turned to nibbling them after giving up smoking. He ate five bunches per day and couldn't stop. A woman who developed a craving for carrots during pregnancy ate a whole bed of young carrots in a fortnight – and started turning yellow. The pigment **carotene** can accumulate in the tissues to simulate jaundice.

Food Diaries

Keeping a food diary is an excellent way to analyse what you are eating and why. They are very simple to devise, e.g.

DAY 1

Time	What was eaten	Where you were	Mood when eating
....			
....			
....			
....			
....			
....			

Remember to record your periods too, in case you have PMS.

Do you overeat:
- At a certain time of the day, e.g. evening?
- When you are lonely or bored?
- When you are stressed?

- In the two weeks before a period?

Increased appetite and food intake in these circumstances are easily overcome.

Do you suffer from these?

- a constant preoccupation with food
- using food to reward or punish yourself, e.g. 'I won't eat chocolate today'.
- bingeing behaviour followed by guilt?
- misuse of laxatives, diuretics or vomiting?
- feelings of guilt if seen eating in public?
- hiding food from others or from yourself?
- is food or your appetite making you miserable?
- do you feel fat, unlovable and stop eating so people will like you more?

These are signs of a more serious food addiction or eating disorder. You need professional help and guidance to overcome these (see Useful Addresses).

- Food diaries will help you and your dietitician/physician pinpoint what you are eating, when you are eating it, and why.
- By spotting situations when you are more likely to indulge in a naughty nibble, you can avoid them.
- If you eat when stressed, you can be taught various techniques to help you relax.
- Flotation therapy is an excellent and healthy way of lowering all the stress indicators in your body. It can also be combined with audio tapes to retrain your eating habits and reinforce your determination to lose weight.

How to Beat Your Cravings

- Drink a glass of sparkling mineral water fortified by the juice of half a lemon.
- Clean your teeth slowly with a strongly flavoured, 'tingling' toothpaste.

- Go for a jog, a workout or a long, brisk walk – avoiding tempting shops.
- Recognize that appetite is often a craving for carbohydrate. Indulge it by giving your body what it wants – not a fatty snack that just piles on the calories. Have a crispbread and an apple or a slice of wholemeal bread, rather than a sausage roll, a cream cake or a doughnut.
- Try eating carbohydrate little and often, especially if your appetite cravings are pre-menstrual. Remember to clean your teeth regularly or your dentist will not be impressed with your sudden increase in tooth decay!
- When you do eat, chew slowly and pause between each mouthful. Your serotonin-induced feelings of satiety will then occur before you've eaten your whole meal.
- Some researchers believe that true carbohydrate addicts should only eat carbohydrate during a one-hour period each day. They believe that eating carbohydrate little and often produces an over secretion of insulin in a few people, triggering the excess insulin-craving cycle. This may work for you.
- If you think you suffer from SADs during the winter months, try hiring a light box and treating yourself to a longer day. This involves sitting in front of the light box from 7–9 a.m. every morning. Most people who are going to benefit will notice a response over the first four days of treatment.
- Follow a wholefood diet with plenty of fresh fruit and vegetables and complex carbohydrates. Abstain from all added sugar.

It is important to feel good about your appetite, yourself and your food. People who can successfully practise self-restraint are shown in studies to be more psychologically healthy, to feel better about food and eating, to have more energy and, interestingly, to have a higher sex drive. Perhaps the next time you fancy a cream cake, you should hop into bed with your nearest and dearest instead.

Appendix 8: Food Analysis Chart

Per 100g of food

	Protein	Fat	Carb	Kcal
Anchovies	25	20	–	280
Apples, eating	–	–	12	48
Apple juice	–	–	10	40
Apricots, raw, stoned	1	–	7	32
dried, stoned	4	1	35	165
Asparagus	3	1	2	29
Aubergine	1	–	2	12
Avocado, flesh only	2	20	2	196
weighed with stone	1	14	1	134
Banana	1	–	23	96
Beans, blackeye, raw	24	2	54	330
blackeye, boiled	9	1	20	125
Beans, green, runner, French	2	–	4	24
Beans, kidney, raw	22	1	44	273
kidney, boiled	8	–	17	100
Beans, mung, raw	24	1	46	289
mung, boiled	8	–	15	92
Beansprouts	3	–	4	28
Beetroot, boiled	2	–	10	48
Blackberries	1	–	5	24
Blackcurrants	1	–	7	32
Bran	14	6	27	218
Bread, ciabatta	9	4	47	260
Bread, focaccia	9	13	44	329
Bread, French baguette	10	3	55	287
Bread, granary	9	3	46	243
Bread, naan	9	13	50	353
Bread, pitta	9	1	58	277
Bread, pugliese	10	6	54	310

	Protein	Fat	Carb	Kcal
Bread, rye	8	2	46	234
Bread, wholemeal	9	2	44	230
Broccoli, boiled	3	1	1	25
Butter	–	82	–	738
Cabbage	1	–	2	12
Carrots	1	–	5	24
Cauliflower	3	1	2	29
Celery	1	–	1	8
Cheese, Brie	20	27	–	323
Camembert	21	24	–	300
Cheddar	25	34	–	406
Cottage	14	4	2	100
Feta	16	20	1	248
Gouda	24	31	–	375
Mozzarella	26	25	–	329
Parmesan	40	33	–	457
Stilton	23	36	–	416
Cherries, weighed with stone	1	–	9	40
Chicken meat, lean, raw	20	4	–	126
meat only, roast	25	5	–	145
Cod, raw	19	–	–	76
Courgette	2	–	2	16
Crab meat, boiled	20	5	–	125
Crispbread, rye	9	2	70	334
Cucumber	1	–	2	12
Dates, raw, with stones	1	–	27	112
dried with stones	3	–	54	228
Egg, whole	13	11	–	151
Figs, dried	4	2	50	234
Filo pastry	8	3	56	283
Florence fennel	1	–	2	12
Fromage frais, plain	7	7	6	115
very low fat	8	–	7	60
Garlic	8	1	15	101
Grapefruit	1	–	7	32

	Protein	Fat	Carb	Kcal
Grapefruit juice	–	–	8	32
Grapes	–	–	15	60
Grape juice	–	–	12	48
Guava	1	1	5	33
Haddock, raw	18	–	–	72
Halibut, raw	18	2	–	90
Herring, raw	17	19	–	239
Kiwi fruit	1	–	10	44
Lamb, lean meat, raw	20	9	–	161
lean meat, roast	25	17	–	253
Leeks	2	–	3	20
Lemons	1	–	3	16
Lemon juice	–	–	2	8
Lentils, raw	24	2	50	314
boiled	8	1	17	109
Lettuce	1	–	2	12
Lobster meat, boiled	22	3	–	115
Mackerel	19	16	–	220
Mango	1	–	14	60
Marrow	1	–	2	12
Melon	1	–	4	20
Milk, semi-skimmed	3	2	4	46
Milk, skimmed	3	–	5	32
Milk, whole	3	4	5	68
Muesli	10	7	64	359
Mushrooms, raw	1	1	–	13
Mussels, flesh, boiled	18	2	–	90
boiled with shells	5	1	–	29
Nectarine, weighed with stone	1	–	8	36
Nuts, almonds, shelled	21	56	7	616
brazils, shelled	14	68	3	680
chestnuts, shelled	2	3	37	183
hazelnuts, shelled	14	64	6	656
peanuts, shelled	26	46	13	570
pecans shelled	9	70	6	690

445

	Protein	Fat	Carb	Kcal
Nuts, pine kernels	14	69	4	693
walnuts, shelled	15	69	3	693
Okra	3	1	3	33
Olives, green, flesh only	1	11	–	103
Olive oil	–	100	–	900
Olive oil spread	–	60	–	540
Onions, raw	1	–	8	36
Onions, spring	2	–	3	20
Oranges	1	–	6	28
Orange juice	1	–	9	40
Parsnip	2	1	12	65
Pasta, white (raw)	12	1	74	353
Pasta, white (boiled)	3	–	19	88
Pasta, wholemeal (raw)	13	1	66	325
Pasta, wholemeal (boiled)	5	–	23	112
Peaches, weighed with stone	1	–	7	32
Pears	–	–	10	40
Peas, boiled	7	2	9	82
Peas, chickpea, raw	20	5	50	325
chickpea, boiled	8	2	18	122
Peas, mangetout, boiled	3	–	3	24
Peppers, capsicum, green	1	–	3	16
capsicum, red	1	–	6	28
chilli, green	3	–	2	20
Pineapple	–	–	10	40
Pineapple juice	–	–	10	40
Plaice	18	2	–	90
Plums, weighed with stones	–	–	8	32
Potatoes (raw)	2	–	17	76
Potatoes, baked (inc skin)	4	–	30	136
Potatoes, baked, flesh only	2	–	18	80
Potatoes, roast	3	5	26	161
Prawns, peeled, boiled	23	2	–	110
shell-on	9	1	–	45
Prunes	3	–	34	148

	Protein	Fat	Carb	Kcal
Radish	1	–	2	12
Raisins	2	–	66	272
Raspberries	1	–	5	24
Rice, brown (raw)	7	3	77	363
Rice, brown (boiled)	3	1	30	141
Rice, white (raw)	7	4	80	384
Rice, white (boiled)	3	1	31	145
Safflower oil	–	100	–	900
Salmon, raw	18	12	–	180
Satsumas	1	–	6	28
Sesame oil	–	100	–	900
Sesame seeds	18	58	1	598
Sole, raw	18	1	–	81
Soya oil	–	100	–	900
Spinach	3	1	2	29
Strawberries	1	–	6	28
Sweetcorn, on-the-cob, boiled	3	1	12	69
Tahini (sesame) paste	19	59	1	611
Tangerines	1	–	6	28
Tomatoes, raw	11	–	3	16
Tomato juice	1	–	3	16
Tomatoes, purée	5	–	12	68
Trout, weighed with bones	17	3	–	95
Tuna, drained from oil	27	9	–	189
drained from brine	24	–	–	96
Walnut oil	–	100	–	900
Watercress	3	1	–	23
Watermelon	1	–	7	32
Wheatgerm	26	8	44	352
Yogurt, Greek strained	6	9	2	113
sheep's milk	4	7	6	103
wholemilk natural	6	3	7	79
low calorie, natural	4	–	6	40
low-fat, natural	5	1	7	57

ALCOHOLIC DRINKS per 100ml

	Kcal
Champagne	75
Port	160
Sherry, dry	115
medium	120
sweet	135
Wine, red	68
rosé	70
white, dry	66
white, medium	75
white, sweet	95

Each gram of protein supplies	4 kcals energy
Each gram of fat supplies	9 kcals energy
Each gram of carbohydrate supplies	4 kcals energy

You can work out the percentage of energy you obtain from your diet by adding up the total number of grams of protein, carbohydrate and fat you eat each day and calculating the proportion of each,

e.g. if you consumed 50g protein, 40g fat and 200g carbohydrate:

50g protein at 4 kcals per gram	=	200 kcals
60g fat at 9 kcals per gram	=	540 kcals
200g carbohydrate at 4 kcals per gram	=	800 kcals
TOTAL	=	1540 kcals

% calories as protein	$= 200 \div 1540 \times 100 = 13\%$
% calories as fat	$= 540 \div 1540 \times 100 = 35\%$
% calories as carbohydrate	$= 800 \div 1540 \times 100 = 52\%$

Don't forget to include alcohol in your calculations. Some British males obtain as much as 17 per cent of their daily calories in the form of alcohol.

Useful Calorie Counter, per Average Portion of Foods

Food	Kcals
Avocado, one half	235
Bacon, well grilled, 1 rasher	80
Bagel, medium	215
Banana, medium	100
Bread, one medium slice	75
Bread roll, average	130
Bread stick, each	15
Celery, one stick	5
Champagne, one glass	95
Chicken leg, grilled	160
Coffee, mug without milk	2
mug with skimmed milk	10
mug with semi-skimmed milk	15
mug with whole milk	20
Corn-on-the-cob, medium	155
Cottage cheese, 1 tbsp	15
Courgettes, each	10
Croissant, each	250
Dates, fresh, each	15
dried, each	15
Egg, size 4	80
Fig, fresh, each	30
dried, each	30
French dressing, 1 tbsp	75
French toast, 1 slice	55
Garlic bread, 1 slice	155
Gherkin, each	10
Honey, 1 tbsp	60
Jam, 1 tbsp	45
Kiwi fruit, each	35
Leeks, each	25
Lettuce, half	10
Mackerel, each	320

Food	Kcals
Mandarin, each	20
Mango, each	100
Mango chutney, 1 tbsp	40
Marmalade, 1 tbsp	45
Mayonnaise, 1 tbsp	120
low-fat, 1 tbsp	40
Melon, half	50
Milk, whole, 600ml	380
semi-skimmed, 600ml	300
skimmed, 600ml	195
Mussels, each	10
Mustard, 1 tsp	10
Nectarine, each	75
Oatmeal, 1 tbsp	40
Oil, 1 scant tbsp	120
Olives, black, each	5
Orange, each	50
Parmesan cheese, grated, 1 tbsp	40
Passion fruit, each	10
Peach, each	40
Pear, each	70
Pepper, each	30
Pitta bread, medium, each	180
mini, each	80
Plums, each	20
Potato, large, baked	175
Salad cream, 1 tbsp	50
low-fat, 1 tbsp	20
Soy sauce, 1 tbsp	15
Spring onions, each	5
Strawberries, each	3
Sugar, 1 tsp	20
Tangerine, each	40
Tea, mug without milk	1
mug with skimmed milk	10

Food	Kcals
Tea, mug with semi-skimmed milk	15
mug with whole milk	20
herbal, without milk	1
Tomato, average, each	15
beef tomato	30
Trout, each	150
Yogurt, low-fat natural 150ml carton	80
very low-fat, natural 150ml carton	60

Appendix 9:
Body Awareness Self-assessment Chart

Fill in the following Body Awareness Assessment Chart at the beginning of your weight loss or healthy eating programme. Then reassess yourself weekly and see how much you have improved.

Age:		....	years
Weight (kg):		....	kg
Height (m):		....	m
BMI $\dfrac{\text{Weight (kg)}}{\text{ht (m)} \times \text{ht (m)}}$		....	kg/m²
Grade of obesity:		....	
Skinfold measurements:	triceps	....	cm
	suprailiac	....	cm
	thighs	....	cm
TOTAL:		**..........**	**cm**
Body measurements:	bust	....	cm
	chest	....	cm
	left upper arm	....	cm
	right upper arm	....	cm
	waist	....	cm
	hips	....	cm
	left thigh	....	cm
	right thigh	....	cm
TOTAL:		**..........**	**cm**

Waist/hip ratio:	....
Apple/pear	....
Ectomorph/mesomorph/endomorph	....
Suppleness score:	....
Resting pulse rate:	....

Maximum pulse rate (220–age): ....

65% maximum pulse rate: ....

Target pulse range (60–80% max.): ....

10 second pulse range: ....

Blood pressure: .... mm Hg

Make sure you have recently been medically screened. This includes having your urine tested for protein or traces of blood, and having your breasts examined plus an up-to-date cervical smear.

Men should have their testicles checked regularly for lumps.

Optimum weight range for health

fine tuning: .... to ....

coarse tuning: .... to ....

Estimated calorie intake to maintain weight: ....

Estimated calorie intake to lose weight: ....

Type of diet you wish to follow:

Food Exchange/Mediterranean Slim Diet/Maintenance Diet

Daily portion allowances:

Complex carbohydrates: ....

Vegetables, Fruit: ....

Milk, yogurt, cheese: ....

Fish, beans, seeds, nuts: ....

Meat, eggs: ....

Smoker/non-smoker ....

Units of alcohol drunk per week: ....

Conversion Charts

LIQUID MEASURES

U.S. MEASURES	FLUID OUNCES	IMPERIAL MEASURES	MILLILITRES
1 teaspoon	⅙	1 teaspoon	5
2 teaspoons	¼	1 dessertspoon	10
1 tablespoon	½	1 tablespoon	15
2 tablespoons	1	2 tablespoons	30
¼ cup	2	4 tablespoons	56
⅓ cup	2⅔		80
½ cup	4		110
⅔ cup	5	¼ pint/1 gill	140
¾ cup	6		170
1 cup/½ pint	8		225
1¼ cups	10	½ pint	280
1½ cups	12		420
2 cups/1 pint	16	generous ¼ pint	450
2½ cups	20	1 pint	560
3 cups/1½ pints	24		675
3½ cups	27		750
3¾ cups	30	1½ pints	840
4 cups/2 pints	32		900
4½ cups	36		1000/1 litre
5 cups	40	2 pints/1 quart	1120
6 cups/3 pints	48	scant 2½ pints	1350
7 cups	56	2¾ pints	1600
8 cups	64	3¼ pints	1800
9 cups	72	3½ pints	2000/2 litres
10 cups/5 pints	80	4 pints	2250

SOLID MEASURES

U.S. and IMPERIAL	METRIC EQUIVALENT
1 oz	25 grams
1½oz	40
2 oz	50
3 oz	60
3½oz	100
4 oz/¼lb	110
5 oz	150
6 oz	175
7 oz	200
8 oz/½lb	225
9 oz	250
10 oz	275
12 oz/¾ lb	350
16 oz/1lb	450
1¼lb	575
1½lb	675
1¾lb	800
2lb	900
2½lb	1000/1 kilo
3lb	1kg 350g
4lb	1kg 800g
4½lb	2 kilos
5lb	2kg 250g
6lb	2kg 750g

Useful Addresses

Please send a stamped, self-addressed envelope if writing to any organization for information leaflets.

Alcohol Counselling and Prevention Services
34 Electric Lane
London
SW9 8JT

Tel: 071–737 3579

Help and advice for those worried about their drinking.
Leaflets; counselling.

Anorexia Anonymous
24 Westmorland Road
Barnes
London
SW13 9RY

Tel: 081–748 4587

Counselling and advice for those with eating disorders.

Anorexia and Bulimia Nervosa Association
Annex C
Tottenham Town Hall
London
N15 4RX

Tel: 081–885 3936

Information and helpline for those with eating disorders.
Leaflets; newsletter.

Centre for Pregnancy Nutrition
The University of Sheffield
Dept Obstetrics and Gynaecology
Clinical Sciences Centre
Northern General Hospital
Herries Road
Sheffield
S5 7AU

Tel: 0742 434343 ext. 4888

Eating for Pregnancy Helpline: 0742 424084

Flotation Tank Association (UK)
PO Box 168
Rickmansworth
Herts
WD3 5TY

Tel: 0923 285868 (24 hours) for details on how to obtain
a list of accredited float centres.

The Vegetarian Society
Parkdale
Dunham Road
Altrincham
Cheshire
WA14 4QG

Tel: 061 928 0793

QUIT
102 Gloucester Place
London
W1H 3DA

Smokers' Quitlines:

UK   071–487 3000 (09.30 a.m. – 17.30 p.m. daily)
Scotland: 0800 848484
N. Ireland: 0232 663281
Wales: 0222 641888

Advice and counselling on giving up smoking.

Index